ENVIRONMENT, SOCIETY AND THE BLACK DEATH

An interdisciplinary approach to the late-medieval crisis in Sweden

edited by

Per Lagerås

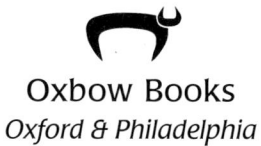

Oxbow Books
Oxford & Philadelphia

Published in the United Kingdom in 2016 by
OXBOW BOOKS
10 Hythe Bridge Street, Oxford OX1 2EW

and in the United States by
OXBOW BOOKS
1950 Lawrence Road, Havertown, PA 19083

Paperback Edition: ISBN 978-1-78570-054-5
Digital Edition: ISBN 978-1-78570-055-2

A CIP record for this book is available from the British Library

Printed in the United Kingdom by Short Run Press, Exeter

For a complete list of Oxbow titles, please contact:

UNITED KINGDOM
Oxbow Books
Telephone (01865) 241249, Fax (01865) 794449
Email: oxbow@oxbowbooks.com
www.oxbowbooks.com

UNITED STATES OF AMERICA
Oxbow Books
Telephone (800) 791-9354, Fax (610) 853-9146
Email: queries@casemateacademic.com
www.casemateacademic.com/oxbow

Oxbow Books is part of the Casemate Group

Front cover: Wall painting from 1437 in Tensta Church, Sweden.
(Photo: Per Lagerås)
Back cover: Traditional agricultural landscape at Åsens by, in the South-Swedish Uplands.
(Photo: Per Lagerås)

Contents

Part III. Conclusions in a wider perspective

Preface

The studies of the late-medieval crisis presented in this book build on the work of many colleagues from different disciplines. We have had the privilege to compile and explore data produced during innumerable hours in the field and behind the microscope. In many cases the original investigations did not primarily deal with the late-medieval crisis, but due to their high quality and careful documentation, they make important contributions to the compilations and discussions presented here. To interpret and reinterpret old and new data from new perspectives have been a truly exciting and rewarding endeavour.

While completing this book we have benefited from valuable discussions with many colleagues and friends. First of all we want to thank Janken Myrdal at the Division of Agrarian History, Swedish University of Agricultural Sciences. His research on the late-medieval crisis is of major importance and has been a great source of inspiration for us. Several others have shared their expertise and we want to especially thank Torbjörn Ahlström at the Dept. of Archaeology and Ancient History, Lund University, Frank Götmark at the Dept of Biological & Environmental sciences, University of Gothenburg, Olof Karsvall and Alf Ericsson at the Division of Agrarian History, Swedish University of Agricultural Sciences, Örjan Kardell at the Dept. of Language Studies, Umeå University, and Ola Magnell at the Swedish National Heritage Board.

We also want to thank Conny Johansson Herven and Lars Salminen at the Kulturen Museum in Lund for giving access to skeleton material, Emma Foberg at ATA Swedish National Heritage Board for providing archived data, Jesper Boldsen at the Institute of Forensic Medicine, University of Southern Denmark, and Chatarina Ödman at Malmö Museer for providing unpublished archaeological data, Timothy Hatton at the Australian National University for providing modern stature data, Adam Bolander and Katja Meissner for tree-ring data handling, and Henrik Pihl and Staffan Hyll for help with graphics. We also want to thank Hélène Borna-Ahlkvist at the Swedish National Heritage Board, UV Syd, for hosting our project and providing excellent research facilities.

The research was funded by the Swedish Research Council and the Swedish National Heritage Board.

Per Lagerås
Lund, January 2015

PART I

INTRODUCTION

1.

An interdisciplinary approach

Per Lagerås

The late-medieval crisis was one of the most dramatic episodes in Europe's history. Characterised by significant population drop, land desertion and social unrest, it was a true societal crisis with few counterparts before and after. The crisis started in the fourteenth century and lasted for several generations, in many areas for more than a century, before the negative chain of events was broken and society slowly started to recover. In one way or the other the crisis affected every corner of society, from town to countryside and from agricultural farmlands to the most remote and sparsely populated woodlands. In a long-term perspective it was an anomaly to the predominant trend of expansion of settlement and agriculture and a break in the exponentially rising graph of population numbers. But to see the late-medieval crisis only as an interruption – as a temporary phase before things went back to normal – would be to diminish its historical role. The crisis had long-lasting consequences for society, for instance by changing the economic and political relationship between social classes, by agricultural change and by stimulating technological development and increased consumption and trade. In a wider perspective it laid the foundation for the strong expansion that characterised many countries in the sixteenth century, and in the long run the transition from the Middle Ages to the Modern Period.

Closely linked to the crisis was the Black Death, the plague pandemic that ravaged Europe, the Middle East and North Africa in 1346–1353. Even though parts of Europe witnessed decline already some centuries before, in particular after a series of crop failures and famines in 1315–1322, most authors agree that the Black Death was the single most important factor behind the dramatic population drop and its social and economic consequences. Killing about half of the population in only a few years, the pandemic for good reason has been called the worst disaster that has ever hit Europe. The first strike was followed by several recurring outbreaks during the late fourteenth and the fifteenth centuries, and sporadic outbreaks continued to haunt the population until the early eighteenth century. In spite of these later outbreaks, of which some were devastating but often of a more local or regional character, the Black Death of the mid-fourteenth century was to be remembered as something special, unrivalled in force and mortality.

Obviously the story of the late-medieval crisis and the Black Death is a sad story – a story about disease, death and abandonment. But it is also a story about survival, new strategies and systemic change. Over the years the plague pandemic itself, as well as the

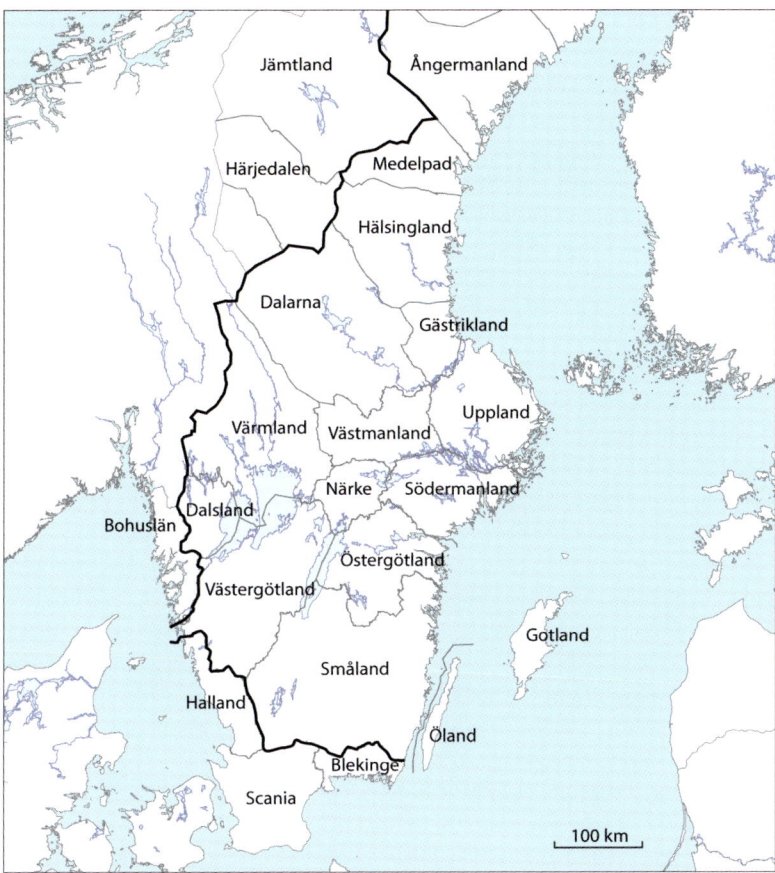

Fig. 1. Map showing provinces in present-day Sweden. During most of the Middle Ages the provinces of Halland, Scania and Blekinge belonged to Denmark whereas Bohuslän, Härjedalen and Jämtland belonged to Norway. The study presented in this book uses material from within present-day Sweden, including these provinces

wider context of the late-medieval crisis, has attracted a lot of research, and in particular the possible relationships between different changes and processes during and after the crisis are the subject of continuous debate. Research has so far mostly been based on historical sources, i.e. written documents of different kinds. These range from literary chronicles giving colourful testimonies of the plague, via letters and charters to manorial accounts and land registers. Most documents are of an economical character, providing evidence on transactions, rents and expenses, which may be used to interpret different aspects of the crisis. The character and amount of the written sources vary greatly between countries and influence the direction of the discussion. To some degree non-documentary evidence, in particular from archaeology, has contributed to the discussion, but still research on the late-medieval crisis in most countries is very much based on written documents and the dominant approach is that of economic history.

In this book we take a deeper look at some non-documentary sources and what they may contribute to the discussion on the late-medieval crisis. Our studies focus on southern Sweden (Fig. 1), but our interpretations and conclusions are discussed in a wider European context. In Sweden the impact of the late-medieval crisis has been upgraded during the last 15 years. According to earlier research, for instance within *The Scandinavian Research Project on Deserted Farms and Villages*, Sweden was hit by the plague and experienced a severe crisis, but in comparison to other parts of Western Europe it seemed to have come off relatively well.[1]

Later research, in particular by Janken Myrdal, emphasises that Sweden was hit hard and that it witnessed significant population drop during the late fourteenth and early fifteenth centuries.[2] However, in comparison to most European countries the documentary source material from the time is scarce. Myrdal's conclusions are based on a broad spectrum of fragmentary medieval sources from the time. Other researchers have used much later sources, in particular cadastral registers and maps from the sixteenth century onwards, to study the late-medieval decline and in particular to estimate the degree of farm abandonment.[3]

Hence, in Sweden like elsewhere present knowledge on the late-medieval decline is much based on the historical record – both scarce documentary records from the time and later more plentiful records used in retrogressive analysis. There have been interdisciplinary attempts, and in particular historical geography has played an active role in some earlier studies, but non-documentary sources have so far made only minor contributions to the discussion. In the studies presented in this book we examine four types of non-documentary evidence: pollen records, dendrochronological data, settlement archaeology and human skeletons.

Pollen records reflect vegetation development and indirectly the development of agricultural land-use and settlement. Sweden has a wealth of pollen-analytical studies and many of them, in particular from the last two decades, are detailed and with good chronologies. In an earlier study, Lagerås showed that late-medieval farm abandonment was possible to detect in South-Swedish pollen diagrams.[4] The conclusion was based on the interpretation of individual diagrams. In the present study we use a data set of 28 pollen records to make quantitative estimations and more thorough interpretations. We provide new evidence on late-medieval abandonment and reforestation, but also on changes within the agricultural system. We discuss the environmental responses to the crisis as well as the possible influence of environmental change on the course of the crisis and the recovery that followed.

Another type of data that we take a deeper look at comes from dendrochronology, i.e. the dating of old wood by tree-ring analysis. In a pioneer dendrochronological study on old farm buildings, Thomas Bartholin showed that there was a significant drop in construction activity soon after the Black Death – a break that lasted for about 100 years.[5] His study areas were situated in Middle and Northern Sweden where medieval log houses are still standing. Inspired by Bartholin's work, we have compiled dendrochronological dates from southern Sweden – 1882 dates, representing churches as well as profane buildings and other constructions from both towns and countryside. Because there are very few buildings from the Middle Ages still standing in southern Sweden, except for the churches, much of our material derives from archaeological excavations. Our aim is to reveal possible changes in the building activity during the Middle Ages and also to discuss the utilisation of woodlands and their possible recovery during the crisis.

Archaeology of medieval settlement is of course an important source of information in this context. Since *The Scandinavian Research Project on Deserted Farms and Villages*, which published its final report in 1981, there has been a strong development of medieval archaeology in Sweden. In addition to theoretical and methodological advances, the number of excavated sites has increased dramatically. However, in relation to the high level of investigation activity and the large amount of documentation, archaeology has made only minor contributions to the discussion on the late-medieval crisis. Abandoned farms have been investigated but few studies have focused specifically on the crisis. In this book we review evidence in Swedish archaeology of the late-medieval decline and also take a closer look at three rural settlement sites. The sites represent settlements that survived in one way or the other and our focus is on how individual households adjusted to the crisis by developing new strategies.

The last of our empirical studies is based on human skeletons. We have compiled osteological data from 65 different medieval churchyards, three execution sites and two military mass graves. Based on estimations of stature on 4876 adult individuals we discuss possible changes in health, diet and the standard of living during the Middle Ages. Stature is an established indicator of diet and welfare both in historical studies and of populations living today. In particular we compare stature before and after the Black Death, but also between town and countryside and between different social classes. To further investigate possible changes in diet and also to look for indications of migration we have performed stable-isotope analysis on teeth from 104 medieval individuals. In addition to the osteological analyses we discuss the burial customs during the plague epidemics.

Our general aim in this book is to present accessible compilations and conclusions that shed new light on different aspects of the late-medieval crisis. To use non-documentary sources may be particularly rewarding in Sweden, because of the scarcity of written documents from the time. Also important is that Sweden has a strong research tradition in both medieval archaeology and palaeoecology. However, a similar interdisciplinary approach has the potential to make major contributions also in countries with abundant documentary material. To use a diversity of source materials and techniques opens up for new perspectives and brings different academic disciplines together.

Notes

1   Gissel *et al.* 1981
2   Myrdal 2003; 2006; 2009; 2012a. Also Dick Harrison (2000) and Lennart Andersson Palm (2001) came to similar conclusions
3   This retrogressive method was used within *The Scandinavian Research Project on Deserted Farms and Villages* (Gissel *et al.* 1981) and has been further developed in later research (e.g. Antonson 2009; Karsvall 2011)
4   Lagerås 2007
5   Bartholin 1989a; 1990

2.

Current knowledge on the late-medieval crisis

Per Lagerås

Society during the Middle Ages was by and large an agricultural society. Even though towns, trade and non-agrarian production were expanding, the vast majority of the medieval population lived in the countryside and made their living from agriculture. In Sweden, where towns were few and small in a European perspective, still by the end of the Middle Ages about 95% lived in the countryside.[1] The most densely populated areas were the fertile plains, which offered good natural conditions for agriculture and where settlement was characterised by villages and hamlets. Uplands, with their poorer stony soils and shorter vegetation period, had a more dispersed rural settlement characterised by smaller hamlets and single farms. The agricultural system was however principally the same in both types of environment, being based on a combination of crop growing and animal husbandry (Fig. 2). The dominating crop was barley, which was used for baking flat bread and making porridge, as well as for brewing beer. Rye, oats and wheat, and occasionally peas complemented it. The number of animals depended of course on social standard, but, if possible, farms had a combination of cattle, pigs, sheep and goats, and they used horses or oxen as draft animals. Because of the relatively harsh climate of northerly latitudes animals were kept indoors during the winter.

Villages and hamlets as well as single farms organised their land into infields and outland. The infields contained arable fields for crop growing and hay meadows for producing winter fodder. They were situated close to the settlement and were protected from grazing animals by fences. During the Middle Ages many villages on the plains practised a two- or three-field crop rotation system, while most upland settlement stuck to a one-field system. Animals grazed in open pastures in the outland, watched over by a herder, and on fallow land in the infields. The combination of crop growing and animal husbandry was important because animals produced manure for the arable. A certain balance between arable, meadows and pastures was therefore aimed at. However, the balance differed between regions and also changed through time. In areas with fertile soil and dense population a larger proportion of the land was put under the plough at the expenses of pastures. In the most heavily cultivated areas there was a shortage of outland pastures and therefore grazing was much restricted to fallow land in the infields. This contrasts to upland areas where more weight was put on animal husbandry – a consequence of excess of pastures in combination with great demands for manure to get decent grain yields from naturally poor soils. The vast outlands of the uplands were also used for slash-and-burn cultivation as a complement to infield cultivation

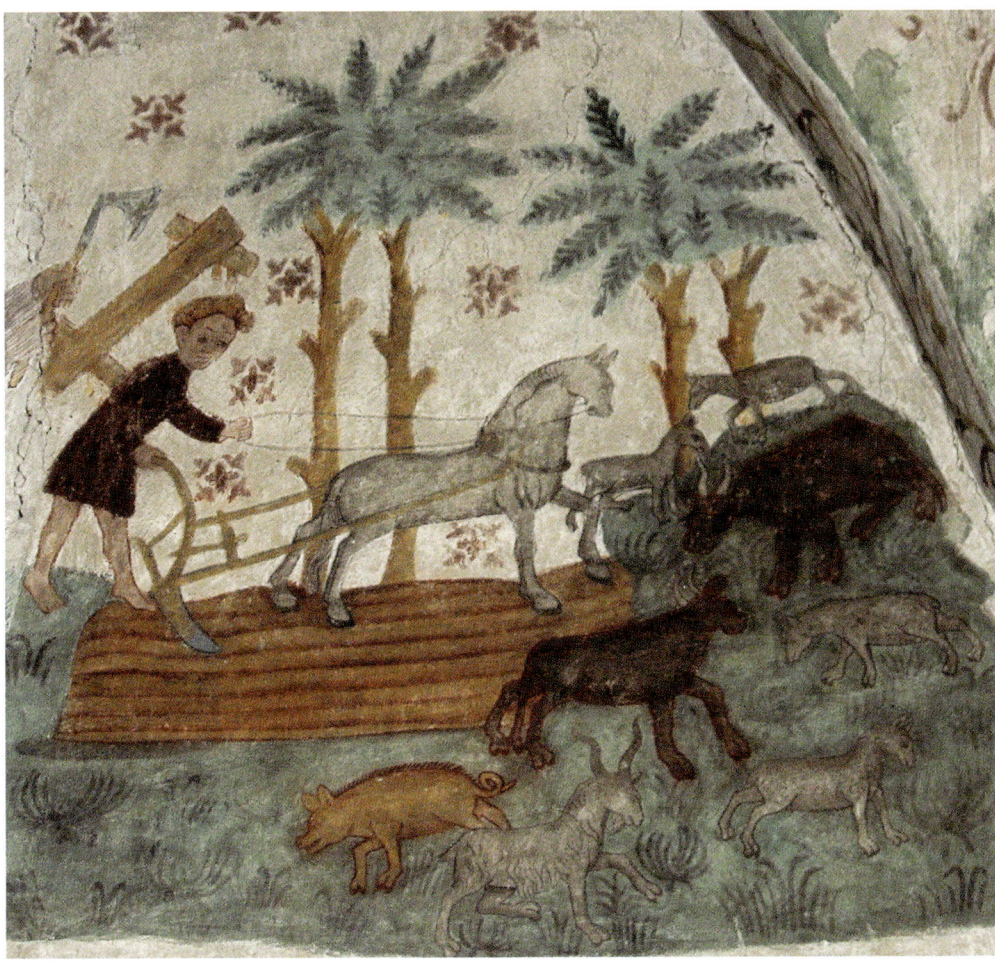

Fig. 2. Wall painting from the fifteenth century in Tensta Church, the province of Uppland, middle Sweden. A man (probably Cain) is plowing the field with an ard pulled by a horse. In the pasture we see two cows, four sheep, a goat and a pig. Trees in the background are pollarded, probably for leaf fodder. The painting gives a good summary of medieval agriculture in Sweden (photo: Per Lagerås)

and for the collection of leaf fodder. Furthermore, upland agriculture was often combined with non-agricultural production, in particular of iron and timber.

Land ownership varied and did not necessarily affect the agricultural practice. Most important from a social point of view was the shift from an estate system based on slavery to a system of manors based on rent-paying tenants and crofters.[2] This process was gradual but finally completed during the thirteenth century. From then on the great landowners were the nobility, the Crown and the church, but there were also numerous freeholders who owned their own land and only paid taxes to the Crown. Demesnes with farms dispersed over large regions now replaced the earlier large estates with continuous land. It was not unusual that farms in the same village paid rent to different landowners, and farms of freeholders were mixed with tenant farms. Because of scarcity of documentary sources the distribution of land ownership cannot be estimated with accuracy before the early sixteenth century. However, by then the nobility in Sweden owned 24%, the church 25%, the Crown 6% and peasants (freeholders) as much as 45%.[3] In Denmark the nobility had a stronger position and peasants owned a much smaller part of the land. This was true also for Scania, which today is the southernmost province of Sweden (and included in the studies presented in this book) but during the Middle Ages belonged to Denmark.

The agricultural society as outlined above was far from static through time. Before the crisis of the fourteenth and fifteenth centuries it was characterised by strong expansion all over Europe. The European population doubled between 1100 and 1300 and Sweden was no exception.[4] Population increased, partly because of expansion of arable land and partly because of increased land productivity (production per hectare). The latter was due to seemingly small but important technological innovations and improvements.[5] In particular the more widespread use of iron for agricultural tools increased the productivity. Iron was used for cutting tools like sickles and scythes already during the Iron Age but during the Middle Ages they became longer and more efficient. More important however was the development of heavy and large ard shares of iron that facilitated deeper and more efficient tilling. (Mouldboard ploughs were introduced to Denmark, including Scania, but were rare in Sweden where the ard was used throughout the Middle Ages.) Also iron-shod spades was an important improvement. Hence, the agricultural expansion went hand-in-hand with expanding iron production.

In Sweden the agricultural expansion started already in the Viking Period but was stronger from the eleventh century onwards. This time also saw the foundation of towns and the building of more than a thousand stone churches. New farms and fields were established in the already densely populated lowlands and particularly during the twelfth and thirteenth centuries there was a strong expansion also in marginal uplands. In some areas this meant the colonisation of uninhabited land, for instance along the old boarder zone between medieval Sweden and Denmark, but most of the uplands were sparsely settled already since the Iron Age or before.[6] The upland environment was completely different from the agricultural plains. It was to a larger degree covered by woodland and the Quaternary deposits were dominated by sandy till, rich in stones and boulders. To clear new land among roots and stones was not an easy task. Today millions of moss-covered clearance cairns in the woods bear testimony of the sweat and hard work invested in the land by early settlers.[7] However, soils may have been more fertile in the initial phase than later, due to nutrients that had accumulated slowly but steadily in deciduous woodland, and the settlers were also favoured by the good climate of the Medieval Warm Period.[8] Later, in the course of the Little Ice Age, climate and soils deteriorated and deciduous woodland was gradually outcompeted by spruce and pine.

During the fourteenth century the agricultural expansion that had characterised much of Europe for several centuries came to an end. A major factor was the Black Death, which ravaged Europe in the mid-fourteenth century, but many areas saw stagnation and decline already before that. The reason for this has been much debated, in particular for England, which has a wealth of documentary sources from the time. According to an influential interpretation by Michael Postan, the stagnation was due to overpopulation combined with a lack of technological innovations and investment.[9] Most of the fertile soils of England were put under the plough already in the eleventh century. Continued population growth during the twelfth and thirteenth centuries resulted in a reduction in the average amount of land per head. The numbers of small cottagers increased and so did the number of landless. Land reclamation continued but now on poor soils that had hitherto been avoided. To add to the burden, the expansion of arable at the expense of pastures resulted in fewer animals per farm and consequently a shortage of manure. All together, land productivity dropped and living standards declined, producing poverty and malnutrition.

The impoverishment of the population was also due to the inequality of medieval society.[10] Even under normal conditions, heavy burdens of taxes, rents, tithes and labour duties left little surplus for ordinary people. The number-one priority for the upper classes and the central power was to keep up their luxury consumption and life style while little resources were invested back into the agricultural system. When they experienced declining incomes due to poor yields their immediate reaction was to compensate by further raising taxes and rents. This counterproductive reaction is partly to blame for the stagnating economy and the non-sustainable agriculture.

For the above-mentioned reasons people were on the edge of starvation. When bad weather resulted in a series of harvest failures in 1315–17 the consequences were disastrous. Both crop and hay harvests failed due to constant raining leading to widespread famine – maybe the worst food shortage ever recorded in Europe. The harvest failures were accompanied and followed by livestock epidemics, first among sheep and later among cattle. In 1320–21 harvests failed again and it was not until 1322 the situation slowly started to improve.[11]

The famines of 1315–22 put a definitive end to the medieval expansion in much of Western Europe. In Sweden there is however no evidence of the Great Famine. The lack of evidence may simply be due to the scarcity of documentary sources from the time. But it is important to note that Sweden was not as densely populated as England and there was still room for expansion, in particular in wooded uplands. Even though the years of bad weather in England and on the Continent may have resulted in harvest failure also in Sweden, the agricultural society was probably still expanding and therefore not as vulnerable.

How troublesome the early part of the fourteenth century may have been, the real disaster came with the Black Death. This very deadly pandemic swept through Europe in a few years in the mid-fourteenth century, leading to immense suffering and killing a large part of the population. The symptoms as far as can be judged from historical documents showed similarities with those of later outbreaks of bubonic plague, in particular the one that struck Canton and Hong Kong in 1894. (The most characteristic symptom of bubonic plague is swollen lymph nodes, buboes, in groins and armpits.) In Hong Kong the plague bacteria *Yersinia pestis* was identified for the first time and the role of rats as transmitters was observed.[12] Further research in connection to the plague outbreaks in India in the beginning of the twentieth century confirmed that *Yersinia pestis* lives in the blood of rats and may be transferred between rats and from rats to humans by the bloodsucking oriental rat flea, *Xenopsylla cheopis*. Hence, most historians have concluded that the Black Death probably was an outbreak of plague, spread by the black rat and its fleas. However, in the absence of firm evidence, some have argued that it may have been some other disease.[13] In particular the very fast spread and high mortality of the Black Death seemed to differ from later plague outbreaks. Furthermore, the oriental rat flea – which was the documented transmitter of the disease from rats to humans in India – is today restricted to areas with high temperatures and would not have managed in medieval Northern Europe.[14]

It was not until recently that the plague hypothesis finally proved to be correct. Evidence came from advances in genetics and the identification of *Yersinia pestis* DNA in skeletons of Black Death victims.[15] However, the question still remains of how the plague was spread. If the oriental rat flea was not present in Europe, or at least restricted to its southern parts, other fleas may have been responsible for the transmission from rats to humans. Best candidates are the European rat flea (*Nosopsyllus fasciatus*) and the human flea (*Pulex irritans*), both of which can stand lower temperatures than the oriental rat flea.[16] But were the rats and their fleas really necessary as transmitters or could the pathogen spread directly from human to human? Here Iceland gives us an important example.[17] The Black Death of the mid-fourteenth century never reached Iceland because ship trade broke down in the wake of the plague and Iceland fell into isolation. Luck lasted for some decades but eventually in 1402–04 and in 1494–95 Iceland was struck by two severe epidemics. These outbreaks resulted in a population drop of 50–60% and 30–50%, respectively, and showed great similarities with the Black Death and its succeeding outbreaks in the rest of Europe. But Iceland during the Middle Ages had no rats, at least as far as we know from present evidence. It therefore seems that medieval plague epidemics could spread without rats.

Based on the Iceland example it has been suggested that the Black Death perhaps should be associated with the type of plague called pneumonic plague. It is caused by the same bacteria as bubonic plague but infects the lungs and may easily spread human-to-human by respiratory droplet transmission through coughing. It is extremely lethal and usually leads to death within one or a few days. The Black Death was certainly a combination of both bubonic and pneumonic plague, since they are just two different symptoms of the same disease, but if the latter has played a larger role than what is generally believed it may help to explain the very fast spread and high mortality. Occasionally the disease may have been transmitted directly human-to-human also by the human flea.[18]

An additional explanation to the force of the Black Death may be the fact that *Yersinia pestis* was new to the medieval population, which therefore had a very low level of immunity. Also for other epidemic diseases, like measles, smallpox and syphilis, the very first outbreak was much more virulent, fast spreading and deadly than later ones.[19] This is because exposure to a deadly pathogen leads to natural selection by which succeeding generations become more resistant. Recently it was proved also that the so-called Justinian Plague, which hit the Mediterranean and much of Europe in 541–543, was caused by *Yersinia pestis*.[20] Therefore this species of bacteria was not entirely new to Europe at the time of the Black Death. However, the reconstructed draft genomes show that the branch of *Y. pestis* that caused the Justinian Plague – referred to as the first plague pandemic – has no known contemporary representatives and that it is genetically distant from the strains associated with the second pandemic (from the Black Death to the early eighteenth century) and the third pandemic (late nineteenth and twentieth centuries). While the branch of the second pandemic via rodent populations lead on to the third, the branch responsible for the first pandemic probably became extinct when the pandemic died out in Europe in the eighth century.

Finally, social factors certainly played an important role in the fast spread of the Black Death. In medieval society the strong traditions of religion and charity aided the spread of diseases. Neighbours and relatives visited the sick and they also visited houses where someone had died to mourn the diseased and to comfort the bereaved family. Clergy went from house to house to the give the last rite and people gathered at funerals. Relatives inherited not only houses but also clothes and other personal belongings. In spite of the circumstances people held on to their traditions, and possibly these traditions became even more important in difficult and uncertain times. Cemeteries from the years of the Black Death testify that plague victims as far as possible were buried in a decent way according to religious customs. In the few cases when mass graves were dug, bodies were placed orderly side by side, sometimes in coffins (see Chap. 6 for further discussion.).[21] All together the impression is gained of a population who desperately tried to keep the social and religious structures intact and to a large degree succeeded. There is no doubt, however, that this facilitated the spread of the plague.

Many questions remain regarding the dissemination mechanisms and the complexity of factors that resulted in the fast spread of the Black Death. There is less controversy on the geographical pattern of spread, at least for Europe. The pandemic originated in the Black Sea region or possibly further east – its very origin is not known[22] – and arrived in Europe in 1347. It was introduced to Europe by ships from Caffa on the Crimean peninsula, via Constantinople to Greece and Italy, but there may also have been other routes, both on land and by sea. The arrival of the plague by ships to Messina on Sicily was described by the Franciscan friar Michael of Piazza, and is frequently referred to as a starting point for the Black Death's conquest of Europe:

> twelve Genoese galleys were fleeing from the vengeance which our lord was taking on account of their nefarious deeds and entered the harbour of Messina. In their bones they bore so virulent a disease that anyone who only spoke to them was seized by a mortal illness and in no manner could evade death …[23]

Also some other seaports like Marseille, Genoa and Venice were hit the same year, but it was in 1348 that larger areas were affected. Within a few months that year the plague spread through the entire Mediterranean region, including Italy, the Balkans, Spain, France, the Middle East and North Africa and even reached as far north as the Netherlands and southern England. In 1349–50 it advanced to the north and north-east, through Germany and Scandinavia, and in 1351–52 it continued eastwards through Poland and Russia.[24]

This was the first strike – the Black Death *sensu stricto* – which swept through Europe from 1347 to 1352. It was followed by several recurring outbreaks, some of them almost as devastating as the first one. In particular major outbreaks in 1358–62 and 1367–71 added significantly to the death tolls in northern Europe.[25] The plague stayed in Europe with sporadic outbreaks all the way up to the early eighteenth century. Some of the later outbreaks, for instance during the seventeenth century, were very devastating but usually more patchy than the medieval ones.

The Black Death, together with recurring outbreaks, resulted in an unprecedented population drop. Already by the first outbreak population numbers fell dramatically and they continued to fall, although more slowly, throughout the fourteenth and early fifteenth centuries. It was not until the mid-fifteenth century that population numbers slowly started to increase again. However, to quantify the population drop is difficult. Most authors estimate it to have been 30–50% on a European scale and as much as 40–60% in northern Europe.[26] All calculations have to be tentative, in particular because pre-Black Death population numbers are very hard to estimate. Even in England, where the documentary evidence is particularly good, recent estimates of the population drop range between 40% and 60%.[27]

An important character of the Black Death was that it hit towns and countryside alike. While many other diseases and parasites, in the past as well as today, spread effectively only in towns and other densely populated areas, this seems not to have been the case with the medieval plagues. Towns were hit hard, but to reach exceptionally high mortality in medieval Europe, where on average no more than 10% lived in urban areas, the Black Death must have spread effectively also in the countryside. Even in a sparsely populated country like Norway, which had no large urban centres, the Black Death had catastrophic consequences and resulted in a population drop of 60% or more.[28]

From this European background we may now look closer at the Black Death in Sweden. In a letter by Magnus Eriksson, king of Sweden and Norway, written in the autumn of 1349 to the diocese of Linköping, he warned for the great mortality that had killed more than half of the population in countries to the west and now was approaching Sweden.[29] Norway was already ravaged and so also the province of Halland, which is situated on the west coast of present-day Sweden but belonged to Denmark at the time. According to the king, people everywhere dropped down dead without any previous notion of disease, leaving too few alive to bury the dead. To limit God's punishment he commanded ritual precautions, prayers and donations to the church. There was little else they could do.

The plague spread from Halland and Norway to the western parts of medieval Sweden possibly already in 1349, but it was in 1350 that the whole country was ravaged (Fig. 3). From scattered indications it appears to have spread from west to east and to have reached the eastern coast, including Stockholm, in the autumn. An exception is the Baltic island of Gotland, which was hit by the plague already in springtime, possibly infected by Hanseatic ships directly from abroad.[30]

The Black Death swept fast and unstoppable through Sweden and by the autumn the disaster that Magnus Eriksson had predicted and warned about was all over the country. In another letter by him, this one written in the late summer or autumn of 1350 and sent to the pope in Avignon, he explained that he was not able to crusade against Russia because the plague had already emptied his country of able men.[31] Obviously, Sweden was hit hard by the plague, but due to the paucity of documentary evidence it is difficult to estimate the impact of the disaster and to quantify population drop. An ambitious attempt was made by *The Scandinavian Research Project on Deserted Farms and Villages*. The project resulted in several detailed studies on selected areas throughout the Nordic countries and the major results were summarised in a comprehensive book in 1981.[32] It was concluded that more than 40% of the farms in Norway were abandoned, while large parts of Sweden (including Scania) only showed a desertion frequency of less than 15%.[33] However, the resulting difference between the two countries was partly due to different criteria used within the project. While the Norwegian historians included circumstantial evidence to estimate the desertion frequency, their Swedish colleagues counted only deserted farms that were securely documented in the scarce sources. That these different approaches may lead to different results, and in particular to an underestimation of farm desertion in Sweden, was realised already in the project.[34] Still, the final conclusion was that Norway was hit particularly hard while Sweden came off relatively well.

This picture remained unchallenged for two decades during which the Black Death and the late-medieval crisis gained little attention in Swedish research. Renewed interest started with a publication by Janken Myrdal in 1999, in which he argued that Sweden was hit hard by the plague.[35] It was followed by publications on the Black Death by Dick Harrison and Lennart Andersson Palm, which were much in line with Myrdal's argument.[36] Palm presented a study of medieval population numbers in present-day Sweden and concluded that the late-medieval population drop, from a maximum in the early fourteenth century to a low stand in the early fifteenth century, was at the same level as in Norway, approximately 60–70%.[37] He based his study on two provinces in particular, Halland and Uppland, from which there are unusually detailed household and tax registers.[38] Two years later Janken Myrdal presented a study based on a broader spectrum of documentary sources: charters and letters (including wills and donations), death registers, Peter's Pence and other tax registers, annals, chronicles, etc.[39] Similar to Palm he concluded that Sweden was hit hard by the Black Death, maybe not as hard as Norway, but with a population drop at the same level as in much of Western Europe. Peter's Pence indicates a population drop of 50% between 1350 and 1370, and based on several different sources Myrdal concluded that the average drop within medieval Sweden was about 40–50%.[40] Because of the scarcity of documentary sources all estimations of the late-medieval population drop in Sweden have to be tentative. It is most difficult to establish the size of the pre-Black Death population, but also population numbers during the presumed low stand in the fifteenth century are uncertain. It is not until 1571 that we have detailed population numbers on a national level. However, the important conclusion from these later studies is that the Black Death was a disaster also in Sweden, with major consequences for society, and that earlier conclusions of a more modest crisis seem to reflect a paucity of sources rather than the true picture.

In Sweden like elsewhere the Black Death (Sw: *digerdöden*) was succeeded by several outbreaks.[41] The first strike in 1350 was followed by two severe outbreaks in 1359–60 and 1368–69. Together the first three outbreaks were probably a demographic and social catastrophe. Later outbreaks by the end of the fourteenth century had less impact until a series of new major outbreaks occurred in the fifteenth century. Years of major outbreaks were 1413, 1420–21, 1439–40, 1455, 1464–65 and 1495. Plague continued to haunt the population also during the sixteenth and seventeenth centuries, but outbreaks were often more of a regional character and did not lead to overall population drop (although the force of the plague increased again during the war-torn seventeenth century). The last outbreak of plague in Sweden was as late as in 1710–13.[42]

Thus people of the fifteenth to early eighteenth centuries were familiar with plague, by own experience, from eyewitnesses or by hearsay. In spite of this the Black Death of the mid-fourteenth century was to be remembered. For example, the Swedish king Gustav Vasa wrote in a letter in 1555, two centuries after the Black Death, that it affected the people badly and that two-thirds of the population died.[43] Gustav Vasa, together with several other writers, connected it with the remains of abandoned farms that could be found in forests and other marginal areas. A general opinion that prevailed for a long time was that the population was larger before the Black Death. Carl Linnaeus, for example, the famous botanist, wrote on his travels through southern Sweden in 1749 that the ancient clearance cairns that he found in the forests were reminders of a larger population before the Black Death.[44]

The sudden population decline due to the Black Death resulted in the abandonment of farms. Abandoned (or deserted) farms are frequently and specifically mentioned in early records, such as cadastral registers and other documents.[45] Some historians have raised doubts about what the term "abandoned farm" in the old records really stands for, i.e. if

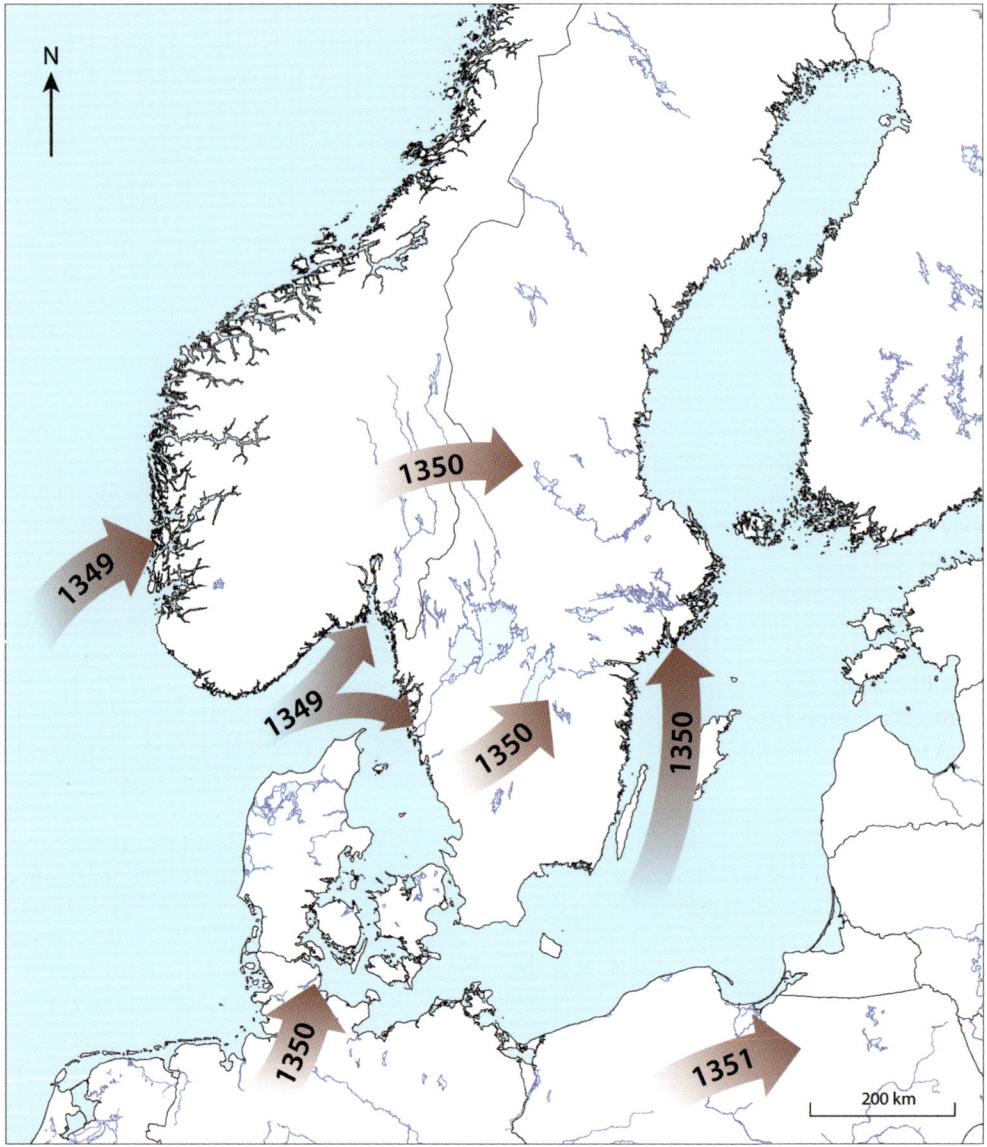

Fig. 3. Map of Scandinavia showing the first strike of the plague, the Black Death (based on Benedictow 2004, 173 and Myrdal 2009, 82)

such a farm was uninhabited or only declared exempt from tax. However, this may be a problem connected to registers from the sixteenth century onwards, but not to medieval ones in which the word abandoned (Sw: *öde*) really stands for uninhabited.[46] Abandoned farms are also identified on maps. Sweden has a wealth of detailed maps from the early seventeenth century onwards that may be used for retrogressive analyses of late-medieval farm abandonment.[47] In addition to written documents and maps, sometimes the physical remains of abandoned farms are found in the field, in particular in forest or heathland outside modern cultivation areas. In Sweden such remains are found in different parts of the country and some of them have been investigated archaeologically (see Chap. 5 for a discussion on the archaeological evidence).[48]

At present little is known about the spatial pattern of farm abandonment and its regional distribution. However, two maps attempting to show regional variations in farm abandonment in Scandinavia have been published, one by *The Scandinavian Research Project on Deserted Farms and Villages* and one later by Janken Myrdal.[49] According to Myrdal, in much of Sweden as well as in parts of Finland, Norway and Demark, between one-third and two-thirds of the farms were abandoned. In the most fertile agricultural plains, situated in the provinces of Uppland, Östergötland and Scania in Sweden and on the Danish islands, the extent of abandonment was less than this and in the most marginal areas it was larger. Areas with an extent of farm abandonment greater than two- thirds were the uplands of southern Sweden, the uplands and mountains of Norway and the sandy heathlands of Jutland. The map from the earlier study differs from Myrdal's map by showing generally lower desertion frequency for Sweden. However, similar to his map, it suggests that within Sweden farm abandonment was most extensive in the southern uplands, and on a Scandinavian level it was most extensive in Norway. Hence, despite the controversy on the extent of farm abandonment in Sweden, both agree that it was most extensive in marginal upland areas. This conclusion is in line with observations from other countries, like England, Germany and Austria, where farm abandonment was most widespread in upland areas and on sandy soil.[50]

A somewhat different view on marginal uplands have been put forward based on studies in the forest regions of middle and northern Sweden, in particular within the *Ängersjö Project*,[51] but also in some other studies.[52] Even though these studies have found evidence of farm desertion, they argue that societies in forested regions may have escaped the crisis better than those on the agricultural plains. This is because they were based on a more diverse economy, which enabled flexible strategies of resource utilisation and land use.[53] In particular iron production seems to have expanded in some areas during the crisis.[54] However, if the more diverse economy of uplands should be regarded as more resilient than the agrarian economy of lowlands is debated.[55] For the time being most evidence on late-medieval farm abandonment – from documentary sources as well as from archaeology and pollen analysis – comes from uplands and other agriculturally marginal areas. Even though non-agricultural economies typical of uplands (iron production, coaling, tar production, logging, etc.) may have expanded in the wake of the crisis, most evidence indicate that there was extensive abandonment of farms in upland areas and probably more extensive than in the lowlands.

The fact that farms on marginal land, where poor soils or climate made agriculture troublesome or at least less productive than elsewhere, were the first to be deserted also seems logical at first. This is particularly so if the underlying cause was the kind of overpopulation and unsustainable land use that Michael Postan suggested for marginal areas in early-fourteenth-century England. According to him the hunger for new land lead to reclamation of poor soils, which after a few decades of cultivation were depleted of nutrients and eventually abandoned.[56] However, the model is not directly applicable for Sweden, which had a much lower population density than England. Furthermore, the soils of the South-Swedish Uplands were poor in relation to those of the fertile plains, but due to the still large extent of pastures and access to manure, they probably gave decent yields.[57]

Also if the underlying cause was climatic deterioration, abandonment of marginal uplands would perhaps be expected. Climate deterioration as a cause of abandonment has been suggested elsewhere, and cannot be entirely ruled out for upland areas also in Sweden.[58] Based on a reconstruction of average temperatures for the Northern Hemisphere the peak of the so-called Medieval Warm Period was reached during the tenth to twelfth centuries, while the lowest temperatures of the Little Ice Age were reached in the sixteenth to seventeenth centuries.[59] The transition from warm climate to colder was gradual, and in the absence of local palaeoclimate data it is difficult to identify any specific period of dramatic climate deterioration, even though such periods may have existed. Short periods of bad weather during the fourteenth century may have been troublesome enough, but it was not until the fifteenth century that climatic deterioration became significant and long lasting. Therefore, at the present state of knowledge, it is unlikely that farm abandonment during the mid-fourteenth century was due to climate. Furthermore, an interesting fact that speaks against a simple relationship between the extent of upland agriculture and climate is that during the sixteenth century – when the Little Ice Age reached its lowest temperatures – there was a strong movement of colonisation and agricultural expansion in the South-Swedish Uplands.

If farm abandonment was not due to soil deterioration or a shift to colder climate, but actually to the Black Death, it is more difficult to understand why upland societies suffered particularly badly. Even though the plague seems to have spread effectively in the countryside we may expect it to have spread faster and more severely in towns and on the densely populated agricultural plains than in sparsely settled uplands. This paradox of plague-ridden lowlands and abandoned uplands is usually explained as an effect of migration.[60] The plague may very well have hit the population of fertile lowlands harder than upland societies, but farms on good soil were not allowed to stay abandoned for long. Survivors of the Black Death adapted to the new situation of a smaller population and were concentrated in fertile areas where better conditions for agriculture made living easier. The details of this process are not known but it is likely that succession rights were followed, even when one or several heirs in line were swept away by the plague. In this way an upland farmer may suddenly and unexpectedly have inherited a farm in a better setting, and probably did not hesitate to take the opportunity. In the case of large landowners, they could redirect their tenants to better farms, leaving less productive units abandoned.

Extensive farm abandonment in upland areas and other marginal areas in the wake of the Black Death could thus be an effect of migration. Still, the possibility that the plague itself also reached remote settlement should not be excluded. People living on single farmsteads in the woods or in other sparsely settled areas were not socially isolated. They belonged to communities and gathered with their friends, neighbours and relatives at home, in church, at market places as did everybody else. Furthermore, many upland farmers were involved in trade with lowland societies, exporting timber, iron and animal products while importing grain. The latter may have been particularly fatal in a time of plague, because grain was usually accompanied by rats and their fleas.[61]

In addition to the geographical variation in the spread of plague and in the extension of farm desertion, there were important differences in how social classes were affected. In contrast to tuberculosis, cholera and some other diseases, plague is not restricted to the poor and malnourished. It may infect also the healthy and wealthy leaving nobody safe. However, the plague of the mid-fourteenth century did hit the poor people harder than the upper classes.[62] The major reason for this was probably different living conditions, where poor people lived in small and unhealthy houses, close to each other and closer to rats. However, poor people who survived the plague had good possibilities to improve their economic and social status. The sudden and dramatic population drop gave small-holders the possibility to move to better and larger holdings, crofters to become tenant farmers, and the poor and landless to gain possession of farms. Because vacant farms were taken over by the previously landless, the process of farm desertion may have been somewhat delayed in relation to the population drop. According to documentary evidence, farm abandonment became widespread not immediately after the Black Death but rather in connection with the following plague outbreaks and later, when society was running out of landless and thus the 'reserve' of the agricultural labour force was used up (see however new results on the suddenness of farm abandonment in Chap.4).[63]

These two factors – the very high mortality from the plague among poor people and the opportunities for the survivors to improve their status – resulted in a general decrease in the number of poor. Another factor that contributed to a higher standard of living for common people, at least in the long run, was the shortage of manpower. The large landowners, the nobility, the church and the Crown, who depended on agricultural production, saw their incomes reduced when tenants died and farms and fields were abandoned. To keep their tenants on the land and to attract new ones to take over vacant farms, landowners had to offer better conditions. Tenants had a good negotiating position and landowners had to accept lower rents and less day labour. But they did so only reluctantly. Their immediate reaction was to increase rents to compensate for declining numbers of tenants, which lead to disputes and conflicts during which many tenants left their holdings, leading to further reduction of the incomes of the landowners. In desperation parts of the nobility turned to a robber economy, plundering the countryside, which lead to counter reactions and resistance. That the latter part of the fourteenth century was a time of conflicts and riots is evident from the building of castles. In spite of the shortage of manpower the building of castles and fortifications, both noble and royal, in southern Sweden increased significantly after the Black Death.[64]

After decades of conflicts and revolts the situation finally improved for tenant farmers and freeholders in the early fifteenth century. Tenant farmers got better conditions with lower rents, and slightly later – in particular after the major uprising of the 1430s – national taxes for free-holding peasants were significantly reduced. This line of development has for Sweden been most explicitly described by Janken Myrdal, who identifies the following phases: the catastrophe *c*. 1350–1370, the dysfunctional societal reaction *c*. 1350/60–1430/1440, and the social and economic recovery and reconstruction *c*. 1440/50–1520/30.[65] More or less the same development has been identified also in other European countries after the Black Death.

When taxes and rents had finally settled on a lower level in the fifteenth century, living standards improved and consumption increased. In Sweden like elsewhere increased popular consumption stimulated non-agrarian production, craftsmanship and trade.[66] Iron production increased and the price of iron fell, making iron tools readily available. Also the import of Flandrian textiles increased together with other commodities from abroad. Although the documentary sources do not provide any details on the consumption of food among ordinary people in medieval Sweden, it is likely that they were, on average, able to eat and drink more and better than before. According to Ole Benedictow, people in general in Western Europe after the Black Death '… ate more meat and butter, drank more beer and wine, socialized more and spent more time in taverns and inns.'[67] (See Chap. 6 for further discussions on living conditions and possible dietary changes.)

Food and drink now lead us to the agricultural production – the economic basis for medieval society. It is obvious that total agricultural production decreased when population numbers were cut by half and farms were abandoned. However, there were probably also changes within the agricultural system that contributed to the rising economy and improved living standards after the Black Death. Many factors may have influenced agricultural development but there is one that seems to have been most decisive, namely the changed relationship between the amount of available land and the number of hands to cultivate it.

When people died in unprecedented numbers of the plague, this naturally affected the everyday work on the farms. Sometimes the whole household was swept away by the plague, but also if only one or a few were killed it usually had severe effects on the family's economy and their possibility to keep the farm going. Temporary losses and gaps in the family structure could be filled by landless – usually disinherited relatives – and possibly this labour reserve may, to some degree, have prevented farm abandonment in the initial phase. Eventually, however, population drop resulted in a shortage of labour. Those who survived the plague were left with an excess of land and a reduced labour force. The relative excess of land was not only due to the shrinking sizes of families and households, but also due to the fact that many farmers took the opportunity two expand their holdings by incorporating the land of abandoned farms. A lot of work had been invested in the land during the centuries, from the initial clearing of woodlands to the continuous tilling, clearing of stones, manuring, fencing, etc. This investment – the so-called landesque capital – was at risk of getting wasted if land-use ceased and arable fields and meadows were left to become overgrown and return to woodland.[68] As far as possible, farmers tried to keep the land open.

One way to adapt to the shortage of manpower was to shift to more extensive cultivation, for instance by sowing seed more thinly and to cut down on labour-intensive weeding and manuring. It would lead to decreased land productivity (yields per hectare) but also to an increased labour productivity (yields per head).[69] Also slash-and-burn cultivation was an efficient way to get decent yields with a dwindling labour force and became common in some Swedish upland areas during the crisis.[70]

Another way to adapt to the new situation was to turn more to animal husbandry. Because of the basic principle of the loss of energy (typically 90%) in each step of the food chain, the possible food production per hectare of animal husbandry is only about one-tenth of that of cereal growing.[71] While animal husbandry is land demanding, cereal growing on the other hand is more labour intensive. In a period characterised by an excess of land but a shortage of labour we would therefore expect an increase in animal husbandry in relation to cereal growing. That such a change indeed happened in the Late Middle Ages is evident from documentary sources, in particular from England, which has a wealth of detailed records.[72] Also in Sweden there are indications of a relative increase in animal husbandry. One such indication is the mentioning of deserted farms in cadastral registers from the fifteenth century and later. According to these records deserted farms were frequently used by neighbouring farms for pasture or hay meadows.[73] Another indication is the increased production of butter, reflected in gradual declining prices of butter relative to grain prices.[74] That abandoned farms in some cases were used for pastures has also been shown by pollen analysis (see Chap. 4 for new results).[75] However, it is still difficult to quantify the importance of animal husbandry and there may have been regional differences.

Even though animal husbandry was less labour intensive than cereal growing the number of people available to take care of the animals was still a limiting factor. In particular the collection of grass hay for winter fodder was labour intensive and the time of hay harvest was one of the busiest during the year. The development during the Late Middle Ages of longer scythes and better rakes – the two important tools for hay mowing – helped to make fodder collection more efficient and less time consuming but it still remained a bottleneck for the possible number of animals that could be kept.[76] Another change that may have facilitated animal husbandry in a time of labour shortage is reflected in the way herding was organised.[77] In Sweden, as in the rest of Europe, herding before the Black Death was carried out mostly by adult men. In Continental Europe this situation persisted into later periods, but then with a higher degree of collaboration, usually with a common village herder. In Sweden most villages and hamlets were too small to employ a village herder and there were still many single farmsteads. Instead the herding task in late-medieval Sweden was taken over by children and women. By so doing, adult men became increasingly available for other duties. This shift from male herders to children and women started in the fifteenth century and probably reflects an adaptation to the shortage of manpower after the Black Death. However, the system with female herders became so well established that it continued all the way up to the early twentieth century, until the very end of traditional herding. In addition, other aspects of animal husbandry, in particular milking but also for instance summer farming in northern Sweden, became strictly female domains.[78]

The plenty of land together with low rents in the mid-fifteenth century meant the beginning of the end for the crisis. Society slowly started to recover and although there were still outbreaks of plague, population numbers were gradually starting to increase. Plague outbreaks during the fifteenth century could still be locally disastrous but on a larger scale the plague had lost some of its former force. This was probably due to a more resistant population shaped by natural selection but also to better awareness of how to avoid the disease. The agricultural expansion that went hand-in-hand with population recovery started slowly but took off during the sixteenth century. To a large degree this expansion meant the reoccupation of farms abandoned in connection with the Black Death and its aftermath. However, many deserted farms remained uninhabited in spite of the rising population numbers and the increased demand for land. This was because the deserted farms were now owned by and incorporated to other farms, which used them for pasture and as hay meadows. The land of deserted farms was regarded as an important resource and the possession of such land was specifically mentioned in cadastral registers. Above all it was a resource for grazing and mowing but eventually also for cultivation. New research show that many deserted farms that were used for cultivation, mowing and pasture, remained uninhabited even into the seventeenth century.[79]

The opportunity to incorporate land of abandoned farms did not only result in larger holdings. In some areas it may also have facilitated the introduction of crop-rotation systems. In parts of the South-Swedish Uplands a three-field system was introduced in the sixteenth century, in connection with agricultural recovery after the crisis.[80] In this system one-third of the infields were fallowed each year, while the other two-thirds were used for growing barley and some other crop, usually rye. The excess of land that followed upon abandonment may thus have facilitated the introduction of systematic fallow in the infields. The same was probably true for the large-scale establishment of summer farms in northern Sweden during the sixteenth century.[81] Although the causal relationships are far from clear on a general level, it is evident that summer farms in some cases represent a secondary use of permanent farms abandoned in the Late Middle Ages.[82]

The sixteenth century was characterised by strong agricultural expansion and the establishment of new settlement. In spite of the relatively harsh climate of the Little Ice Age, expansion was particularly strong in marginal upland areas that had suffered from extensive farm desertion during the crisis. The agricultural expansion was to some degree the result of successful politics by the increasingly strong state. By declaring outlands to be state property and by offering tax exemption for new holdings, the colonisation of remote woodlands was stimulated. However, the foundation for the expansion were the agrarian and social changes of the preceding century. The shortage of manpower after the Black Death had stimulated the development of more efficient agricultural tools and better techniques, and the larger holdings with emphasis on stock farming had resulted in increased labour productivity. Abandoned farms and the excess of land had facilitated the establishment of agricultural systems based on crop rotation, fallowing and transhumance, which in turn were the foundation for a more sustainable agriculture. And, in addition, the improved living standards and increased consumption by the majority of the population had stimulated non-agricultural production, craftsmanship and trade.

These changes laid the foundation for societal development and the strong economy of the sixteenth century. However, little is known about the more long-term effects of the late-medieval crisis. Hypothetically, the profound changes may have had long-lasting effects – not only within agriculture, economy and consumption – but also in a wide range of areas, from the genetics of European population to social structure, culture and religious belief.[83] Less speculatively, however, population drop and farm abandonment also had major impact on the landscape development. Vegetation and fauna naturally changed in response to changes in agriculture and settlement, both in times of expansion and decline, but there may also have been long-term effects on biodiversity. So far little attention has been paid to the ecological and environmental aspects of the late-medieval crisis.

Notes

1   Myrdal 2012a, 228
2   Myrdal 2011, 89ff
3   Myrdal 2012a, 211. These numbers refer to medieval Sweden excluding Finland (which belonged to Sweden until 1809). In Finland peasants owned almost all land
4   For Europe: Livi Bacci 2000, 6; Ponting 2007, 95; for Sweden: Myrdal 2012a, 222
5   Myrdal 2011, 82–86; 2012a, 218
6   For medieval colonisation see Larsson 1975, 97ff; Lagerås 2007, 31ff; Myrdal 2011, 77ff
7   Lagerås & Bartholin 2003; Lagerås 2013a
8   Moberg *et al.* 2005
9   Postan 1972. Principally, Postan's model is based on Thomas Malthus' writings in the late eighteenth and early nineteenth centuries. According to Malthus there was a permanent cycle in history, where human numbers increased until they were too large for the available food supply

and prevailing technology to support. Famine and disease would then reduce population numbers until they were in balance with the food production

10 Christopher Dyer, among others, argues that demographic pressure should not be seen as an independent force but rather as a result of economical and social factors (e.g. Dyers 2002, 246–263)

11 Kershaw 1973, 6–15

12 Benedictow 2004, 9–10

13 Twigg 1984; Scott & Duncan 2001; Cohn 2002; 2003; Knudsen 2009

14 According to a study by Bacot (1914, 645), quoted in Moseng (2009, 32), the oriental rat flea needs temperatures above 13°C to hatch

15 Haensch *et al.* 2010; Schuenemenn *et al.* 2011

16 Moseng 2009, 32ff

17 Karlsson 1996

18 Moseng 2009, 39ff

19 Ponting 2007, 203–216

20 Wagner *et al.* 2014

21 Grainger *et al.* 2008, 12ff

22 Christensen 2009, 15

23 Benedictow 2004, 70

24 For a detailed account on the spread of the Black Death see Benedictow (2004)

25 Myrdal 2012a, 223

26 Livi Bacci 2000, 81; Harrison 2000, 72; Benedictow 2004, 383

27 Dyer 2002, 235; Benedictow 2004, 383; Campbell 2012, 121

28 Livi Bacci 2000, 84; Myrdal 2012a, 227

29 Nordberg 1995, 160

30 Benedictow 2004, 173; Myrdal 2009, 82

31 Nordberg 1995, 161

32 Gissel *et al.* 1981

33 Sandnes 1981, 103

34 Österberg 1981a, 48. The project was later criticised by Janken Myrdal (2003, 165–183; 2012a, 226)

35 Myrdal 1999, 116

36 Harrison 2000; Palm 2001

37 Palm 2001, 28

38 For these two provinces, Palm concluded that there were about one hundred farms per parish in the early fourteenth century and suggested that this was the rule also elsewhere in Sweden

39 Myrdal's thorough research on the Black Death and the late-medieval crisis was first published in Swedish (Myrdal 1999; 2003) and then later in English (Myrdal 2006; 2009; 2012a)

40 Myrdal 2011, 80; 2012a, 227

41 Myrdal 2006, 154; Bisgaard 2009, 97

42 Persson 2001

43 Palm 2001, 27; Myrdal 2003, 9

44 Linnaeus 1751, 79–80. Also Olaus Magnus, who wrote his *History of the Nordic People* in the mid-sixteenth century, saw the overgrown fields as an indication of depopulation due to "plague, war and famine" (Olaus Magnus 1555, Bk 1, Ch. 29, Bk 2, Ch. 21)

45 E.g. Larsson 1970; Österberg 1977; Bååth 1983; Myrdal 2003

46 Myrdal 2003, 168

47 E.g. Antonson 2009; Karsvall 2011

48 E.g. Gauffin 1981; Hansson *et al.* 2005; Åstrand 2006

49   Gissel *et al.* 1981, 103, 107; Myrdal 2012a, 226
50   Abel 1980, 88–89
51   Johansson (ed.) 2002
52   Svensson 1998; Svensson *et al.* 2012; Berglund *et al.* 2009
53   Emanuelsson 2001, 26
54   Berglund *et al.* 2009
55   Cf. Lagerås 2013b for a discussion on these two opposing views on uplands
56   Postan 1972, 26
57   Widgren 1995, 93
58   Lamb (1982) argues strongly for climatically induced farm abandonment in Britain, in particular in upland areas, both during the Middle Ages and later
59   Moberg *et al.* 2005, 616
60   Abel 1980, 88–89; Dyers 2002, 352; Benedictow 2004, 261; Myrdal 2011, 80; 2012a, 225, 227
61   Harrison 2000, 33. According to Ole Benedictow (2004, 20), rat fleas could occasionally live off grain and grain debris, depending on blood only for laying eggs, and thereby survive for a while even when their rat hosts had died from the plague
62   Dyer 2002, 271–272; Benedictow 2004, 382
63   Myrdal 2006, 159; 2012a, 227
64   Lovén 1996; Myrdal 2012a, 230
65   Myrdal 2012a, 232–237
66   Myrdal 2012a, 229; cf. Dyers 2002, 296
67   Benedictow 2004, 390
68   The importance of the landesque capital in pre-industrial agriculture is discussed by Widgren (2007, 61)
69   Campbell 2012, 137; Myrdal 2012a, 222
70   Vestbö-Franzén 2004, 225
71   Redman 1999, 41–42
72   Campbell 2006, 185; 2012, 124
73   Myrdal 2006, 169
74   Söderberg 2007, 143–144
75   Lagerås 2007, 69–77
76   Myrdal 2012a, 221
77   Myrdal 2012a, 217; 2012b, 222
78   Larsson 2012, 20
79   Karsvall 2011
80   Myrdal 2003, 237; Vestbö-Franzén 2004, 225
81   Larsson 2012, 26
82   Hansson *et al.* 2005, 89–90; Antonsson 2009, 636
83   For a discussion on possible long-term effects of the late-medieval crisis in a wide range of areas, see the essays by David Herlihy, published 1997 in *The Black Death and the Transformation of the West*

3.

Societal crisis and environmental change

Per Lagerås

The Late Middle Ages was obviously a period of stress and hardship and the sequence of events that characterises the fourteenth and fifteenth centuries are generally referred to as a crisis, depression or decline. It is important to note, however, that medieval peasants were used to stress and hardship. The agricultural system frequently suffered from small returns and peasants and tenure farmers had to carry heavy burdens of taxes and rents. Agriculture was also sensitive to weather, partly due to the absence of draining and irrigation, and yields could vary significantly from one year to another.[1] To mitigate these difficulties and to secure survival, farmers in medieval society (as in most pre-industrial societies) were oriented to reducing risks rather than to maximise production and profit.[2] In spite of this strategy, poor yields and harvest failures from time to time inevitably resulted in malnutrition, starvation and sometimes famine. Also infectious diseases were common and contributed to the high mortality and low life expectancy of the time. Hence, medieval farmers were all too familiar with small-scale crisis like starvation and disease. For individuals and families these difficulties could be hard enough, but thanks to the social structure with many landless – the reserve of the agricultural labour force – they did usually not lead to farm abandonment or to any significant decrease in agricultural production.

To this background of everyday struggle and of more or less expected setbacks and difficulties, the late-medieval crises stood out as something different. Its widespread distribution and the enormous cost of lives made it a major crisis, challenging the agricultural system and the very structures of society. Why this happened – why familiar problems like harvest failure and disease during the fourteenth century escalated to a major crisis – is the subject of much research and a matter of debate. The complexity of the possible causal relationships has been touched upon in the previous section and may be summarised as a combination of external and internal factors. One of the two major external factors was the rainy summers and harvest failures of 1315–17, which together with epidemics among cattle and sheep and further harvest failures lead to the Great Famine. The other was the Black Death, the plague pandemic of 1347–52, which together with succeeding plague outbreaks caused immense suffering and a dramatic population drop.

There can be no doubt that these two exogenous calamities played leading roles in the crisis. But internal factors like social, political and economic conditions may also have contributed. In particular the Great Famine is frequently interpreted as a combined effect of harvest failures and a stagnated society, although there are different opinions on why society stagnated. Two main directions in the debate may be identified.[3] One of them – usually referred to as neo-Malthusian – focuses on the dynamics of long-term waves in demography and economy. According to this view, a major underlying cause behind stagnation in Western Europe in the late thirteenth and early fourteenth centuries was overpopulation leading to land shortage. The other direction represents a more Marxist view, and criticises the first for being too deterministic and for not paying sufficient attention to class structures. According to this view the major cause behind stagnation was the limitations of the feudal system and its inability (and unwillingness) to change. A major problem of feudalism, apart from the obvious social inequalities, was that too much of the agrarian income was spent on luxury consumption by the elite while too little was invested back into agricultural production. The system left the servants with neither incitement nor financial means to invest in their agriculture.

Without going into this debate, it should be noted that interpretations that identify internal societal factors and their possible contribution to the crisis should not without caution be transferred from one region or country to another. For instance, population density varied greatly across Europe. And even if some areas, like southern England, may have been overpopulated by the late thirteenth century, other areas were definitely not. In much of Sweden and other sparsely populated regions, population density was not a limiting factor and population growth and agricultural expansion probably continued all the way up to the Black Death. Also when discussing the feudal system it is important to note that the system looked different in different countries and regions. Tenants in Sweden during the thirteenth and fourteenth centuries had a better legal position than in many other countries and serfdom proper did not exist.[4] Therefore conclusions on a so-called feudal crisis may not necessarily be transferable, for instance, from France or England to Sweden.

Also when it comes to the Black Death, internal social factors may have contributed to its impact, but the force of the pandemic would probably have been disastrous for any society, stagnated or not. Research have focused on how society changed after the disaster and on the economic processes triggered by the population drop. Again, due to differences in the political systems, social reactions may have differed between countries even though the overall development seems to have been similar on a general level. In Sweden like in some other countries the immediate reaction from the landowning elite, who saw their incomes dwindle when their tenants died and fields were laid wasted, was to increase oppression and to turn to brutal plundering. Janken Myrdal, who used crisis theory to interpret the line of events, called this phase the dysfunctional social reaction.[5] According to him the counterproductive reaction by the elite deepened the crisis. The Black Death started a vicious circle in which internal social factors and reactions (together with recurring outbreaks of plague) played an important role. Thus, the increased oppression did not start the crisis but it acted as a positive feedback to the downward trend.

Oppression and plundering resulted in resistance and peasant revolts, which eventually turned successful. Rents and taxes were reduced and the share of the production that stayed with the peasants increased. This was the start of the recovery phase and once again positive feedback mechanisms may be identified. The starting point was the improved living standard of the large number of common people. It resulted in increased consumption, which stimulated craftsmanship, trade, iron production, etc., which in turn stimulated agricultural expansion. However, this was not only a phase of recovery but also of reconstruction. The crisis changed the power relationship between the classes and paved the way for a stronger state. Myrdal has emphasised that these structural changes were important parts of the late-medieval crisis and at the same time contributed to the strong expansion of the sixteenth century.[6] The societal crisis thus may have had positive effects for economic growth seen in a longer time perspective.

To sum up the discussion so far, the late-medieval crisis had several characteristics typical for a major crisis: a dramatic population drop, a decreased total production and an economic recession, increased oppression leading to riots and conflicts, and changed power relationships, which challenged the political and social structures. On this general level it shows similarities with other major crisis and fits into a broader picture of societal crisis as an inherent part of human history.

Historical examples of societal crises and in particular of what is referred to as societal collapse has gained increased attention during the last two decades, both within the research community and among the general public. This is certainly due to concerns for our own society and problems that we have to face today and in the future. Typical case studies that have been widely discussed are the collapse of great empires and civilisations, like the Western Roman Empire and the Classic Lowland Maya, but also the collapse of much smaller societies in fragile environments, like Rapa Nui on Easter Island and the Norse settlements on Greenland.[7] Naturally, processes and mechanisms have varied greatly between such different societies, and also the definition of collapse may vary between different authors. According to Joseph Tainter, collapse is first of all a political process characterised by a "… rapid, significant loss of an established level of socio-political complexity."[8] Although external catastrophes may have a triggering effect, the underlying cause of collapse is to be found in the structure and organisation of society itself. A single-event catastrophe, like a volcanic eruption or a major disease epidemic, never fully explains collapse. Jared Diamond suggests a similar but wider definition. According to him a collapse is characterised by "… a drastic decrease in human population size and/or political/economic/social complexity, over a considerable area, for an extended time."[9] Similar to Tainter, he finds social factors to be decisive for how societies manage to cope with stress and challenges and to modify their practices in response to perceived crises, and ultimately whether they will collapse or not.

Research on collapse, and particularly the work by Jared Diamond, has been influential within several disciplines, from archaeology and history to human ecology. However, it has also been criticised, most explicitly by the authors of the anthology *Questioning collapse*.[10] They admit that societal crises in a historical perspective certainly existed, but rarely did societies collapse in an absolute or apocalyptic sense. The overriding human story is one of survival and regeneration rather than of collapse and societal failures. Therefore, according to the authors, it would be fruitful to focus more on survival strategies than on collapse and to emphasise resilience of past societies.[11]

Surprisingly, the late-medieval crisis is rarely discussed in this context. It is not included in the lists of historical examples of societal collapse presented by Tainter and Diamond, and it is only rarely discussed in connection to resilience thinking.[12] This is surprising having in mind that the late-medieval crisis is frequently referred to as a major crisis and the Black Death generally regarded as one of the worst catastrophes to have ever struck Europe. The reason may be that medieval society – in spite of the severe crisis and dramatic population drop – did not collapse. This is, however, a matter of definition, and as Diamond points out, it becomes arbitrary to decide how drastic a decline must be before it qualifies to be labelled as a collapse.[13] It seems justified to regard the population drop in connection to the Black Death as a collapse of the European population, but to interpret and quantify the possible decrease in complexity is more difficult. The decades after the Black Death were characterised by increased oppression and conflicts and the previously well ordered but rigid feudal system in Sweden as well as, for instance, in parts of Germany, was replaced by a plunder economy with robber barons raiding the countryside.[14] Obviously this was a period of decreased economic and socio-political complexity. On the other hand, in spite of chaos and political instability, social structures remained surprisingly intact even in the most difficult of times. As Christopher Dyer points out for England in the years of the plague, everywhere officials, clerks and tenants died, but substitutes were usually found, and where fields were harvested, rents were collected.[15] Royal courts and other institutions were robust enough to withstand the stress and soon resumed their work after a brief interval. Even feudalism in a wider sense survived but with a stronger state and somewhat weakened nobility.

Regardless of whether the late-medieval crisis should be classified as collapse or not, it may be fruitful to borrow research perspectives from the modern field of studies of historical collapse. Several such studies have a human-ecological approach with an interest in the relationship between society and the environment. Special attention has been paid to historical examples where overexploitation resulted in environmental destruction, which in turn was unfavourable for society. Environmental destruction may be deforestation, soil depletion, desertification, salinisation, etc. The paramount example is Easter Island, where environmental degradation was brought on by human deforestation, leading to societal collapse and dwindling population numbers.[16] Frequently the fate of Easter Island and other historical examples of human mismanagement of the environment are used as a lesson and a warning to our own time:

> The metaphor is so obvious. Easter Island isolated in the Pacific Ocean – once the island got into trouble, there was no way they could get free. There was no other people from whom they could get help. In the same way that we on Planet Earth, if we ruin our own [world], we won't be able to get help.[17]

Even though one may be pessimistic about our ability (or willingness) to learn from the past, there is no doubt that concerns about our own environment have resulted in an increased interest in historical studies of how different societies have coped with environmental problems.

In the case of the late-medieval crisis, present knowledge indicates that it was not caused primarily by environmental mismanagement. The model proposed by Postan for the late thirteenth and early fourteenth centuries involved environmental aspects: population pressure resulted in land reclamation of too poor soils, leading to decreasing land productivity, starvation and abandonment.[18] This may have been a contributing factor in some areas, but on a European scale it was probably of minor importance. However, even if human impact on the environment was not the underlying cause of the crisis – but rather the plague pandemic in combination with harvest failures and social factors – the immense population drop and land-use changes certainly had significant consequences for the environment. It is important to note that the landscape already during the Middle Ages was strongly affected by human impact and in particular by agriculture. The original woodland cover of Europe was much reduced by clearing and by the thirteenth century the woodland that existed before the onset of the medieval expansion in the sixth century was reduced by at least 50%.[19] Thus, the medieval landscape was a cultural landscape influenced and shaped by humans and their agricultural land use. Most ecosystems were anthropogenic ecosystems, tightly linked to human actions and society.

Because of the important human role in the ecosystems and for shaping and maintaining cultural landscapes, the dramatic decrease in human numbers in connection with the Black Death – perhaps a halving of the European population – must have had significant ecological consequences. We may expect reforestation of abandoned fields, meadows and pastures, but also other vegetation changes when new agricultural strategies were developed. A few attempts have been made to reveal vegetation change in connection with the late-medieval crisis by using pollen analysis and this is further elaborated in Chapter 4.[20]

The ecological consequences of the late-medieval crisis in Europe are an intriguing but still much under-researched area. However, parallels may be drawn with America. Infectious diseases like smallpox and measles, brought by Europeans in the sixteenth century, caused catastrophic drops in population numbers and massive disruption in society.[21] Settlements were abandoned and fields and grasslands were reforested. It was not until relatively recently that it was realised to what large extent the pre-Columbian landscape had been affected by humans, shaped not only by agriculture but also by hunting and fire. The forests that the European colonists thought were primeval and enduring were actually in a state of swift change. The massive decrease in human population not only caused vegetation changes but also large-scale changes in the fauna. Many question marks remain, but it appears that the "land of plenty", with its enormous populations of bison, passenger pigeons, etc., to some degree was actually a temporary effect of the sudden disappearance of humans.[22]

According to a hypothesis by Urban Emanuelsson, historical periods of decreased human impact were beneficial for biodiversity, not only in the short run, but also in a long-term perspective.[23] He argues that recurrent periods of decreased human impact – due to disease, war and other factors – have contributed positively to the high biodiversity that characterised many traditional cultural landscapes of Europe before the agricultural revolution. To put it drastically, periods of hardship for humans may have been periods of relief for some species of both plants and animals. But the relationship is complicated, because many species are favoured by agricultural land use and other kinds of human disturbance.

What makes environmental changes particularly interesting in this context is that they may not just passively reflect the societal crisis – they may also in turn have affected the development and the course of the crisis. A bold and much debated hypothesis was proposed by William Ruddiman. According to him anthropogenic global warming due to the greenhouse effect is not a late phenomenon restricted to modern times, but may be traced back to the very beginning of agriculture when humans started to deforest the Earth. Gradual deforestation for millennia resulted in slowly increasing levels of carbon dioxide in the atmosphere and a warmer climate than what would have been expected without the interference of humans. During periods of population drop, this long-term trend of a gradually increasing greenhouse effect was temporarily broken: abandonment of agricultural land resulted in a reversed development, with reforestation, decreased levels of carbon dioxide in the atmosphere and cooler temperatures. Along this line of reasoning, Ruddiman argues that the population drop in Europe during the late fourteenth and fifteenth centuries, together with the similar but even sharper population drop in the Americas in the sixteenth and seventeenth centuries, contributed to the low temperatures of the Little Ice Age. Hence, disease did not only kill millions of people, indirectly it changed the climate.[24]

The Ruddiman hypothesis has been criticised and climate modelling indicates that human impact is not necessary to explain the observed changes in carbon dioxide concentrations and temperature.[25] Furthermore, we still know very little about the degree of reforestation in the wake of the pandemics. Still, the hypothesis has resulted in a fruitful debate on past human impact on the climate. And, more importantly, by pointing to the possibility that past societal change caused climatic change, which in turn may have had major consequences for society even on a global scale, it has drawn attention to the two-way relationship between society and the environment in a long-term perspective.

On a more local scale, the environmental and ecological aspects of the late-medieval crisis are tightly linked to strategies developed on individual farms. Decisions made by the survivors – for instance, to stay or to move, to change the balance between crop growing and animal husbandry, or to turn to non-agrarian activities – were decisive for their economy and for their general standard of living. The decisions also had environmental consequences, both short-term and long-term, which influenced the course of the crisis and the later expansion. In the following chapters we will investigate environmental and agricultural change in the wake of the Black Death, we will present examples of strategies developed at household level, and we will discuss possible changes in living conditions and diet.

Notes

1   Frank 1995, 228
2   Redman 1999, 450
3   See the different contributions to the so-called Brenner debate, compiled in Aston & Philpin (eds) 1985. In this debate the neo-Malthusian view is represented by Postan & Hatcher and Le Roy Ladurie while the Marxist view is represented in particular by Brenner and Bois
4   Myrdal 2012a, 209
5   Myrdal 2012a, 205
6   Myrdal 2012a, 235–237
7   See comprehensive introductions by Tainter (1988) and Diamond (2005)
8   Tainter 1988, 4
9   Diamond 2005, 3
10 McAnany & Yoffee (eds) 2010, see in particular the introductory chapter by the editors
11 Societal resilience is the ability of a society to absorb disturbance and still retain its basic function and structure
12 Svensson *et al.* 2012
13 Diamond 2005, 3
14 This was the "dysfunctional social reaction" according to Myrdal (2012a, 234–235). For Germany see Abel (1980, reprinted 2013, 76)
15 Dyer 2002, 272–273
16 Diamond 2005; 2007
17 Diamond 2005
18 Postan 1972
19 Williams 2006, 87ff
20 Lagerås 2007; Yeloff & van Geel 2007
21 The pioneer work was written by Crosby (1972, reprinted 2003). See also e.g. Cronon 1983 (reprinted 2003, 85ff); Redman 1999, 195–199; Ponting 2007, 211–214
22 Mann 2006, 350–366
23 Emanuelsson 2009, 225ff
24 Ruddiman 2003; 2005, 115–146
25 Claussen *et al.* 2005; Broecker & Stocker 2006; Olofsson & Hickler 2008

PART II

EMPIRICAL STUDIES

4.

Abandonment, agricultural change and ecology

Per Lagerås, Anna Broström, Daniel Fredh,
Hans Linderson, Anna Berg, Leif Björkman,
Tove Hultberg, Sven Karlsson, Matts Lindbladh,
Florence Mazier, Ulf Segerström & Eva Sköld[1]

A palaeoecological approach to a societal crisis

The medieval landscape in Sweden as in much of Europe was a cultural landscape. It was shaped by agriculture and most of the ecosystems were greatly influenced by human activities. When the human population was drastically reduced after the Black Death, and also when those who survived developed new strategies, we may expect environmental consequences. In fact, any large-scale change in society during the Middle Ages is likely to have resulted in changes in the environment, particularly in the vegetation.

Because of this strong relationship between vegetation and agriculture, studies on vegetation change may contribute to our understanding of the late-medieval crisis. However, documentary sources from the Middle Ages give us very little information about the vegetation. This is true for many countries but particularly so for Sweden, which has a rather scanty record of medieval documentary sources. Most preserved documents are of an economical character and tell us about taxes, rents, transactions and expenses, and they rarely give us any direct information on vegetation. Some glimpses may be gained from letters, legal documents (e.g. the landscape laws of the thirteenth and fourteenth centuries) or religious texts (like the visions of Saint Bridget), but they never explicitly describe the vegetation or the agricultural landscape. Preserved wall paintings in medieval churches may, when deciphered from their religious symbolism, provide some information on agricultural tools and practices (Fig. 2 in Chapter 2). But again, they give us glimpses and details and not the large picture. Old maps are perhaps the best documentary sources to past vegetation and to agricultural landscapes in general. Sweden has a wealth of such maps, in particular cadastral maps of hamlets and villages, but the oldest ones are from the seventeenth century, more than two centuries after the Black Death.

Hence, documentary sources give us no direct evidence on vegetation or environmental change in connection with the Black Death and the crisis. But indirectly they point to large-scale and profound changes. In countries with richer documentary sources, changes in rents, taxes and prices indicate changes in the agricultural production that must have been connected to vegetation change. In Sweden, the many deserted farms and the significant population drop (reflected in *Peter's Pence* and several other sources) in particular indicate a social crisis that must have had major environmental and ecological consequences. In this way, we may use historical evidence of the societal crisis to discuss its possible environmental consequences, but much of the reasoning would be hypothetical.

A different approach is to use pollen analysis or other palaeoecological techniques to study vegetation changes more directly. In the study presented in this chapter pollen data from southern Sweden are used to interpret vegetation and agricultural change in the wake of the Black Death. Pollen analysis is a widely used method for studying vegetation change,

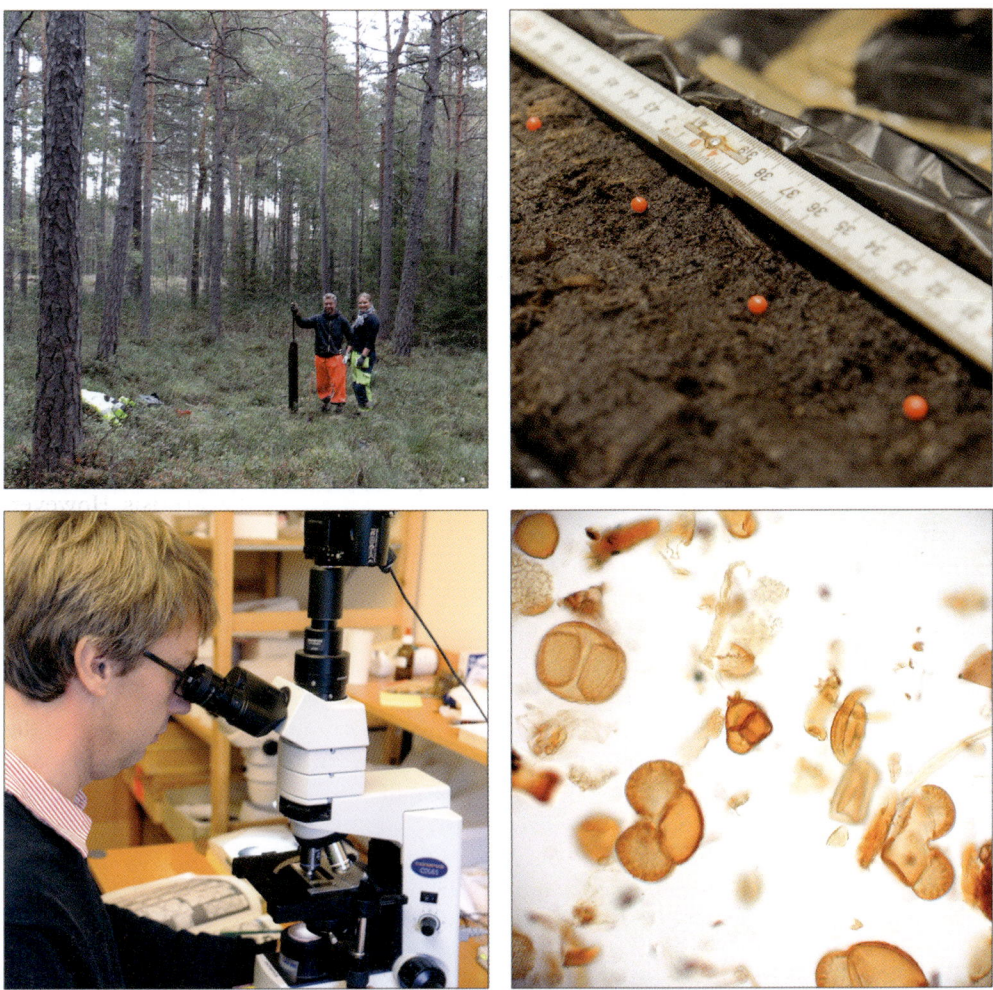

Fig. 4. The basic steps of pollen analysis, from peat coring on a bog, via subsampling to microscoping. The pollen photo is taken at magnification ×400 (photos: Per Lagerås and Henrik Pihl)

but its potential is still rather unexplored in the context of the late-medieval crisis. In general it is used to study long-term vegetation changes of a distant past, in particular of prehistoric periods from which we have no written sources. However, also from later periods, like the Middle Ages and later, pollen analysis and other palaeoecological techniques have the potential to make important contributions.

Some earlier studies, both in Sweden and other countries, have shown that reforestation and other vegetation change in connection to the Black Death may be identified in pollen diagrams.[2] However, studies are few and usually based on only one or a few sites, which have made it difficult to draw general conclusions. In this study a large set of pollen data based on numerous individual pollen studies is used. The aim is to look beyond local variation to identify possible regional changes in vegetation and land use that may be associated with a large-scale societal crisis.

The method of pollen analysis will be presented below but one principally important difference from the use of written sources should be mentioned here. Pollen data first of all reflect vegetation. But because vegetation in a cultural landscape is much influenced by agricultural land use, pollen data also reflect agriculture. Furthermore, because agriculture and, in particular, crop growing indicates nearby settlement, pollen data may be used to interpret not only vegetation and agriculture, but also settlement dynamics. And when large sets of pollen data are compiled, like in this study, the observed settlement dynamics may even be discussed in terms of population dynamics. Thus, the line of reasoning is from pollen to vegetation, from vegetation to land use, from land use to settlement dynamics, and finally from land-use and settlement dynamics to population dynamics. This is opposite to the line of reasoning offered by written documents. They primarily deal with social and societal matters, which indirectly may provide hints on vegetation change.

Hence, a palaeoecological approach offers new perspectives by taking changes in vegetation and agricultural landscape as starting points for discussion. In so doing it highlights the environmental and ecological dimensions of the social crisis.

Data and methods for this study

Pollen analysis is the most widely used method for studying past vegetation. The method was introduced already a century ago,[3] and even though there has been considerable development in data processing, modelling and in dating techniques, the basic principle remains the same (Fig. 4).[4] Pollen is released during flowering and in particular wind-pollinated plants disperse enormous amounts of pollen, of which the majority does not fulfil its mission of pollination but just falls to the ground. The pollen grains are very robust to decay and if they get embedded in wet, anaerobic environments, like peat or lake mud, they may be preserved for thousands of years. One cubic centimetre of such sediment may contain as many as hundreds of thousands of pollen grains. Since pollen carries information on past vegetation and landscapes, peat bogs and lake-bottom sediments with their microscopic content of pollen are nature's own historical archives.

From cores retrieved from such archives several small samples are taken out at various depths representing different times of deposition. The samples are treated with chemicals to extract and concentrate pollen and thereafter analysed using a high-magnification microscope.

The identification and counting of pollen grains is a time-consuming task and takes skill and patience. Usually between 500 and 1000 pollen grains are identified in each sample to get a statistically significant result. Some characteristic pollen grains can be identified down to species level but most of them only to so-called pollen types, which may include several species, or to plant genera or family. After identification, the raw pollen counts from each sample are transferred to percentage values and usually presented in a diagram with individual graphs for each pollen taxon. The diagram can be used to interpret past vegetation around the site, and the changes in pollen percentages observed throughout the stratigraphic sequence reflect vegetation change through time. Peat or other plant remains from the analysed core are radiocarbon dated to obtain an absolute chronology.

After its introduction, pollen analysis was for long used only to study what was regarded as natural vegetation development, in particular changes in forest composition, and how it may have reflected climate. This was partly due to the limited knowledge on pollen identification at the time, which was much restricted to tree pollen, but partly also to the general opinion during the early twentieth century that past human impact on the vegetation was small and not measurable. However, from the 1940s onwards, with the first identification of pollen from cereals and from plants thriving in pastures, pollen analysis gradually became a method also to study past agriculture.[5] After an influential paper by Björn E. Berglund,[6] pollen diagrams in the 1970s and 1980s were frequently used to identify periods of agricultural expansion and decline, which were discussed in relation to Ester Boserup's model of a stepwise societal development and to ideas on carrying capacity in relation to different agricultural techniques.[7]

Until the 1980s pollen analysis was mostly used to study long-term trends over several millennia and the pollen diagrams that were produced had a rather poor time resolution. They also had a poor spatial resolution since they used cores from large lakes and bogs with a large pollen source area, and aimed at describing the regional development rather than the local. This changed in the 1990s. From then onwards there has been an increasing interest in Sweden and in many other countries for more detailed pollen studies of local vegetation development with a shorter time perspective. Some of these local pollen diagrams have been produced within the context of forest ecology, with the aim to answer questions on tree successions and woodland dynamics at stand scale.[8] Others have been produced in connection with archaeological excavations in order to interpret local vegetation and land use that may be linked to the investigated remains.[9] In both cases a detailed picture of local conditions with a high temporal resolution is preferred before a more general picture of long-term trends over a large region.

Hand in hand with this development, there has been an increasing awareness of problems connected to radiocarbon dating. Chronologies of most early pollen diagrams were based on radiocarbon dating of bulk lake sediments, which due to the so-called reservoir effect may provide erroneously old dates (the error is usually 100–300 years but occasionally much larger).[10] In modern studies radiocarbon dating of bulk samples from lake sediments is usually avoided. Instead bog moss and other macro-remains (fruits, leafs, etc.) from terrestrial plants are used which has resulted in more accurate chronologies.[11] This advance has been facilitated by the AMS technique (Accelerator Mass Spectrometry), by which very small samples can be dated.

Sweden has a long tradition of pollen analysis and a wealth of pollen data, and in particular during the last two decades several high-resolution pollen records have been

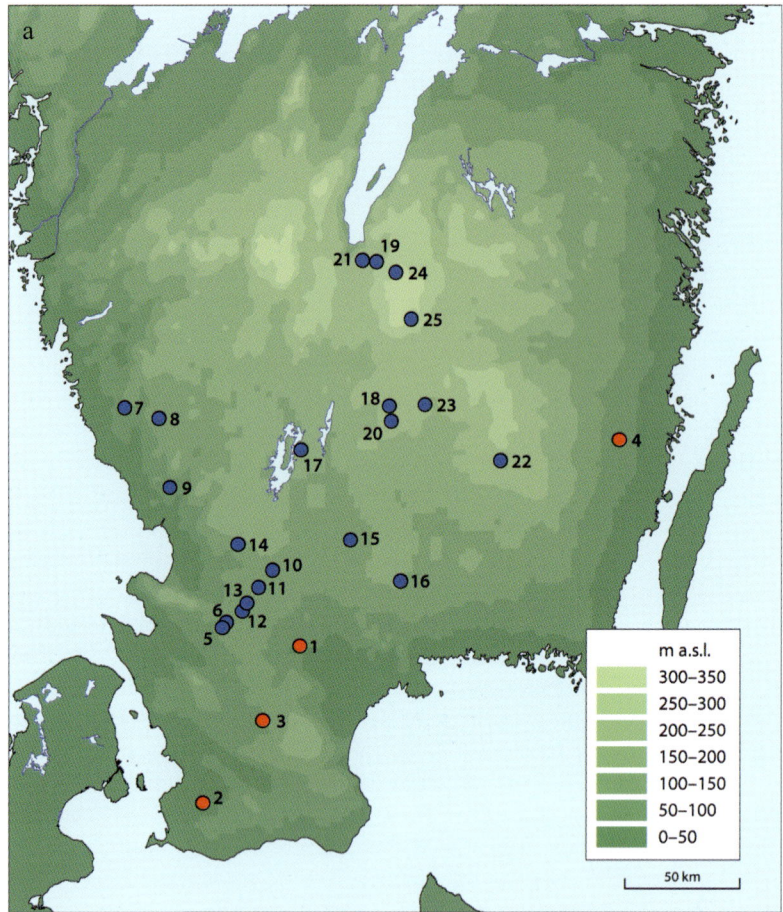

Fig. 5a. Map showing pollen sites in southern Sweden used in the present study. Symbol colours distinguish between lowland sites (< 100 m a.s.l.) (red dots), and upland sites (>100 m a.s.l.) (blue dots). Sites: 1 Skeakärret, 2 Torup, 3 Häggenäs, 4 Skärsgölarna, 5 Östra Ringarp, 6 Grisavad, 7 Bocksten, 8 Yttra Berg, 9 Trälhultet, 10 Exhult, 11 Köphult, 12 Rosts täppa, 13 Bjärabygget, 14 Baggabygget, 15 Råshult, 16 Siggaboda, 17 Flahult, 18 Lindhultsgöl, 19 Öggestorpsdalen, 20 Åbodasjön, 21 Store mosse, 22 Storasjö, 23 Skärpingegöl, 24 Bråtamossen, 25 Mattarp

published. These detailed, local records are the foundation for the present study. Because the aim is to reveal possible vegetation changes connected to the late-medieval crisis, which in a palaeoecological perspective is a rather sudden and short-lasting event, care has been taken to use pollen records that have a reasonably high resolution (i.e. many pollen-analysed levels) for the last 1000 years and have good and independent chronologies. Pollen records with chronologies based on radiocarbon dating of lake sediments or on pollen-analytical correlation with other sites have been excluded.

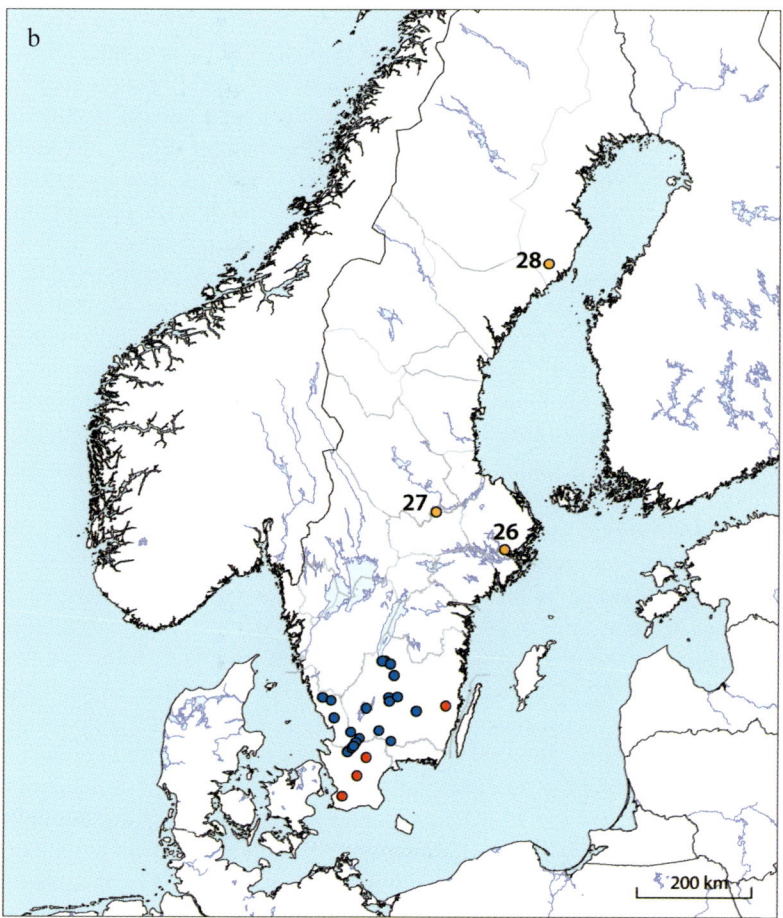

Fig. 5b. Map showing the pollen sites used in the present study including three sites in middle and northern Sweden (yellow dots). Sites: 26 Fjäturen, 27 Kalven, 28 Kassjön. For site descriptions and references to original publications see Appendix 1

Based on the above criteria a set of pollen data from 25 sites from southern Sweden (Fig. 5a) has been established. The vast majority of them (21 sites) are situated in the South-Swedish Uplands (Sw: *Sydsvenska höglandet*), and therefore much of our conclusions and discussions will focus on these uplands. One reason why the uplands have attracted so many pollen-analytical studies is that they are rich in well-preserved peatlands. In contrast, the agricultural plains of the lowlands have very few preserved peatlands, due to cultivation, drainage and peat cutting, and hence there are only a few useful pollen records (four sites) from the lowlands in the data set. In addition to records from the uplands and lowlands of southern Sweden, there are three sites from further north – two of them from middle Sweden and one from the northern part of the country (Fig. 5b) (for details about the pollen sites see Appendix 1).

The South-Swedish Uplands range *c.* 100–377 m above sea level and today they are, to a large degree, covered by forest, in particular planted spruce and pine forest. The high degree of forestation is due to the relatively poor natural conditions for agriculture. In comparison to the lowlands of Scania in the south, the mean annual temperature of the uplands is *c.* 1–2° lower and the growing season is 10–20 days shorter.[12] The Quaternary deposits are dominated by sandy till, rich in stones and boulder, reflecting the hard gneissic bedrock, whereas the agricultural plains of the lowlands are characterised by more fertile, calcareous clay and silt.

The strong bias in our pollen data to marginal uplands makes it difficult to draw general conclusions on a national scale or to make comparisons between lowlands and uplands. However, because settlements of marginal areas were not isolated, ups and downs in marginal areas in one way or the other reflect changes in central areas too. Furthermore, marginal areas appear to be most suitable for studies of environmental responses to societal change. In comparison to central areas they show a more discontinuous land-use and settlement history, which makes it relatively easy to distinguish periods of agricultural expansion from periods of stagnation and decline. In particular semi-open landscapes characterised by a mosaic of woodlands and agricultural land are suitable for a palaeoecological approach, because in such landscapes changes in human impact are likely to result in vegetation changes that are distinct enough to be detected by pollen analysis. Therefore studies on marginal areas may be used to take the temperature on society as a whole.

In addition to pollen records, conclusions presented in this chapter are drawn from dendrochronological dating. The basic principle of this technique is the counting and measuring of tree rings for comparison with reference tree-ring series of known age.[13] Trees, timber or any wooden objects that contain tree rings can be dated with very high precision, even down to a single year if the outer tree ring is preserved. In Sweden the construction of reference tree-ring series and systematic dendrochronological dating started in the 1970s.[14] Since then a lot of dating has been performed, in particular of timber from churches and other standing buildings but also of wooden objects from archaeological excavations.

In middle and northern Sweden well-preserved extant log buildings (mostly small barns and storage buildings) have attracted a lot of dating activity, and many of them have turned out to be very old.[15] The oldest ones are from the late thirteenth century and quite a few are from the first half of the fourteenth century. What is most interesting for the scope of this book is that the dates show a gap of about 100 years between the 1360s and the 1460s. The gap obviously reflects a pause in building activities due to stagnation and population decline in connection with the late-medieval crisis.[16] To investigate if building activities also show a similar break in southern Sweden, a large number of dendrochronological dates have been compiled and analysed. Our data set includes all dates from the provinces of Småland and Östergötland performed by the Swedish National Laboratory for Wood Anatomy and Dendrochronology at Lund University (all together 1882 dates). Since southern Sweden has very few standing profane buildings from the Middle Ages the data represent first of all planks, posts and other wooden objects documented during archaeological excavations, but also standing churches.

Dendrochronological data from Småland will be used in this chapter as a complement to pollen data from the same region, first of all to discuss the dating of the late-medieval decline, but also in relation to woodland development.[17]

Abandonment of fields and farms

Among the different aspects of the late-medieval crisis, abandoned farms are probably the most acknowledged. In fact the mentioning of abandoned or deserted farms in written records from the centuries after the Black Death is one of the strongest indications of the societal crisis and of the associated drop in population numbers. Also the physical remains of them are sometimes preserved. The archaeological study of deserted farms and villages is a well-established field of research in several countries, particularly in England but also for instance in Germany, where they are referred to as *Wüstungen*. Even though farms may be abandoned for different reasons, and have so been from time to time throughout history, the Late Middle Ages appear to have been a period of unusually extensive abandonment.

In Sweden relatively few have been archaeologically investigated and conclusions on late-medieval farm abandonment are based mainly on documentary evidence.[18] In particular cadastral registers have been extensively studied.[19] However, the earliest of these registers are from the late fifteenth century and most of them are from the sixteenth or seventeenth centuries, i.e. several centuries after the Black Death of 1350. Therefore they do not catch the actual process of abandonment and they do not show the original number of deserted farms. What the cadastral registers do show is that many farms were still deserted one or several centuries after the Black Death.

The reason why abandoned farms are mentioned in these records in the first place is that they were still someone's property. They were uninhabited but owned by other farms in the vicinity or by big landowners and they were regarded as a resource (or a potential resource) with an economical value. When they were registered they were uninhabited and probably had no buildings left, but their land was owned and managed by other farms, usually for pasture or mowing. The term "abandoned farm" (Sw: *ödegård*) in the cadastral registers thus means a piece of land that once belonged to a farm that is now uninhabited. Because the registers are not from the nadir of the societal crisis, but rather from afterwards when there was strong expansion of agriculture and settlement, many once abandoned farms were probably already re-inhabited and therefore no longer deserted. In the records they will appear as ordinary tax paying farms, undistinguishable from farms that were never abandoned. Furthermore, there were probably many abandoned farms in particular in distant areas that were never reclaimed or registered. They were simply deserted, overgrown and forgotten and therefore missing in the historical record.

For these reasons it is not possible to say, based on the historical documents, how many farms that were originally abandoned in the wake of the Black Death and this is why different scholars have arrived at different conclusions. According to the cautious estimation by *The Scandinavian Research Project on Deserted Farms and Villages*, only about 15% or less of the farms in several parts of Sweden were abandoned.[20] However, for one study area, situated in the uplands of southern Sweden, they suggested a more extensive desertion, about 25–40%.[21] Janken Myrdal presented a quite different conclusion. According to him, in many areas of southern Sweden 30–60% of the farms was abandoned and in marginal uplands even more.[22]

From this background we will now turn to pollen data and look specifically for indications of farm abandonment. Because crop growing is closely associated with settlement, cereal pollen may be used as an indicator of settlement. In Figure 6 the cereal pollen graph for

Lagerås et al.

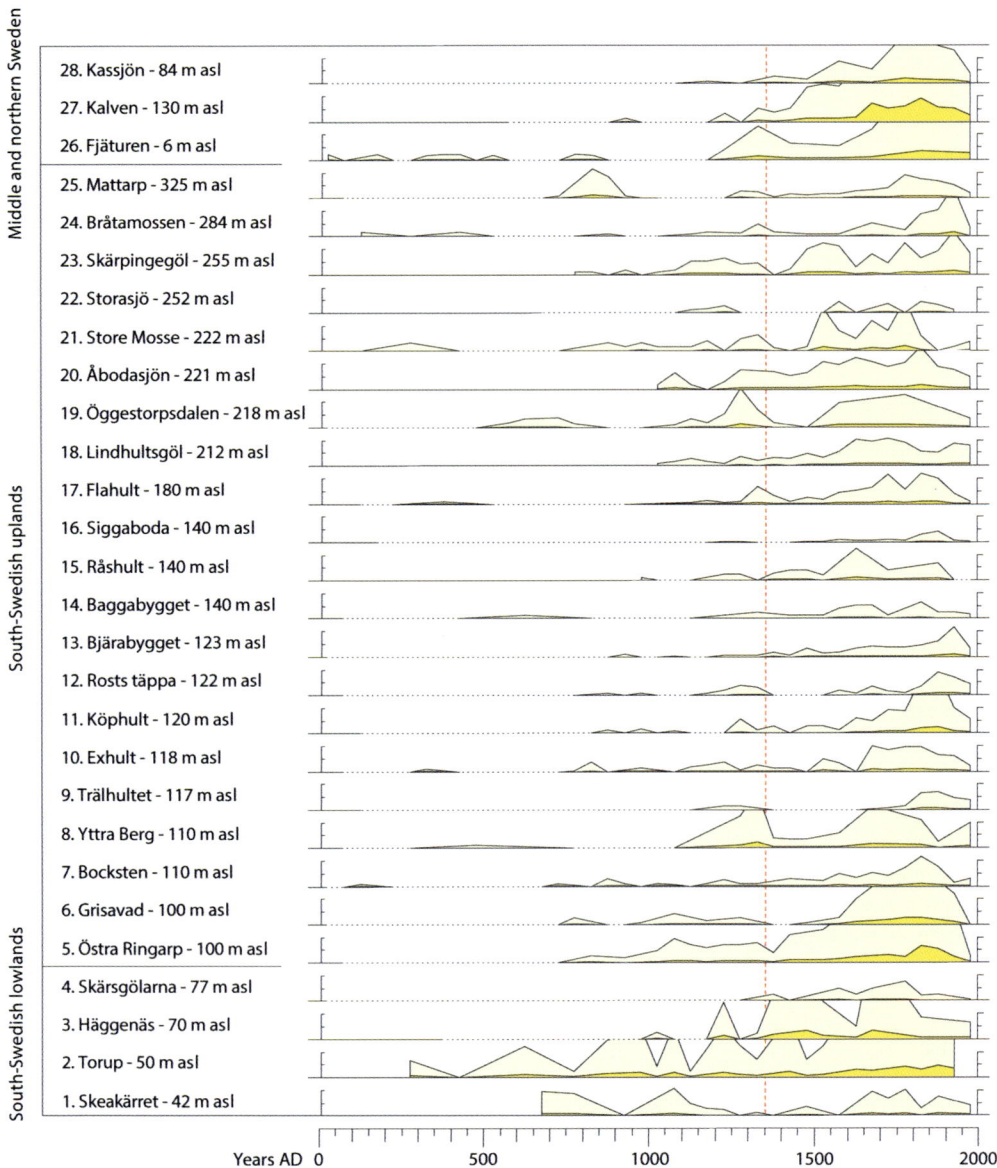

Fig. 6. Graphs showing cereal-pollen percentages from each individual pollen site plotted on a time scale (site numbers refer to Fig. 5 and Appendix 1). Dark-yellow graphs show percentages of the pollen sum (the length of the vertical scales is 10%), whereas light-yellow graphs show an exaggeration by ×10. The year 1350 is indicated by a red line

each individual site in the data set is presented. Except for the three sites from middle and northern Sweden, presented at the top the diagram, the sites are presented in order of altitude, starting with the lowermost site at the bottom. The graphs are plotted on a time scale and

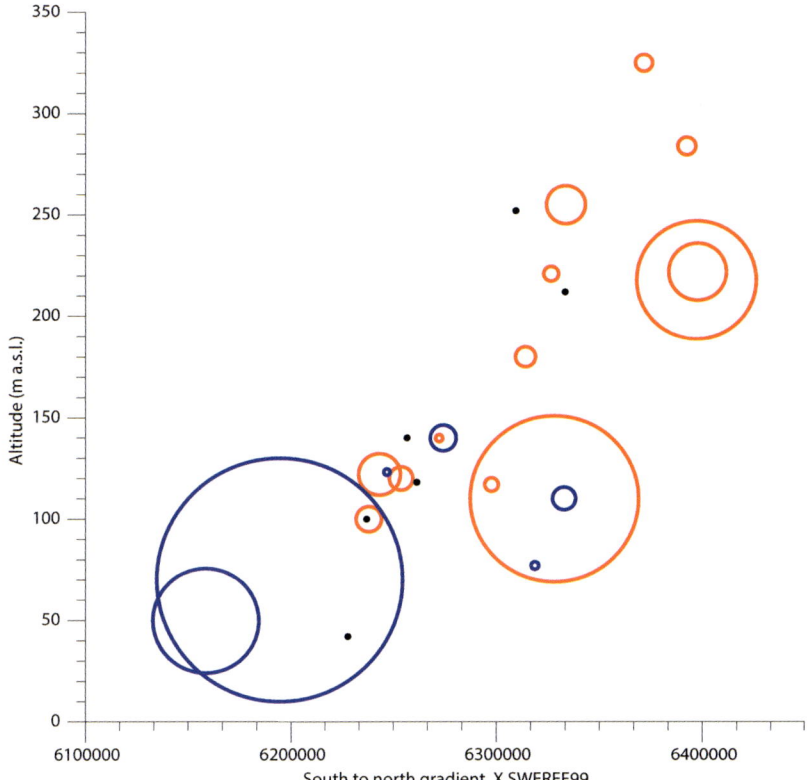

Fig. 7. Bubble graph showing the change in cereal-pollen percentages around 1350, based on a comparison between the two periods 1250–1350 and 1350–1450. Each site is represented by a circle or a dot, plotted against altitude (vertical axis) and south-to-north position (horizontal axis). Blue circles represent sites that show an increase in cereal-pollen percentages from 1250–1350 to 1350–1450, and red circles represent sites that show a decrease. The sizes of the circles are proportional to the size of the increase or decrease, respectively. Black dots represent sites with no change

most of them cover the last 2000 years. Because cereals do not survive in the wild, cereal pollen is the best pollen indicator of crop growing and indirectly of agricultural settlement. With the exception of rye, all cereals are poor pollen producers, and even though the pollen grains are dispersed by wind, they are relatively large and heavy and do not travel long distances. Consequently, cereal pollen in most pollen diagrams reach only low percentages of the pollen sum (i.e. of the total number of identified pollen grains in the sample), but even low percentages may be used as indications of arable fields in the vicinity.

In some of the original diagrams, different types of cereal pollen have been distinguished. However, with the exception of rye, the distinction between different cereal-pollen types is difficult and sometimes arbitrary, and different analysts may use different identification criteria. Therefore, to enable comparison between the sites and calculations of mean values, they are all put together here into one common graph including all types of cereal pollen from each site.

The first impression from Figure 6 is that all the graphs look different. The differences reflect differences in the history of cereal growing between the sites, but that is not the whole truth. The pollen percentages are also influenced by other factors, like the size of the sampled basin (i.e. the peatland or lake) and the distance between the basin and the past cereal growing. Furthermore, the cereal-pollen percentages are affected by vegetation structure, which may have differed from site to site and also through time.

Hence, the graphs all look different, partly because of differences in their local agriculture and settlement histories and partly because of pollen-dispersal factors. Still it is possible to find patterns beyond the site-to-site variation. For instance, all sites show higher cereal-pollen percentages from the last millennium than from the previous one. Furthermore, most of the sites show a decrease during the last one or two centuries, reflecting the farm abandonment and forest plantation that characterised the uplands in the late nineteenth and twentieth centuries. Hence, the comparison of cereal graphs from different sites reveals both local variations and common regional trends. Also a closer look at the time of the Black Death and the late-medieval crisis, indicates great variation between the sites, but some important conclusions can be made. Of the 25 sites from southern Sweden, 11 show decreasing cereal-pollen percentages around 1350 (Grisavad, Östra Ringarp, Yttra Berg, Trälhultet, Rosts täppa, Flahult, Öggestorp, Store mosse, Skärpingegöl, Bråtamossen and Mattarp), others show little change, whereas only five sites show increasing values (Torup, Häggenäs, Skärsgölarna, Bocksten and Råshult). Thus, the number of sites showing decreasing cereal-pollen percentages around 1350 is higher than the number of sites showing increasing values.

Furthermore, from the same figure it can be concluded that the few sites that show increasing cereal-pollen percentages around 1350 are situated at relatively low elevation. This relationship is also evident from the bubble graph in Figure 7. The graph reveals clearly that two sites at low altitudes (Torup and Häggenäs) deviate strongly from the others by showing significantly increasing cereal-pollen percentages. These two sites are also the two southernmost sites, situated not far from the agricultural plains of Scania (sites 2 and 3 in Figs 5 and 6).

To summarise the evidence so far, pollen sites that show decreasing cereal-pollen percentages around 1350 are common in the South-Swedish Uplands, whereas two lowland sites in southernmost Sweden, on the contrary, show a distinct increase. The difference between lowland and upland sites is intriguing, but because of the low number of lowland sites any interpretations regarding the development in the lowlands have to be tentative and do not allow for any detailed analysis.

The same is true for much of middle and northern Sweden. Only three sites with detailed chronologies were available for the present study, and they represent rather different ecological and climatic zones. They are here used only as examples of agricultural development in different regions. Site Fjäturen, which is situated in a low-lying agricultural area north of Stockholm, has a cereal-pollen graph similar to many sites in the South-Swedish Uplands. It shows an increase in cereal-pollen percentages in the thirteenth century followed by a decrease in the fourteenth century. The latter indicates a late-medieval agricultural decline. It was followed by a second expansion in the seventeenth century. Lake Kalven is situated in an upland forest region and mining district of middle Sweden. It shows an increase in cereal-pollen percentages immediately before 1350, reflecting the first agricultural expansion in the area. The expansion was soon followed by stagnation and possibly decline after 1350.

A renewed expansion started in the fifteenth century, later followed by a much stronger expansion in the seventeenth century. Lake Kassjön is the northernmost site, situated outside Umeå in northern Sweden. A continuous cereal-pollen graph begins in the fourteenth century. There is no clear indication of decline but rather a slow step-wise increase in cereal pollen, reflecting expansion periods in the sixteenth and eighteenth centuries.

The two sites from middle Sweden – Fjäturen and Kalven – show indications of late-medieval agricultural decline. In particular Lake Fjäturen is interesting, since it is the only lowland site in the data set that shows strong indication of agricultural decline in connection to the Black Death. Lake Kassjön in northern Sweden shows no such decline, but rather indicates an establishment of continuous crop growing at the same time. Written records are scarce and it is still an open question if the Black Death reached that far north.

Similar to lowland sites from southern Sweden, the sites from middle and northern Sweden provide interesting examples but are too few to allow for any representative analysis. In contrast, the South-Swedish Uplands are very well represented. As many as 21 pollen sites in the data set are from this relatively homogeneous upland region, which makes a solid basis for interpretation. Therefore the rest of this chapter will focus on the uplands. (Hopefully future research will provide more pollen sites from lowland areas as well as from regions further north.)[23]

We may now look at the average development in the South-Swedish Uplands by calculating mean cereal-pollen percentages for all the 21 upland sites together. This was done for 50-year time slices and the result is presented in Figure 8a. As evident from the diagram mean cereal-pollen percentages from upland sites are very low during much of the first millennium after Christ. Following an initial increase in the late eighth and early ninth centuries a significant increase starts in the late eleventh century and continues to the early fourteenth century. This increase reflects medieval colonisation and expansion, which is well known from other sources, like settlement remains, written documents, place names, etc. The expansion was part of a general agricultural expansion over much of Europe.[24] The upward trend in the graph is broken in the mid-fourteenth century by an abrupt decrease in mean cereal-pollen percentages. There can be no doubt that this decrease reflects a significant decrease in cereal growing in the uplands after the Black Death. After the decline, values remain low for at least a century, until they start to increase slowly during the late fifteenth century onwards. In the sixteenth century they reach the same level as before the decline. Except for a possible stagnation in the early eighteenth century they continue to rise until the early nineteenth century. From the late nineteenth century onwards, cereal-pollen percentages decline, which reflects depopulation of the countryside and large-scale introduction of modern forest plantations in the uplands.

The fact that the mean cereal-pollen percentages for the upland sites drop sharply in connection to the Black Death is a strong and independent indication of agricultural decline. It shows that in spite of the site-to-site variation, and in spite of the very low cereal-pollen percentages in general from upland sites, the regional trend is clear. The mean value decreases from 0.4% to 0.2% of the pollen sum, i.e. a halving.[25]

In order to estimate what this change in mean pollen-percentage values represents in the landscape, past vegetation cover for each 50-year time slice has been modelled using the so-called Landscape Reconstruction Algorithm.[26] This modelling technique uses pollen counts, pollen-dispersal characteristics (pollen production and fall speed of pollen grains)

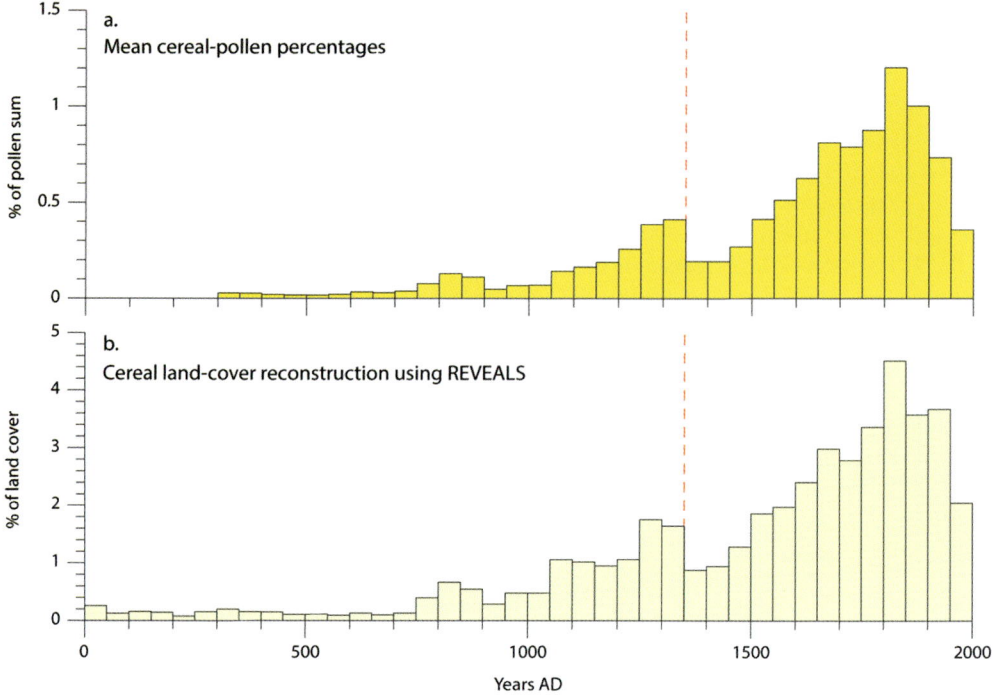

Fig. 8. Bar charts showing (a) the mean cereal-pollen percentages for each 50-year time slice based on all the 21 upland sites, and (b) the corresponding cereal land-cover reconstruction using the Landscape Reconstruction Algorithm, submodel REVEALS. The year 1350 is indicated by a red line

and site characteristics (basin size) to translate the fossil pollen record to vegetation cover. Thus, the model enables us to describe the actual extent of cultivated fields, pastures and woodland. The model corrects for over- and under-representation of strong and weak pollen producers, respectively (for instance, most trees are over-represented in the pollen record and most herbs under-represented). Some of the problems connected with the interpretation of pollen percentages, for instance the over-representation of plants growing on the sampled peatland, also affects the model output, but the technique is the best available to reconstruct vegetation cover from pollen data. For this study pollen data and site characteristics for all the 21 upland sites have been used.[27]

The graph in Figure 8b shows the reconstructed land cover of cereal vegetation in the upland region for each 50-year time slice.[28] The shape of the graph is similar to the one for cereal-pollen percentages, with only small differences. Most important in this context is that the reconstruction allows us to tentatively discuss not only pollen percentages but also the land cover of arable fields. According to the reconstruction, cultivated arable fields (excluding fallows) covered approximately 2% of the upland region in the late thirteenth and early fourteenth centuries. After a drop around 1350 they covered approximately 1% in the late fourteenth and early fifteenth centuries. After the late-medieval nadir they expanded to reach the maximum distribution of all time in the nineteenth century, when they covered

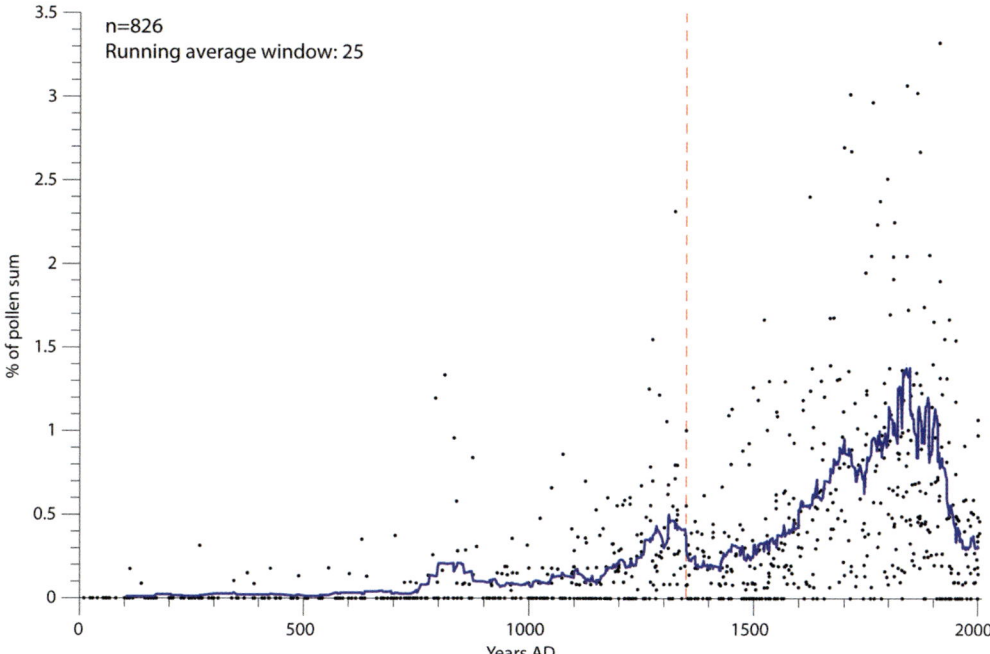

Fig. 9. Cereal-pollen percentages from all the 21 upland sites. Each dot represents an original pollen sample with its corresponding cereal-pollen percentage (vertical axis) and original dating (horizontal axis). The samples were sorted chronologically and a running average was calculated (blue line). Four dots with very high values from the nineteenth century were excluded from the picture but included in the running-average. The year 1350 is indicated by a red line

4–5% of the landscape. Thereafter they decreased and in the late twentieth century they covered approximately 2%.

Based on historical documents, the average land cover of arable fields for southern Sweden during the early eighteenth century has been estimated to approximately 5%, and for forested uplands to approximately 2%.[29] The latter figure fits reasonably well with the land cover reconstruction based on pollen records presented here. According to the reconstruction, cereal cultivation covered approximately 3% of the uplands in the eighteenth century (Fig. 8b). The good agreement for the eighteenth century, from which there is plenty of documentary evidence, indicates that the pollen-based reconstruction is reliable enough also for earlier periods.

Regarding the drop around 1350, the reconstruction shows a halving of cereal cropland, from *c.* 2% to 1% of the land cover. Thus the pollen record – both pollen percentages and pollen-based land-cover reconstructions – gives support to earlier interpretations of historical records that suggest extensive farm abandonment in upland areas during the late-medieval crisis. Even though a halving of cereal production, as indicated by the pollen record, does not necessarily reflect a farm-desertion frequency of 50% (farms may have survived but reduced their acreage), it indicates that a desertion frequency of that size is not at all unlikely.

Some earlier pollen studies have similarly shown a decrease in cereal-pollen percentages after the Black Death. Evidence comes from several parts of northern and western Europe, for instance from Sweden, Norway, Denmark, Estonia, France, Netherlands, England and Ireland.[30] Many of these studies are of high quality, with high-resolution analysis and detailed chronologies, but most of them are based on single pollen sites or occasionally a few sites. Dan Yeloff and Bas van Geel reviewed pollen-analytical evidence on late-medieval farm abandonment in Europe.[31] Their review considers only positive evidence of abandonment and they emphasise that there are also many other pollen diagrams from Europe that instead show continuity. They arrived at the conclusion that the effect on the European rural landscape of the Black Death varied geographically. They also concluded that abandonment in some areas started already before the Black Death, for instance in France and England.

In spite of these earlier studies, it is difficult to draw any general conclusion on the late-medieval decline based on pollen data, in particular on a European scale but also on national and regional scales. However, the method used in this study – to combine a large number of local pollen studies from one region at such high time resolution – is a step forward. With this approach it has been possible to interpret the regional development and at the same time reveal local variation within the region.[32] Also, the technique of landscape reconstruction modelling used here enables us to discuss the actual extent of arable and how it has varied through time.

Sudden impact of the Black Death

The late-medieval crisis was a complex and multifaceted process that lasted for more than a century and several different factors may have contributed to the circle of events. The Black Death of 1347–52 was certainly a major factor, but in some parts of Europe there was stagnation and even farm abandonment already before that period, in particular after the harvest failures leading to the Great Famine of 1315–22. There is no evidence of the latter from Sweden but that may very well be due to a paucity of documentary records.[33] If the harvest failures struck Sweden, farm abandonment might be expected, not only connected to the Black Death, but also before.

Furthermore, abandonment may have continued long after the Black Death. Based on documentary evidence, Janken Myrdal suggested that widespread farm abandonment did not begin until the 1360s and 1370s. Before that time, vacant farms were probably taken over by the many landless and poor. Abandonment started when this reserve of the labour force was used up and it continued well into the fifteenth century. It was most extensive in the 1420s or somewhat later. According to Myrdal the prolonged process of abandonment was due to recurring outbreaks of plague in combination with social oppression and conflicts.[34]

The pollen data presented here may contribute to the discussion of timing. In the diagram for upland sites in Figure 8a, mean cereal-pollen percentages decrease exactly at 1350, but this is partly due to the construction of the diagram. To enable the calculation of mean values, the original samples from the different pollen sites were adjusted by interpolation to 50-year time slices.[35] Therefore changes in the diagram are restricted to 50-year intervals. All that can be concluded from the diagram, regarding the time of the Black Death, is that the mean cereal-pollen percentages decrease significantly from the 1300–1350 time slice to the 1350–1400 time slice.

In an attempt to obtain a finer resolution than 50 years, a different type of diagram is presented in Figure 9. This diagram is also based on all the 21 upland sites, but instead of showing calculated mean values based on time slices, it shows all the original pollen samples from the different sites. In large measure the curve of the running average resembles the graph of mean values in Figure 8a. The important difference is that this one is not limited by the 50-year intervals of the time slices. Therefore it is interesting to note that it falls sharply exactly at 1350.

The chronologies of the different pollen diagrams included in the data set are all based on radiocarbon dating. Even though only pollen diagrams with chronologies that are regarded as sufficiently reliable have been included, radiocarbon dating is still a rather blunt technique in this context. Even if the radiocarbon dates are correct themselves they have a statistical error. Furthermore, the construction of the time/depth models used to calculate sample ages in the original studies include errors connected to interpolation.[36] In spite of these possible chronological errors, which probably blur the picture, the mean cereal-pollen graph shows a distinct decline around 1350 (Fig. 8a) and, more important, the running-average curve for the original samples falls steeply at exactly 1350 (Fig. 9). Hypothetically, the fall in the latter would be even more concentrated to 1350 if the underlying chronologies were perfectly correct.

In conclusion, pollen data from the uplands indicate an immediate effect of the Black Death, which we know from other sources ravaged Sweden in the year 1350. They do not indicate a delayed effect, as suggested by Myrdal based on documentary evidence. However, the running-average curve seems to support his conclusion that abandonment continued into the early fifteenth century. Regarding the Great Famine in the early fourteenth century, the curve shows a slight decline from approximately 1320, but perhaps not strong enough to prove abandonment already at that time.

This conclusion of the timing of the decline based on pollen data may be compared with an entirely different type of source material, namely the dating of wood by dendrochronology. This dating method is very precise. If the outermost tree ring is preserved, the very year when the tree was cut down can be identified. If the outer tree rings are not preserved, the felling year may be estimated. The precision of this estimation varies, and depends on how much of the tree trunk that is preserved, but it is usually higher than for radiocarbon dating.

In Figure 10, a compilation is presented of all the dendrochronological dates from the Province of Småland performed by the National Laboratory for Wood Anatomy and Dendrochronology at Lund University (dates later than 1800 were not included). Småland covers most of the upland region that is covered by the pollen data. The diagram is based on 702 individual dates, representing 96 dating projects in 47 different parishes (Fig. 11). The dated objects were standing buildings (in particular churches) as well as posts, planks and other construction details revealed by archaeological excavations. They represent both churches (142 dates) and profane contexts (560 dates).

The diagram (Fig. 10) shows a more-or-less gradual increase in the number of dates per 50 year slice from 1100 to 1350, which reflects medieval settlement expansion, and, in connection to that, the establishment of numerous churches.[37] Around 1350 the number of dates decreases distinctly, and from 1350 to 1600 there are very few dates per 50 years. The

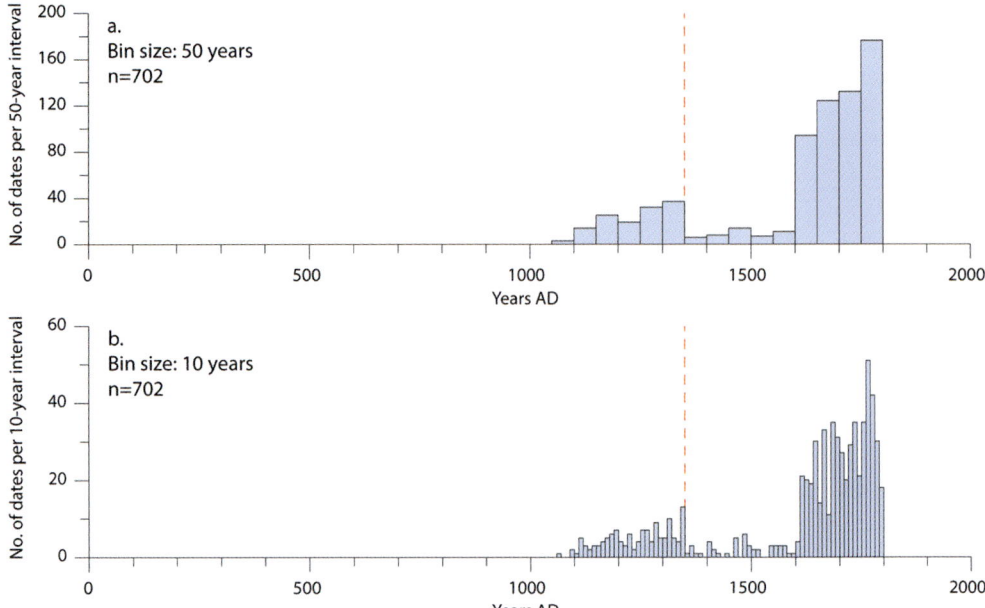

Fig. 10. A compilation of all dendrochronological dates (felling years) from Småland performed by the National Laboratory for Wood Anatomy and Dendrochronology at Lund University. Bars show the number of dates per (a) 50-year and (b) 10-year time slices, respectively. Dates later than 1800 are not included. The year 1350 is indicated by a red line

low number of dates after 1350 indicates a distinct drop in building activity in connection with the late-medieval crisis. At 1600 the number of dates increases sharply. The sharp increase in the number of dates in the early seventeenth century is partly due to a bias in the dating activity. Whereas very few post-medieval rural settlements have been investigated, there have been intense archaeological investigations in the early-modern towns of Jönköping and Kalmar, which have well-preserved timber constructions from the sixteenth century onwards.

Also, in some earlier studies a decrease in building activity in connection with the late-medieval crisis has been inferred from dendrochronological data. In middle and northern Sweden a compilation of dates from standing log buildings showed a gap of about 100 years starting in the 1360s, interpreted as reflecting a pause in building activity.[38] Similarly, a compilation of dendrochronological dates from Norway showed that the Black Death of 1349–50 more or less halted the building activity in Norway for 60 years.[39] The data from Småland fits into this picture by indicating a marked decrease in building activity after the Black Death. Also a new compilation from the province of Östergötland shows a similar pattern (see Chap. 5).

The temporal distribution of dendrochronological dates from Småland may be compared with the pollen record of the uplands presented above. A comparison of Figure 10 with Figure 8 reveals striking similarities. The gradual increase in the number of dendrochronological dates from 1100 to 1350 corresponds with a similar increase in the cereal-pollen percentages during the same time period. The two different types of data thus provide independent

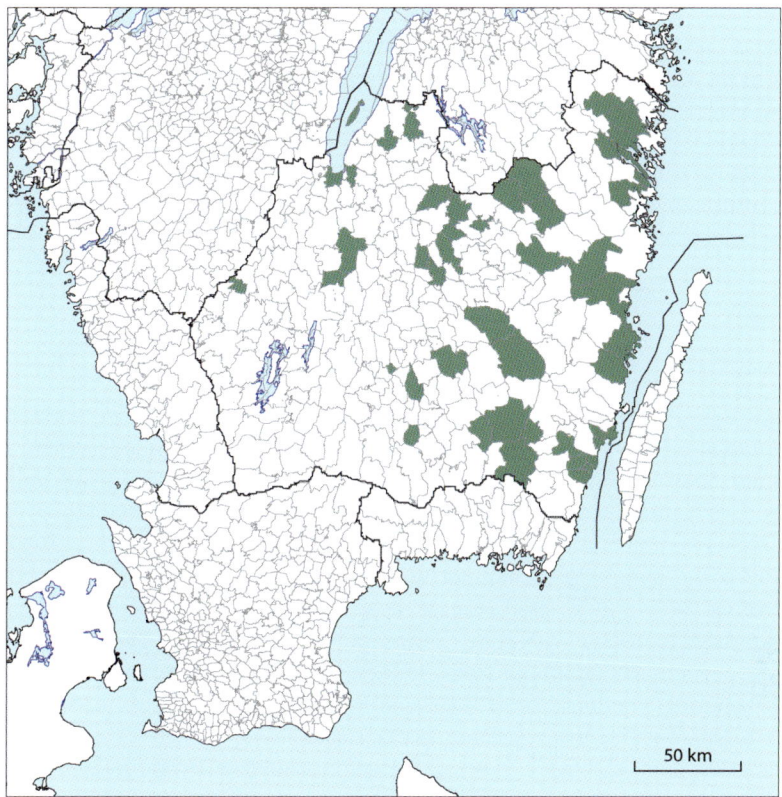

Fig. 11. Map of southern Sweden with parishes. Green indicates parishes in Småland from which we have dendrochronological dates

evidence of the medieval expansion in the uplands, reflecting construction activity and cereal growing, respectively. Both types of data also show a decrease around 1350, providing independent evidence of the severe effect of the late-medieval crisis in the uplands. It is fascinating how similar are the pictures obtained of the medieval development from these two completely different types of data.

In Figure 10a the dendrochronological dates are grouped in 50-year intervals for easy comparison with the cereal-pollen percentages. To get a higher resolution the same dendrochronological dates are grouped in 10-year intervals in Figure 10b. Although the diagram shows considerable variation from one decade to the other, it indicates that the most marked decrease in building activity followed directly upon the first struck of the plague in 1350. Even though a larger number of dates may change the picture in the future, at present dendrochronological data from Småland support the interpretation of a sudden decline in close connection to the Black Death.

To sum up the discussion on timing, both cereal-pollen percentages and the compilation of dendrochronological dates show a clear drop from the period 1300–1350 to the period 1350–1400. They provide independent evidence of a distinct decrease in crop growing and building activity in the South-Swedish Uplands in the mid-fourteenth century. It is not possible from these two data sets to prove or disprove a smaller decline already in connection to the Great Famine of the early fourteenth century. And, likewise, it is difficult to judge the effect of later plague outbreaks, during the late fourteenth and early fifteenth centuries. However, the high-resolution diagrams in Figures 9 and 10b strongly indicate that the major decline was close to the year 1350. The conclusion that can be made is that the first struck of the plague – the Black Death *sensu stricto* – had a significant and immediate effect on upland settlements.

Plague victims or lucky emigrants?

The data presented above suggest that the uplands of southern Sweden were hit hard by the late-medieval crisis. It may be concluded that there was a population decline and that population numbers remained low for more than a century. Furthermore, the decline seems to have been very sudden – as far as can be judged from our chronologies the decline happened in close connection to the year 1350. The timing and the suddenness point to the Black Death as the major factor behind the decline. If for instance climatic deterioration were the driving force a more gradual process would have been expected.

Our conclusion is in line with some earlier studies that have suggested extensive farm abandonment particularly in upland areas. Janken Myrdal suggested that farm abandonment was extensive (more than two-thirds) in the South-Swedish Upland.[40] Also *The Scandinavian Research Project on Deserted Farms and Villages* came to the conclusion that farm abandonment was most extensive in the uplands,[41] and studies from England, Germany and other countries have come to similar conclusions.[42]

Obviously, population numbers in the uplands dropped in the mid-fourteenth century and the strong temporal correlation with the year 1350 indicates that the Black Death was the major underlying cause. But were the upland people directly hit by the plague? Several authors explain the extensive abandonment in uplands not as a direct effect of the plague, but rather as an indirect effect through migration.[43] According to this line of reasoning, the plague may have ravished the lowlands harder than the uplands, but farms on good soil were not abandoned for long. When lowland farmers on good holdings died there were always those who were eager to take over. This was the rare moment when landless and farmers of poor holdings got the opportunity to improve their living conditions and probably did not hesitate to do so. Also the large landowners had to adapt to the dwindling labour force by redirecting their tenants to the most productive farms.

Pollen records from lowlands are unfortunately few, and therefore it is difficult to make comparisons between lowlands and uplands. In the data set used for this study there are only four records from southern Sweden that represent sites situated below 100 m above sea level. It is interesting to note, however, that the lowland records deviate from the picture revealed by the much more numerous upland sites. Of these four lowland sites, three show increasing cereal-pollen percentages around 1350 and in particular two of them – Torup and Häggenäs – show a strong increase. These two sites are also the two southernmost sites in the data set. Even though they may not be representative for the lowlands, they do indicate that parts of the lowlands of southern Sweden did not witness agricultural decline during the fourteenth century but rather expansion. If the migration hypothesis were correct a decline in crop growing in the uplands and no decline, or at least a smaller decline, in the lowlands would be expected. The pollen records of Torup and Häggenäs give some support to this hypothesis by indicating no decline in crop growing. However, the fact that they indicate an increase in crop growing is difficult to explain.

Turning to the uplands again, it is likely that the decline in cereal growing to some extent was due to migration. But the possibility that upland people were also directly hit by the plague should not be ruled out. No farm was completely isolated. Also inhabitants of the most remote settlements belonged to social networks and gathered for instance in church and at market places. Even though question marks remain regarding the dissemination mechanisms, the fast spread of the Black Death through Europe – where only a minority lived in Urban areas – shows that it spread effectively also in the countryside. Even sparsely populated countries witnessed a dramatic population drop, like Norway in connection with the Black Death of 1349–50 and Iceland in connection to the plague outbreak of 1402–04.[44] Certainly the plague knocked on the door also of farmsteads in the South-Swedish Uplands.

Trade connections were important for the spread of the plague, and, as Dick Harrison has emphasised, settlements depending on imported grain may have been particularly vulnerable.[45] This is because grain was usually accompanied by rats and their fleas. Possibly parts of the uplands depended on such trade. At least this was the case later, from the sixteenth century onwards, when grain was imported to the uplands in exchange for animal products.[46]

The very suddenness of the decline, indicated by both cereal-pollen percentages and dendrochronological dates (Figs 9 and 10b), is interesting in this context. It may indicate that the upland settlements were hit directly by the plague, or, alternatively, that the process of migration started immediately after the plague, with no measurable delay. Regardless of which interpretation is correct (most likely it was a combination of both), it is noteworthy that the Black Death had an immediate impact on upland societies. If the Black Death of 1350 is regarded as the starting point for the late-medieval crisis in Sweden, it can be concluded that marginal uplands were immediately affected by the crisis. There is no indication of any delay from centre to periphery, and, thus, no indication that upland societies were more sustainable or resistant to change. When the Black Death hit southern Sweden it had an instant impact on the entire society, from towns and agricultural plains to remote woodlands.

A turn to animal husbandry

So far the discussion in this chapter has focused on crop growing and been based primarily on cereal pollen. An advantage with such an approach is that crop growing is closely connected to settlement and the results may be compared with previous studies on farm abandonment. Another advantage is that cereals do not grow in the wild and they disappear quickly when cultivation stops. Cereal pollen is therefore the best pollen indicator of crop growing and indirectly of settlement, and it shows an immediate response both to the beginning and end of cultivation.

Although less straightforward, pollen records may also be used to study animal husbandry.

This is because certain plants thrive in pastures and meadows.[47] Humans do not intentionally grow these plants, and many of them are part of the natural flora. But because they are light demanding and well adapted to withstand grazing, they are competitive and dominating in pastures and also in hay meadows. Vegetation changes related to the introduction or cessation of grazing are more gradual than the ones related to crop growing, but they may still appear relatively sudden in a historical perspective. If grazing or mowing stops, a natural succession would lead to overgrowing by shrubs and trees, and shade-intolerant species like heather, grasses and other herbaceous plants would decrease and eventually disappear. Apart from temporary glades, most dry ground in southern Sweden would be forested if it were not for grazing and other agricultural land uses, which hold back the forest. In this respect grazing and mowing (and also crop growing) keeps the vegetation at an early phase of succession.

Consequently, landscape openness as reflected in the pollen record may be used as a measure of agricultural impact on the landscape and in particular of the impact of animal husbandry. Land used for animal production – in particular pastures but also hay meadows – in most pre-industrial agricultural systems was much larger than the one used for crop growing.[48] Landscape openness is therefore strongly related to the impact of grazing and mowing and ultimately to the number of grazing animals. In the uplands of southern Sweden domestic grazers would have been cows, oxen, sheep and goats and to a smaller extent horses.[49]

To quantify landscape openness and how it changed through time we return to the Landscape Reconstruction Algorithm, which was used in a previous section to recalculate pollen percentages to land cover. Figure 12 shows the model output based on all the 21 upland sites. For cereals it is the same output as in Figure 8b, but here all the vegetation types estimated by the model are presented.

Starting from the bottom of the diagram, the lowermost field shows the relative land cover of cereals, which was discussed above. The next field, named Mixed herbaceous, shows the land cover of all herbaceous plants excluding cereals, grasses and sedges. Most of the mixed herbaceous plants grew in pastures and meadows, while some may have grown for instance as weeds in arable fields.[50] Next follow grasses and then sedges and heather. Grasses to a large degree reflect pastures and meadows, even though some species of grass may grow in woodland, at lakeshores (reed), in naturally open wetlands or in mowed wetlands. Sedges are largely restricted to wetlands, mowed as well as natural. Heather thrives in poor pastures (heathland), usually characterised by high grazing pressure and acidic soils, but may also grow in peat bogs. After heather in the diagram follow shrubs (juniper, hazel) and different types of trees. Juniper and hazel may have grown in half-open pastures and meadows. Also birch, which is a shade-intolerant tree, may have grown in wooded pastures. However, it is also an early-succession tree that quickly expands on abandoned land when land use ceases or grazing pressure decreases. After birch in the diagram (as well as in a natural succession) follow the more shade-tolerant trees.

The diagram presents groups of plants separately that in the landscape were often mixed together. For instance, wet meadows may have contained a mix of sedges, grasses and several different herbaceous plants, whereas dry pastures had a mix of grasses, herbaceous plants and heather. Also, arable fields did certainly not contain only cereals, but also different weeds represented in the diagram by mixed herbaceous plants. In the same way most woodland before the introduction of modern forest plantations was a mix of several different tree species. Important to note is also that the transition between open land and

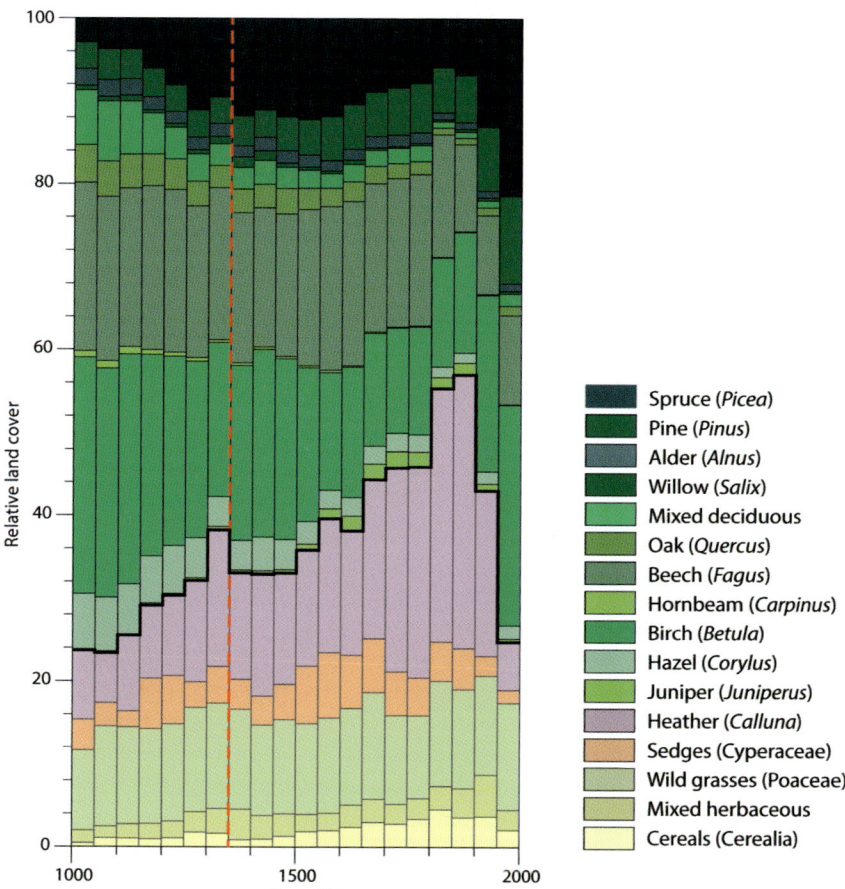

Fig. 12. Vegetation land-cover reconstruction based on pollen data from the 21 upland sites using the Landscape Reconstruction Algorithm, submodel REVEALS. The bold line between heather and juniper marks the boundary between open-land vegetation below that line and the vegetation of shrubs and trees above it. Mixed deciduous include Ulmus (elm), Tilia (lime tree) and Fraxinus (ash). Mixed herbaceous plants include Compositeae SF. Cichorioideae (dandelions, hawk's-beards, etc.), Filipendula (dropwort, meadowsweet), Plantago lanceolata (ribwort plantain), Potentilla type (tormentil, cinquefoil), Ranunculus acris type (buttercups), Rubiaceae (bedstraw), and Rumex acetosa type (sorrel). Cereals include Secale cereale (rye) and Cerealia type (unspec. cereals). The year 1350 is indicated by a red line

woodland in the pre-industrial agricultural landscape was often diffuse and gradual. There was a range from open pastures, meadows and fields, via half-open pastures and meadows with scattered shrubs and trees, to wood pastures and dense woods. Landscape openness usually decreased by the distance to settlement.

Even though the details of these vegetation patterns are not known nor how different plant groups were mixed together, the total land cover of open-land vegetation can be used as a measure of landscape openness. In the diagram the upper limit of heather (bold line) marks the relationship between all the open-land plants below that line and the shrubs and trees above it. It represents a summary of the land cover of all open-land vegetation and gives us a quantitative estimate of landscape openness and how it has changed through time.

The model output based on the 21 upland sites shows that open-land vegetation in the uplands expanded gradually from the eleventh century, when it covered approximately 24% of the landscape, to the early fourteenth century, when it covered 38%. Some open-land vegetation belonged to naturally open wetlands, but the strong expansion of the open landscape at the regional scale was certainly due to agricultural clearance, establishment of new settlements and increasing numbers of grazing animals.

Similar to the expansion of cereal growing, the expansion of open-land vegetation came to a halt in the fourteenth century. The gradual deforestation that had been going on for centuries stopped and from the early to the late fourteenth century landscape openness decreased from 38% to 33%. Although a relatively small decrease, it is the most marked decrease of landscape openness recorded during the last 1000 years, except for the decrease during the twentieth century. After the reforestation in the fourteenth century, landscape openness remained at the same level, about 33%, for a century and a half. In the sixteenth century open land started to expand again and apart for some short-term stagnation periods it continued to expand all the way up to the nineteenth century, when landscape openness peaked at 57%. Finally, during the twentieth century, the extent of open landscape was dramatically reduced, and during the second half of that century landscape openness was only 25%. Hence, landscape openness today in the uplands is back at the same level as by the onset of the medieval expansion one millennium ago. However, it has a very different character because of woodland species composition and how the open land is managed.

The landscape development of the last century is interesting because it gives us an opportunity to test the reliability of the landscape reconstruction. According to the reconstruction in Figure 12, the reduction of open land in the twentieth century was characterised most of all by a strong decrease in heather vegetation. Also the land cover of cereals, mixed herbaceous plants and sedges decreased at the same time. The parallel reforestation was characterised by a strong expansion of spruce, but also of pine and birch. These changes, suggested by the pollen-based reconstruction, fit nicely with the well-known landscape development based on various sources:[51] Much agricultural land in the uplands was abandoned during the twentieth century and in the same process modern forestry was introduced with large-scale forest plantation. In particular heathland and other poor pastures were planted with spruce and, to some degree, with pine.[52] Pastures left for natural succession were colonised by birch and later by coniferous trees. By the turn of the century 1900 open heathlands were still common and widespread, in particular in the western part of the uplands, but today they are all gone.

The good agreement between the land-cover reconstructions based on pollen data and the well-documented landscape development for the last century increases the credibility of the reconstruction also for earlier periods. Furthermore, the fact that modelled land cover of heather vegetation shows a sharp decrease in the twentieth century, when grazed heathland disappeared but natural peat bogs in the uplands changed very little, indicates that most of the heather vegetation, according to the diagram, belonged to pastures.

We may now return to the decrease in landscape openness that took place in the fourteenth century. Apart from cereals, particularly heather decreased whereas birch and some other trees expanded. It reflects how pastures on poor soils were abandoned and gradually became overgrown particularly by birch in a natural succession. Also sedges and grasses show a slight decrease. The only open-land vegetation that increased at this time, according to the reconstruction, was mixed herbaceous plants. It may reflect an expansion of weeds and other plants in abandoned arable fields when crop growing stopped and they were turned into pastures or meadows.

An interesting observation is that the decrease of open-land vegetation from the early to the late fourteenth century was proportionally much smaller than the decrease in crop growing. Whereas the total land cover of open-land vegetation decreased from 38% to 33% (a decrease of 13%), the land cover of cereals was halved. Obviously landscape openness did not decrease as dramatically in the wake of the plague as the extent of arable fields. Even though some of the open-land vegetation grow in natural wetlands that were not affected by agricultural change, the much smaller relative decrease in landscape openness than in cereals indicates that grazing (and possibly mowing) did not decrease as much as crop growing during the crisis.

Hence, in addition to the change in landscape openness, there was also a change in the proportional relationship between different types of agricultural land. In the traditional agricultural landscape of southern Sweden, areas connected to animal husbandry (pastures and meadows) usually covered much larger areas than areas used for crop growing. The relationship between arable fields, meadows and pastures differed between regions and also changed through time, but everywhere, except for in the most densely populated plains, pastures and meadows dominated the agricultural landscape. In the uplands, where animal husbandry played a more important role than in the lowlands, arable fields represented only a minor part of the productive land. The hamlet Lönsboda in the southern part of the uplands is a typical example.[53] According to a map from 1696, it consisted of two households with 2.5 hectares of arable each. The total arable made up less than 2% of the land belonging to the hamlet, whereas the rest consisted of meadows, pastures, woods with clearings, swidden land and bogs. The meadows were more than ten times larger than the arable.

To conclude, animal husbandry has always been important in the uplands, but it became even more so after the Black Death. Population drop and farm abandonment resulted in a distinct and sudden decrease in crop cultivation, whereas land associated with animal husbandry decreased much less. The pollen record thus indicates that animal husbandry gained in relative importance after the Black Death. The same conclusion has been put forward by several authors based on the historical record.[54] In Sweden indications are found in cadastral registers from the fifteenth century onwards. According to them, many deserted farms were used as pastures and meadows.[55] Another indication is the increased production of butter, reflected in declining prices of butter relative to grain prices.[56] Even though it is difficult to quantify the increased importance of animal husbandry, the landscape reconstruction shows that this change of the agricultural system resulted in vegetation changes that were distinct enough to show up in the pollen record on a regional scale. Because animal farming is more land demanding but less labour intensive than crop growing, this relative increase in animal husbandry at the expense of arable appears to have been a strategic, labour-saving change in a time of land excess but shortage of manpower.[57]

It is not possible from the pollen-based landscape reconstruction to distinguish hay meadows for fodder production from pastures. Even though animal husbandry in general was less labour intensive than crop growing, the collection of winter fodder by mowing was rather labour intensive. At the time of hay harvest, mainly in late July to early August, the size of the workforce was a limiting factor. The development during the Late Middle Ages of longer scythes and better rakes made hay mowing more efficient and less time consuming, but fodder production still remained a bottleneck in the animal production.[58] Cadastral registers mention deserted farms used for hay mowing, at least during the late fifteenth century and later, but probably the landscape was kept open first of all by grazing. Fenced-in meadows and arable were grazed after harvest but for most of the grazing season animals roamed freely in the outlands, watched over by herders. The shift from male herders to children and women, which started in the fifteenth century, probably reflects an adaptation to the shortage of manpower after the Black Death, and helped to keep a larger livestock in relation to the number of people.[59]

In the wake of population drop and abandonment, arable fields were turned to meadows and pastures, and some meadows were turned to pastures as well. At the same time, the decrease in land cover of heather vegetation after 1350 indicates that poor, less productive heathlands were completely abandoned and left to reforestation. The only open-land vegetation that increased was the one represented in Figure 12 by mixed herbaceous plants, which increased in the late fourteenth century from 3% to 4% of land cover. It probably reflects an expansion of weeds and other open-land plants when cereal growing stopped and arable fields were turned to meadows or pastures. Such an expansion of grazing indicators at some sites in the fourteenth century has been shown earlier in a few individual pollen diagrams. Examples of plants that expanded were ribwort plantain, cow-wheat, goosefoot, sorrel and grasses.[60] The reconstruction presented here shows that the increase of this type of vegetation is detectable also at a regional scale.

The decrease in land cover of heather and the increase in mixed herbaceous plants indicate that the average quality of pastures and meadows increased. It was the combined effect of two processes – the reforestation of the poorest heathland and the establishment of rich herbaceous vegetation on abandoned arable fields. This appears to have been the result of strategic decisions. By turning arable to pastures and meadows and by leaving the poorest pastures to natural succession, peasants took the opportunity to increase the land productivity of their stock farming.

The changes discussed so far happened in the fourteenth century and were connected to the Black Death and the associated population drop. Eventually, after more than a century, the first signs of agricultural expansion and recolonisation are visible. Both crop growing and animal husbandry (as reflected in landscape openness) started to expand again, but there appears to have been a time lag between the two. According to the landscape reconstruction, cropland reached a nadir in the late fourteenth century (Figs 8b and 12). In the first half of the fifteenth century it remained almost the same with only a slight increase, but for the second half of that century it shows a relatively distinct increase. It marks the beginning of an expansion of arable land that continued more or less uninterrupted to the early nineteenth century. The total land cover of open-land vegetation (Fig. 12) shows a similar development but slightly delayed. After the decrease in the mid-fourteenth century landscape openness remained the same throughout the fifteenth century, and the first marked increase according to the reconstruction was not until the first half of the sixteenth century. From then on, open land expanded to reach maximum openness in the late nineteenth century.

A plausible interpretation of this time lag is that the first agricultural effort, when population numbers had recovered enough to enable expansion, was to increase crop production. Arable fields once abandoned were now put under the plough again. On the stony ground that characterises much of the uplands, it was an obvious advantage to return to old fields that had already been cleared from stones. In this way the great effort once invested in stone clearance was not wasted.[61] The re-establishment of previously abandoned fields is indicated by the pollen-based reconstruction. The increase in cereal cultivation in the late fifteenth and early sixteenth centuries is matched by a decrease of mixed herbaceous plants. This group of open-land plants was the only one to expand in the late fourteenth century (interpreted above as the turn of arable land to pastures and meadows), and it was the first to decrease its land cover when arable started to expand again.

The pollen record from the uplands thus indicates that agricultural expansion after the crisis started by the re-establishment of arable land. By doing so crop production and the total land productivity increased. In other words, more people could be fed on the same land. The introduction of crop growing on the deserted farms was probably associated with the establishment of new buildings and, of course, the moving in of people. Slightly later, in a second step of the expansion, forest clearing begun. This two-step process reflects a difference in the labour input required. To gradually expand pastures in the woods by girdling and fire, for instance by grazing of swidden land, may not have been a very labour intensive task, but to turn woodland to permanent arable certainly was. The felling of trees and clearing of roots to prepare the soil for cultivation was hard work. In contrast, abandoned fields that in the meantime had been used for grazing and mowing would have been relatively easy to put under the plough.

An interesting question in connection to this is to what degree vegetation and land-use during the late-medieval crisis had any influence on the duration of the crisis. As evident from the historical record and further supported by the pollen record, many deserted farms were used for pastures and meadows by other farms. In this way surviving farms got the opportunity to expand their land and in particular their animal production in the wake of the population drop. It is interesting to note that deserted farms used for pasture were frequently registered even though no rent had to be paid.[62] Probably they were not seen only as pastures, but also as land that could be put under the plough in better times. In other words they were a resource for future expansion. Hence, the grazing and mowing of deserted farms did not only provide valuable pastures and fodder – by holding the forest back the threshold for future expansion was lowered. Regardless if this was an intentional strategy or not, it was a land use that facilitated the expansion and recolonisation that followed. If all deserted farms had been left for natural succession and reforestation, the threshold for clearance would have been higher and the recolonisation of the uplands delayed.

Expanding woodlands

Reforestation on abandoned land is frequently associated with social crisis and depopulation in the same way as its opposite – forest clearing and deforestation – is associated with agricultural expansion and population growth. Many of the most famous and well-studied examples of social collapse were followed by reforestation, for instance in Central America after the Maya decline in the tenth century, in North America in the sixteenth century, and in Amazonia after the sixteenth century.[63] Also the late-medieval crisis in Europe is frequently associated with reforestation.[64] According to a much-debated hypothesis by William Ruddiman, reforestation in Europe after the Black Death and in the Americas in the sixteenth and seventeenth centuries was significant enough to result in a reversed greenhouse effect and climatic cooling.[65] Although the hypothesis has been questioned, the possible effect of past land-use changes on the climate has received increased attention during the last decade. However, few empirical studies have focused on environmental changes after the Black Death and we still know very little about the degree of reforestation. Several pollen studies provide individual examples of forest expansion, but there have been no attempts to quantify late-medieval reforestation for larger areas.[66] Here pollen-based reconstructions using LRA, like the one used in the present study, have great potential.[67]

Reforestation throughout most of history – in Sweden before the last two centuries – was not by planting but by secondary succession. It was a natural process of woodland re-growth on abandoned land. The forest was held back by agricultural land use and as soon as the impact of this land use stopped or decreased a secondary succession of shrubs and trees would begin. In the traditional agricultural landscape of Sweden, there were sometimes pollards among settlement and in the meadows (Fig. 2 in Chap. 2), but most trees and woodland were to be found in the outlands. Woodland was the natural vegetation and grazing and continuous clearing was needed to keep the vegetation open and to hold the woodland back. Natural seeding of trees occurred also in open pastures but saplings were bitten off by grazing animals, and in the meadows mowing effectively stopped any sprouting of unwanted tree vegetation. Still, tree saplings that germinated in pastures and meadows could survive for many years even if browsed or cut down, ready to sprout whenever they got the opportunity.[68]

As soon as the impact of people and their animals decreased or stopped, trees would invade the open vegetation by sprouting and seed dispersal. In the uplands the first trees to establish would be birch and rowan.[69] (Rowan is insect-pollinated and therefore poorly represented in pollen records.) Also oak and hazel may be quick to expand, as well as goat willow. Of these early succession trees birch was the most important. It is a typical pioneer tree, which quickly occupies cleared surfaces.[70] It is also fast growing and will soon produce a dense canopy that covers lower vegetation. The process would be quick on barren soil and slower on a well-developed grass sward, but generally it would take 20–50 years for a canopy to develop.[71] Birch and other pioneer trees dominate the first phase of succession. They are, however, shade-intolerant and after a while they will be outcompeted by more shade-tolerant and usually more slow-growing trees. Typical such late-successional trees in the uplands are beech and spruce.

Turning to the result of the pollen-based landscape reconstruction, which was based on all the 21 upland sites, the diagrams in Figure 13 shows the regional land cover for a selection of tree taxa. Of the different trees to expand in the late fourteenth century, birch shows the most distinct increase. It started to expand in connection to farm abandonment in the late fourteenth century and reached a temporary peak in the early fifteenth century. The expansion of birch was a temporary interlude in a long-term declining trend of birch woodland. Oak displays a similar development. A long-term gradual decrease of oak woodland was interrupted by a temporary expansion in the late fourteenth century.

Another tree that shows an increase in land cover in the late fourteenth century is spruce. However, in contrast to birch and oak, the long-term trend of spruce during the Middle Ages was expansion. Spruce is the latest tree immigrant in southern Sweden and the only one to have expanded from north to south.[72] Its slow but steady conquest of the uplands started in the northern parts in eight century and by the nineteenth century it had reached also the southern parts.[73] The increase in the late fourteenth century appears to have been part of this long-term development, but locally the establishment of spruce forest may have been facilitated by agricultural abandonment.

An expansion of birch in connection to late-medieval farm abandonment, which is evident from the landscape reconstruction presented here, is a distinct feature also of several individual pollen diagrams.[74] In at least one of them, the peak in birch-pollen percentages is followed by an increase of pollen from more shade-tolerant trees, reflecting a gradual transition from early to late-successional woodland.[75] Such a complete succession from open land to woodland of shade-tolerant trees certainly occurred locally, but is not evident from the regional landscape reconstruction presented here. Probably the time between abandonment and re-expansion was not always long enough for a complete succession. However, it is interesting to note that oak, which similar to birch starts to expand already in the late fourteenth century, peaks somewhat later. The land cover of birch woodland peaks in the early fifteenth century, 50–100 years after the Black Death, whereas oak peaks in the next 50 years period, in the late fifteenth century. It may reflect the difference in life span and growth rate between the two species. Oak as well as birch quickly colonises abandoned land, but because oak is more slowly growing, birch dominates in the first phase and soon establishes a canopy. However, birch is a short-lived tree that does not usually exceed 100 years.[76] Its short life span together with its inability to regenerate under a closed canopy explains why the birch phase of a natural succession is only temporary. Oak trees grow much older and are more shade-tolerant. Therefore the reforestation of oak woodland is a longer process that continues after the first generation of birch trees has died off.

The strength of the landscape reconstruction presented in Figure 12 is that it is based on a large number of sites from a relatively homogenous region – the South-Swedish Uplands above 100 m above sea level. From the perspective of woodland development, however, this region is not so homogeneous. An important difference within the uplands during the last 1000 years was the different spatial distribution of spruce and beech, respectively. Both species are competitive and shade tolerant, but with different climatic preferences. As mentioned above, spruce is a late immigrant from north to south and did not reach the southern and western parts of the uplands until a century ago.[77] During much of the last 1000 years it was restricted to the northeastern parts of the uplands. Beech is also a late immigrant in a Holocene perspective but expanded from south to north. It reached the southernmost parts of the uplands in the fifth to tenth centuries and slowly expanded northward. Even today beech woodland is much restricted to the southern and western parts of the uplands with only scattered stands further north.[78]

Because of this difference, the pollen sites in the data set were divided into two groups – one for the southwestern parts of the uplands and one for the northeastern (Fig. 14) – and the two subsets were run separately using the LRA. The results are presented in Figure 15. The two reconstructions do not only represent a SW–NE gradient, but also different elevation since the northeastern parts of the uplands are higher. The sites in the southwestern group

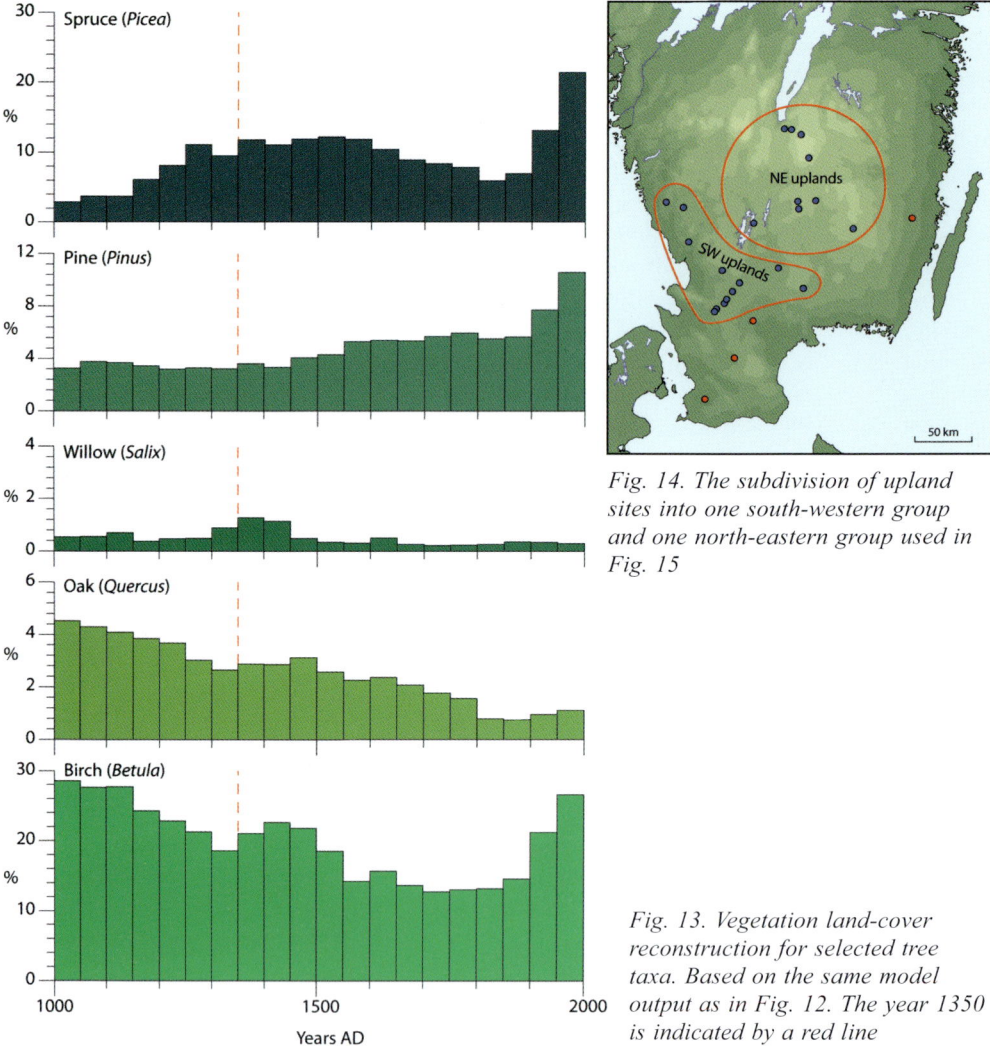

Fig. 14. The subdivision of upland
sites into one south-western group
and one north-eastern group used in
Fig. 15

Fig. 13. Vegetation land-cover
reconstruction for selected tree
taxa. Based on the same model
output as in Fig. 12. The year 1350
is indicated by a red line

range 100–140 m above sea level, whereas those in the northeastern group range 180–325 m. An obvious drawback with this approach is the smaller number of sites underlying each reconstruction, 12 sites in the southeastern group and nine in the northeastern. It leads to a stronger influence of individual sites, and, therefore, a larger variation in the estimated vegetation cover. The subset reconstructions will therefore not be used here to interpret subtle details, but only the major and most apparent differences between the two.

The different distribution of beech and spruce is evident from the reconstructions. Beech woodland had an average land cover of *c*. 25–30% in the southwestern parts during much of the last millennium, but never reached more than 10% in the northeast. Spruce showed a different development. It played a minor role before the eleventh century, but from then

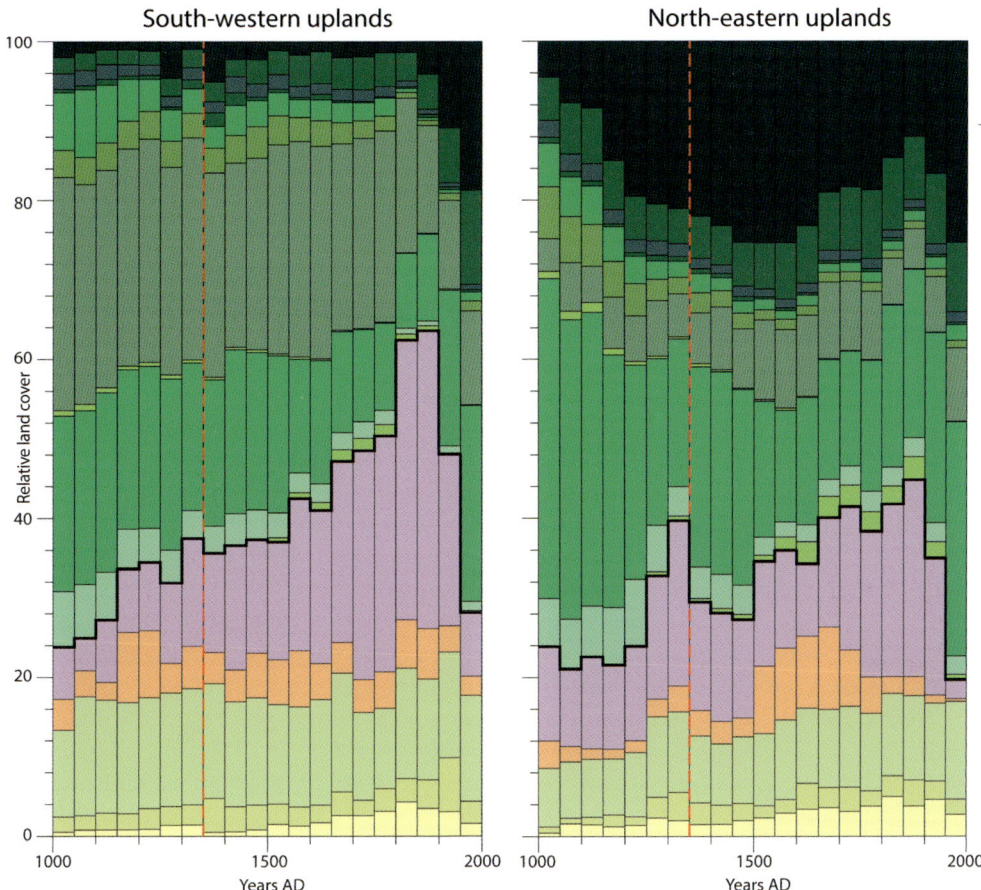

Fig. 15. Vegetation land-cover reconstruction for the lower south-western parts of the uplands, based on 12 sites, and for the higher north-eastern parts of the uplands, based on 9 sites. Cf. Fig. 14. For further details and legend see Fig. 12

on it expanded strongly in the northeastern parts, where it reached a land cover of 25% by the sixteenth century. Spruce forest and other woodlands reached a nadir in the nineteenth century, but they increased strongly again in connection to the reforestation of the twentieth century. In the southwestern parts spruce played a much smaller role, reaching less than 5% of land cover for most of the period. Not until the twentieth century did it expand strongly to reach a land cover of almost 20%. The strong expansion of spruce all over the uplands in the twentieth century was associated with the introduction of modern forestry and spruce planting.

Even though beech and spruce woodlands showed very different development and distribution in different parts of the uplands, none of them seems to have been affected by the late-medieval decline in agricultural activity. Spruce did expand, but this expansion seems to have been part of a long-term expansion that lasted from the eleventh to the sixteenth century. It may be concluded that the land cover of dense, climax woodland did not change in the wake of the population drop, regardless if the dominating tree species was beech or spruce. None of them were able to compete with birch and other early-successional species on abandoned land.

If we now turn to the degree of landscape openness in the uplands, the two diagrams reveal an interesting difference between the northeastern and southwestern parts. In the northeast, there was a very marked decrease in landscape openness after the Black Death. Total land cover of open-land vegetation decreased by one fourth. All types of open-land vegetation decreased, but heather most of all. At the same time, birch woodland expanded strongly. In contrast, the southwestern parts of the uplands show no signs of reforestation. Although some individual diagrams in the southwestern parts do reflect reforestation, the reconstruction presented here based on 12 sites does not.[79] It may be concluded that woodland expansion in the wake of the Black Death was more common in the higher, northeastern parts of the uplands. In the southern and western parts, grazing and possibly mowing to a greater extent kept the landscape open. This difference may reflect the harsher climate of high altitudes, leading to more widespread abandonment and depopulation. On the other hand, land cover of cereal growing shows a smaller decrease after 1350 in the northeast than it does in the southwest. Hence, the results are contradicting. Future studies will hopefully provide a better basis for interpretations of differences within the uplands. At present, what can be said with any certainty, based on the comparison presented here, is that reforestation after the Black Death was more common and widespread in the higher parts of the uplands.

Pollen records provide the best basis for studies of medieval woodland development but interesting information may be gained also from dendrochronology. The most important underlying cause to woodland expansion in some areas in the wake of the Black Death was certainly decreased agricultural impact. However, with dwindling population numbers there was also a reduced demand for fuel, timber and other woodland products. As discussed above, compilations of dendrochronological dates from Småland as well as from other regions show that there was a marked decrease in building activities during the late-medieval crisis.[80] The building of castles and fortifications continued or even increased, probably due to increased repression and riots,[81] but the need for new ordinary buildings and in particular farm buildings was much reduced. Also, there was no need for new churches during the crisis and there were little resources for renovation.[82] On the contrary, many churches decayed during the crisis and some were abandoned.[83]

Compilations of dendrochronological dates, like the one presented here for Småland, clearly reflect the decline in building activities after the Black Death, but they may also provide some insights into the woodland development. It is a routine in dendrochronological dating not only to date the last tree ring, which of course is the one of interest for trying to date the construction of the building, but also when possible to date the innermost tree ring to estimate the year of germination. The latter may provide information on woodland establishment and reforestation. Furthermore, wood dated by dendrochronology is routinely also identified to tree species.

Dated wood from Småland and the rest of Sweden is almost entirely of oak and pine. These two tree species were by far the most important timber trees for building and they are also the ones for which there are long reference tree-ring series.[84] The diagram in Figure 16 shows the temporal distribution of the dates (estimated felling years) from Småland. It is the same data as in Figure 10 but now with oak, pine and spruce separated. The diagram shows that oak was an important building timber during the Middle Ages before the crisis. It was particularly important for large buildings, and much of the dated oak is from churches, but it was also frequently used for profane buildings in towns. No oak has been dated to the period between 1360 and 1464. Some oak timber was used in the late fifteenth and early sixteenth centuries, but after that almost none was used until the eighteenth century. Also pine was used in churches as well as in profane buildings in towns during the Middle Ages (very few profane buildings in the countryside have been dated). Both pine and oak were important as building timber before the crisis. Later, in connection to the very strong expansion of several towns (Jönköping, Kalmar, Eksjö, etc.) in the sixteenth century, only pine timber was used. The regular use of spruce timber started very late, in the eighteenth century.

The shift from oak and pine to a strong dominance of pine may to some degree reflect a change in the composition of woodlands – from the sixteenth century onwards the land cover of oak woodland had decreased whereas pine woodland had increased (Fig. 13). However, the change in woodland composition appears to have been very slow and gradual. More important was probably the fact that all oaks in Sweden were declared royal property (*regale*) in the mid-sixteenth century. Because of their value as mast trees and timber trees for royal shipbuilding, no oak trees wherever they grew were allowed to be felled or cut in any way by peasants.[85]

We may now look not only at the years of tree felling, but also at woodland regeneration as reflected in the dating of the innermost tree ring of each tree. In Figure 17 the temporal distribution of all the estimated germination years is presented. The diagram shows several peaks but one of the strongest is at 1350–1360. It indicates that several of the trees that were later cut and used for building had germinated around the time of the Black Death. Later and stronger peaks are found at 1480–1500 (possibly associated with the plague years 1484 and 1495)[86] and 1670–1690.

More details are revealed by the presentation in Figure 18. In this diagram all the individual dates from Småland are presented. For each of the identified tree species – pine, spruce and oak – the dates are in chronological order based on their estimated felling years (blue dots). In the cases where also the germination year has been possible to estimate (usually with an error of within ±20 years), the life span of the tree is indicated by a black line. Most interesting for the discussion here are the germination years of trees that were cut during and after the late-medieval crisis. Of pine very few were cut during the late fourteenth and fifteenth centuries, and most of them had germinated before the crisis. In the mid-sixteenth century some pines that had germinated soon after the Black Death of 1350 were cut, probably in connection to clearings of secondary woodland on abandoned land. However, not all pines that germinated in association with the Black Death were cut during the sixteenth century – several survived much longer. Still throughout the seventeenth century, pine trees that germinated soon after 1350 were occasionally cut and used for building timber. The last 'Black Death-pines' according to the diagram were actually cut down as late as in the early eighteenth century. In 1704, a pine tree was cut that had germinated approx. 1355. It was by then 350 years old. A little later, in 1712, a few pines were cut that had germinated approx. 1380 (Fig. 19). They were the last reminders of the woodland regeneration of the late fourteenth century.[87] Later on, all trees used for building were much younger.

Oak tells a somewhat different story than pine. Due to the *regale*, very few oak trees

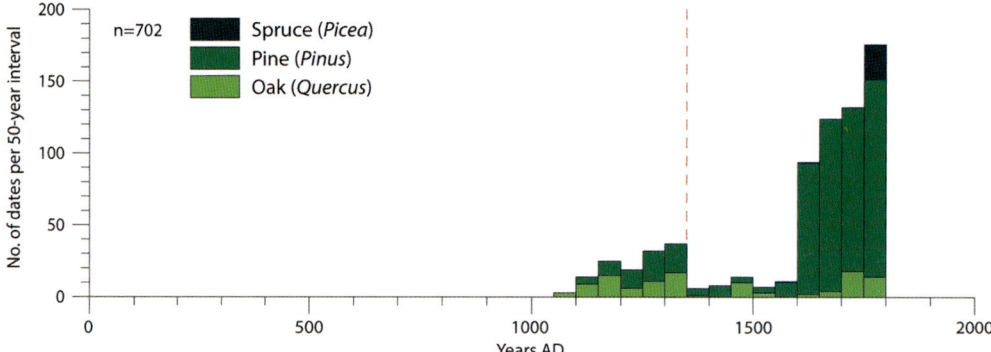

Fig. 16. The same dendrochronological dates (felling years) from Småland as in Fig. 10, but here with tree species distinguished

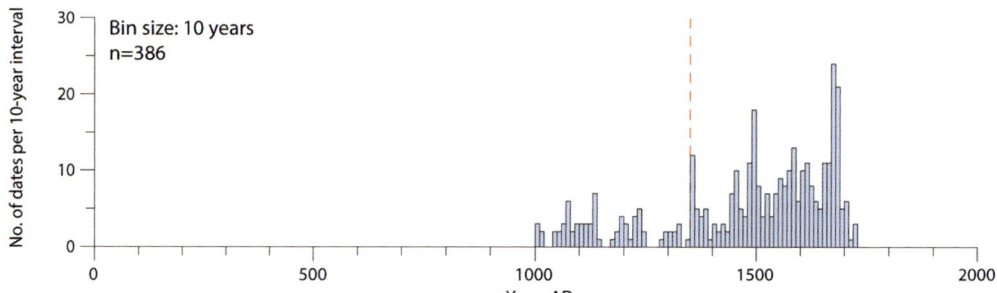

Fig. 17. A compilation of all the dated germination years in the dendrochronological record from Småland. Bars show the number of dates per 10-year time slices

were cut and used for building constructions during the seventeenth century. There may very well have been old oak trees growing in the landscape, of which some had their roots in the Black Death, but since they were not cut and used for building constructions, they do not show up in the data presented here. However, a number of oaks were cut down in 1464–1509, before the regale, in connection to the building of two churches.[88] As shown by the diagram the majority of these oaks germinated in connection to 1350. A plausible interpretation is that secondary oak woodland that once got established on abandoned land in connection to the Black Death, now a century and a half later was cut down. The timber was obviously used for construction but a purpose of the clearing may at the same time have been to re-establish agricultural land. The dendrochronological data thus supports the interpretation of the pollen based land-cover reconstructions, according to which there was a slight expansion of oak woodland in the uplands after the Black Death.

Spruce was not used regularly as building timber until the eighteenth century, and there are only two older samples in the data set. Interestingly, one of them was a very old tree that was cut in 1624 to be used in a house foundation in the town of Jönköping. It had germinated almost 300 years earlier, in approximately 1355.

Hence, the dendrochronological record indicates that there was woodland regeneration

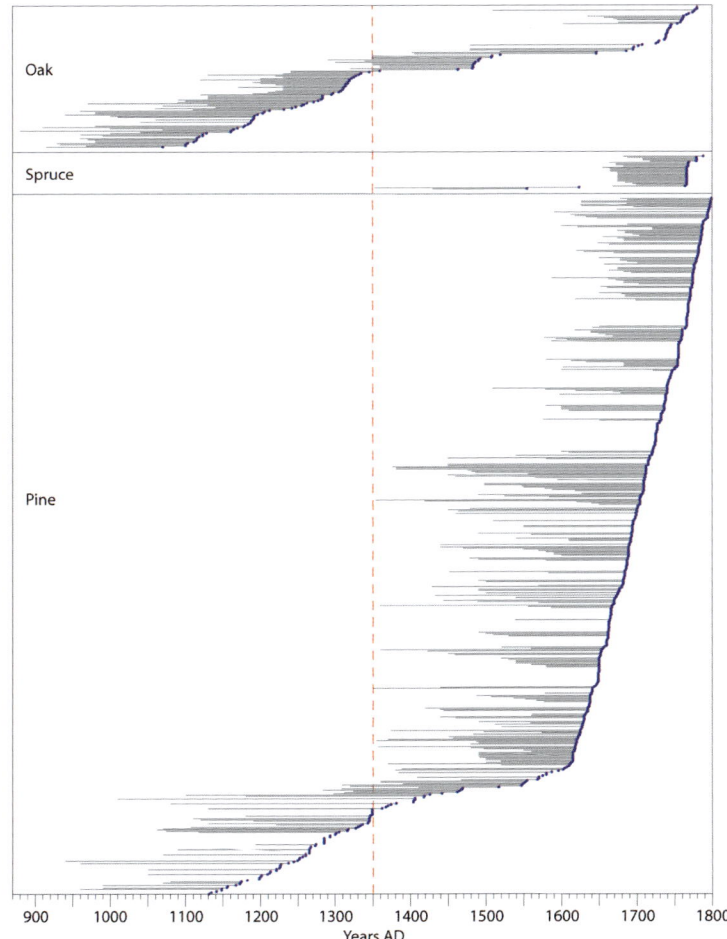

Fig. 18. All the 702 dendrochronological dates from Småland separated into tree species and presented in chronological order based on felling years (blue dots). In those 386 cases where also the germination year has been determined, the life-span of the individual tree is marked by a black line. The year 1350 is indicated by a red line

Fig. 19. Uranäsboden on display at the Kulturen Museum in Lund. It was originally situated in Älghult Parish, Småland, in the eastern part of the uplands. According to dendrochronological dating of the timber, parts of the building originate from the early sixteenth century but it was re-built and enlarged in the early eighteenth century. Some of the timber that was cut and used in the early eighteenth century was from very old pine trees that had once germinated on abandoned land in the wake of the Black Death (photo: Per Lagerås)

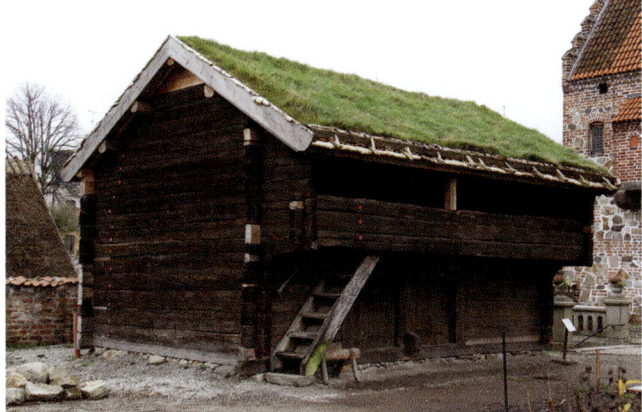

during the late-medieval crisis. Furthermore, it shows that this reforestation started already in close connection with the Black Death of 1350. This result is in line with earlier studies from middle and northern Sweden and from Norway.[89] Whereas the pollen record indicates particularly birch but also oak regeneration, dendrochronology gives examples of oak and pine regeneration. The total absence of birch in the dendrochronological record is due to the fact that birch was not used for building timber. However, it is more difficult to explain why an expansion of pine after 1350 stands out stronger in dendrochronological data than in the pollen record. Probably, large pine trees were valuable for building timber and particularly sought for, leading to over-representation in the dendrochronological record. Even though the dendrochronological record does not allow for any quantification of woodland regeneration, it indicates that there was increased germination of both oak and pine immediately after the Black Death. Much of the secondary woodland of birch, oak and pine was cleared in connection to the recovery and agricultural expansion that followed upon the crisis, but still after three centuries there were old pine trees growing in the woods that originated in the Black Death.

Summary of conclusions

The pollen and dendrochronological records presented in this chapter have provided new insights into the late-medieval crisis. The most important conclusion, which is also fundamental for a broader discussion, is that societal changes in connection to the crisis resulted in environmental changes. These changes were distinct and far-reaching enough to show up in the palaeoecological records on a regional scale. The conclusion is not surprising, because in a cultural landscape there is always interdependence between vegetation and human activities. Still, high-resolution palaeoecological records with good chronologies are needed to detect these changes. The uplands are suitable in this respect because of the numerous lakes and well-preserved peatlands and the large number of high-quality pollen diagrams available. Furthermore, the half-open landscape of the South-Swedish Uplands – characterised by a mosaic of open agricultural land and woodland – may be particularly suitable for this type of study. Trees and woodland were never far away and reforestation after abandonment was less delayed than it would have been in a more tree-less landscape. Also the mixed agriculture with a large element of pastures and hay meadows enabled swift changes, for instance from arable to pastures.

The aim of this chapter has been not only to interpret vegetation changes as such, but to discuss how these changes may reflect several important aspects of the late-medieval crisis, like population drop and settlement abandonment, agricultural strategies developed during the crisis, and also the recovery afterwards. These are the major conclusions:

During the fourteenth century there was a halving of arable in the uplands, which indicates extensive farm abandonment and population drop. From the lowlands, sites are too few to allow any certain conclusions, but two lowland sites, which are also the most southernmost sites in the data set, deviate from all the upland sites by indicating an increase in cereal growing in the late-fourteenth century.

The decline in arable in the uplands during the fourteenth century started already in 1350 or soon afterwards. The conclusion is based on both the pollen record and the compilation of dendrochronological dates. Hence the first struck of the plague – the Black Death *sensu stricto* – had an immediate effect on upland societies. If this was a direct effect of the plague or an indirect effect through migration, is not possible to tell from the palaeoecological records.

Abandonment of agricultural land resulted in woodland expansion, but to some extent the landscape was still kept open by grazing. The decrease in pastures and meadows appears to have been proportionally smaller than the decrease in arable, which indicates that animal husbandry in relation to crop growing gained in relative importance during the crisis.

Land left for reforestation was in particular poor, heath-like pastures characterised by heather vegetation. At the same time, abandoned arable was in many cases transferred to pastures and meadows with herbs and grasses. The reforestation of poor pastures and the establishment of new, probably more productive ones on abandoned arable, suggest that the average productivity of land used for animal husbandry increased during the crisis.

Reforestation by natural succession on abandoned pastures was more common in the higher, northeastern parts of the uplands. In the southern and western parts, grazing was more successful in holding the forest back. Where reforestation occurred, particularly birch but also oak, pine and spruce colonised the abandoned land. Dendrochronological dates show that such woodland regeneration in some cases started immediately after the Black Death of 1350. Due to different ecological preferences and life spans of the different tree species, a fast and strong expansion of birch woodland was followed by a slower and subtler expansion of oak and pine.

In association with societal recovery and agricultural expansion after the crisis, abandoned arable fields were put under the plough again. The landscape reconstruction indicates that there was a slight time lag between the reestablishment of arable and the clearing of secondary woodland. The expansion of arable started in the late fifteenth century and the deforestation in the early sixteenth century. This was the beginning of a strong agricultural expansion and deforestation that continued more or less to the nineteenth century, when landscape openness in the uplands peaked. Today, after substantial reforestation during the twentieth century, forest cover is back at the same level as before the medieval expansion.

Notes

1   Lagerås is main author. Broström and Fredh performed landscape reconstruction modelling based on pollen data. Berg, Björkman, Fredh, Hultberg, Karlsson, Lagerås, Lindbladh, Mazier, Segerström and Sköld contributed with pollen data. Linderson contributed with dendrochronological data
2   Moe 1991; Stebich *et al.* 2005; van Hoof *et al.* 2006; Lagerås 2007; Yeloff & van Geel 2007; Sköld *et al.* 2010; Poska *et al.* 2014
3   The method was introduced by Lennart von Post in a lecture in 1916, which was later published in English (von Post 1967)
4   For a thorough introduction see Moore *et al.* (1991).
5   Iversen 1941 (in English 1949)
6   Berglund 1969
7   Boserup 1965; Berglund 1991, 14
8   Bradshaw 1988; Björkman 1996; Lindbladh 1998
9   E.g. Edwards 1991; Lagerås *et al.* 1995; Lagerås 2007
10 Olsson 1991
11 To avoid the reservoir effect when radiocarbon dating, the important thing is to use remains of plants that, during photosynthesis, get their carbon dioxide directly from the atmosphere (like

most terrestrial plants), and not from lake water (like green algae, which make up the bulk of most lake sediments)

12 Based on instrumental data for the period 1961–90 (Raab & Vedin 1995). Growing season is the part of the year when average temperature exceeds 5°C

13 Cf. Eckstein (1984) for a thorough introduction

14 Bartholin 1987

15 E.g. Bartholin 1989; Raihle 1990; Hovanta 1994

16 Bartholin 1989, 125

17 Dendro data are also presented in Chap.5

18 E.g. Gauffin 1981; Hansson *et al.* 2005; Åstrand 2006. See also discussion in Chap. 5

19 E.g. Larsson 1970; Österberg 1977; Bååth 1983; Myrdal 2003

20 Sandnes 1981, 103

21 Sandnes 1981, 103; Bååth 1983, 199

22 Myrdal 2012a, 226

23 To make a simple and clear definition, all sites above 100 m a.s.l. were regarded as upland sites. Consequently, all sites situated below 100 m a.s.l. were excluded, even though one of them, Skärsgölarna, was situated in a rather poor environment of upland character

24 Cf. Chap. 2 for further background

25 An unpaired *t* test shows that the difference in mean cereal-pollen percentages between 1250–1350 and 1350–1450 is very statistically significant (two-tailed P value equals 0.0099)

26 Broström *et al.* 2004; 2008; Sugita 2007; Gaillard *et al.* 2010; Fredh *et al.* 2012; Mazier *et al.* 2015. Of the Landscape Reconstruction Algorithm we use the submodel REVEALS (Regional Estimates of Vegetation Abundance from Large Sites) presented by Sugita (2007), with the application on small sites tested by Mazier *et al.* (2015)

27 The model has been validated for southern Sweden (Hellman *et al.* 2007;, 2008; Mazier *et al.* 2015, Trondman *et al.* 2014)

28 Because of the different pollen-dispersal characteristics of rye and other cereals, respectively, they were calculated separately and then put together into one graph

29 Gadd 2011, 124

30 Moe 1991 (Norway); Hall 2003 (Ireland); Stebich *et al.* 2005 (France); van Hoof *et al.* 2006 (Netherlands); Yeloff & van Geel 2007 (Denmark and review of published data from several countries); Yeloff *et al.* 2007 (England); Sköld *et al.* 2010 (Sweden); Poska *et al.* 2014 (Estonia)

31 Yeloff & van Geel 2007

32 The strength in combining local pollen studies to regional synthesis has been emphasized for instance by Lagerås (2007) and Woodbridge *et al.* (2012)

33 Cf. Chapter 2 for background and further discussion

34 Myrdal 2012b, 227, 234–235

35 The use of a resolution of 50 years is a compromise – a courser resolution would reveal too few details while a finer resolution would give a more irregular graph due to a smaller number of samples within each time slice.

36 Based on a number of radiocarbon-dated levels, the ages of the pollen-analysed levels in a stratigraphic sequence are calculated by interpolation. Most studies use linear interpolation but also other methods (like cubic spline) are occasionally used. The present study relies on the chronologies of the original publications, with no changes or adjustments

37 Note, however, that the total absence of dates from before the eleventh century does not mean a total absence of settlement. Traces of long houses and other buildings from the first millennium AD have been archaeologically documented in the uplands, but they are too poorly preserved for dendrochronological dating.

38 Bartholin 1989, 125; see Fig. 21a in Chap. 5

39 Thun 2005, 73
40 Myrdal 2012a, 226
41 Gissel *et al.* 1981, 103, 107
42 Abel 1980, 88–89
43 Abel 1980, 88–89; Dyers 2002, 352; Benedictow 2004, 261; Myrdal 2011, 80; 2012a, 225, 227
44 Karlsson 1996; Livi Bacci 2000, 84; Myrdal 2012a, 227
45 Harrison 2000, 33
46 Myrdal & Söderberg 1991, 133
47 E.g. Behre 1981; Gaillard *et al.* 1994
48 Gadd 2011, 123ff
49 Myrdal 2011, 93
50 Mixed herbaceous plants include the following pollen types: Compositeae SF. Cichorioideae (dandelions, hawk's-beards, etc.), *Filipendula* (dropwort, meadowsweet), *Plantago lanceolata* (ribwort plantain), *Potentilla* type (tormentil, cinquefoil), *Ranunculus acris* type (buttercups), Rubiaceae (bedstraw), and *Rumex acetosa* type (sorrel)
51 E.g. Eriksson *et al.* 2002; Bernes 2011, 49ff; Morell 2011, 179ff; Fredh *et al.* 2012
52 Large-scale forest plantations took off after the Forestry Act of 1903 (Bernes 2011, 50)
53 Weimarck 1953; Gadd 2011, 128
54 E.g. Abel 1980, 70; Campbell 2006, 185; 2012, 124; Myrdal 2012, 221
55 Myrdal 2006, 169
56 Söderberg 2007, 143–144
57 See Chap.5 for examples of additional strategies developed during the crisis interpreted from the archaeological record
58 Myrdal 2012a, 221
59 Myrdal 2012a, 217; 2012b, 222; cf. Chap. 2
60 Lagerås 1996; 2007, 73; 2013b, 86
61 Cf. Widgren (2007) for a discussion on the landesque capital.
62 Myrdal 2006, 169–170
63 Redman 1999, 197–199, 202
64 E.g. Williams 2006, 117
65 Ruddiman 2003, 2005, 115–146
66 For pollen diagrams showing late-medieval reforestation in Europe, see for instance Moe 1991; Stebich *et al.* 2005; van Hoof *et al.* 2006; Lagerås 2007; Yeloff & van Geel 2007; Sköld *et al.* 2010; Poska *et al.* 2014.
67 Gaillard *et al.* 2010; Trondman *et al.* 2014
68 Kinnaird 1974, 470
69 Götmark & Kiffer 2014
70 Atkinson 1992; Hynynen *et al.* 2010
71 Götmark & Kiffer 2014
72 Bradshaw *et al.* 2000
73 Björkman 1996a, 13; Giesecke & Bennett 2004; Lagerås 2007
74 E.g. Björkman 1997b, 2003c; Sköld *et al.* 2010
75 Sköld *et al.* 2010
76 Atkinson 1992, 848
77 Björkman 1996a; Lagerås 2007
78 Björkman 1996b; Lindbladh *et al.* 2008
79 Lagerås 2007; Sköld *et al.* 2010
80 Bartholin 1989, 125; Thun 2005, 73
81 Lovén 1996; Myrdal 2012a, 230

82   It cannot be excluded that some old timber was reused for small-scale building and renovation
83   Nyborg 2009
84   Bartholin 1987
85   Proclaimed by King Gustav Vasa in 1558 (Eliasson & Hamilton 1999, 53)
86   Myrdal 2012a, 223
87   The Black-Death-pines cut in the early eighteenth century were found in Uranäsboden (see Fig.
     19), whereas Black-Death-pines cut in the seventeenth century are from Yxenhaga Gammelstuga
     (Svenarum Parish) and from different constructions in the towns of Eksjö and Jönköping
88   The dated samples are from the church of Hakarp and the campanile at the church of Härlöv
89   Bartholin 1989, 127; Thun 2005, 66. A similar conclusion can be drawn from a study in Scotland,
     in which imported building timber from Scandinavia and the Baltic countries was identified (Mills
     & Crone 2012). Many of the logs that were imported during the late fifteenth century and the
     sixteenth century were from trees that had started to grow soon after 1350

5.

Change, desertion and survival
– an archaeology of the late-medieval crisis

Lars Ersgård

Introduction

Historical archaeology in Sweden has not provided any comprehensive approach to the late-medieval crisis. There are several reasons for this. One is that later parts of the Middle Ages have never been perceived as important as the earlier parts of this epoch, often being reduced to just a transitional phase between the High Middle Ages and the Renaissance. Furthermore research on crisis as a general societal process has by tradition not been a topic of primary interest within Swedish historical archaeology compared to phenomena like state formation, urbanisation, Christianisation etc. Finally, earlier influential research by historians, especially within *The Scandinavian Research Project on Deserted Farms and Villages*, which significantly reduced the impact of the crisis on society in medieval Sweden, probably has played a role for a certain lack of interest among Swedish archaeologists.[1]

On the whole the awareness of the crisis has been highly varying in historical archaeological research, also in projects explicitly dealing with the late Middle Ages. The different attitudes represent a wide range from an almost total absence of interest to a more problematising approach to the phenomenon. Usually looked upon as an agrarian crisis, it has been regarded as just a matter of desertion with no closer connection to societal changes during the late Middle Ages. In this respect the crisis has often been referred to as a general historical background and as an explanation to different archaeological phenomena such as deserted farmsteads or discontinuities in the construction of churches etc. The role played by archaeology has often been a confirming one, supporting conclusions by written history.

Such an approach characterised the historical archaeological part of the interdisciplinary research project on the development of the cultural landscape in the southern part of the province of Scania, denominated *The Cultural Landscape During 6000 Years in Southern Sweden* (The Ystad project).[2] Historical archaeology was well represented in this project, collaborating with several disciplines.[3] Formation of villages, establishment of manors and ecclesiastical development being the main problems, no special focus was put on the late-medieval crisis. There was an awareness of the latter, however being just a matter of desertion and regression in the landscape.

A wider and more complex perspective on the late-medieval crisis has been presented by Anders Andrén in his dissertation on medieval towns in Denmark. Including the towns in the discussion on the crisis, he emphasises the period 1350–1400 as a time of stagnation and decline as well as a time of change towards a more uniform urban structure.[4]

This chapter will present an archaeological picture of the late-medieval crisis with a primary starting point in the idea that this discipline may provide an independent contribution to the study of the phenomenon. The following archaeological study will not focus on the crisis only in the traditional way, that is tantamount to desertion of agrarian settlement, and repeat earlier questions, formulated by historians, concerning economy and demography. The crisis will be looked upon in a wider sense, as a movement affecting the society as a whole, not only economically and demographically but also culturally. In this way also the material culture becomes important, as a source for the study of strategies and acting on a cultural and mental level.

Janken Myrdal has considerably vitalised and widened the debate, presenting a three-phase model of the development of the crisis.[5] An initial phase, *catastrophe*, covering the two decades after 1350 when plague raged Scandinavia in three horrific outbreaks, was followed by a phase called *societal reaction,* which lasted up to 1450. This phase was characterised by a dysfunctional acting of the elite, which exacerbated the crisis and highly hampered the recovery of society. The final phase, *recovery and reconstruction*, which lasted 1450–1530, saw the beginning of a new expansion of society accompanied by technological changes and the emergence of a new effective political structure. This model will be of importance for the following analysis, not as a final answer but as a starting point and source of inspiration.

The late-medieval crisis was not only a matter of decline and decrease of population in the later part of the fourteenth century, followed by recovery in the fifteenth century – it was also a matter of change. Hence it is necessary to look upon it in a wider perspective of societal development. Profound changes characterised the early centuries of the Middle Ages, the landscape being successively transformed by population growth, land clearance and agrarian innovations. The large estates of the Early Middle Ages, which were based mostly on labour force of thralls, were replaced by farms based on the single family, and the peasants became either tenants or freeholders. Other important changes were the emergence of landowning nobility, the territorially defined parish and an extensive urbanisation in some parts of the country.

In the thirteenth century a new regionalisation of the country started, the regions from now on developing in different cultural directions. A socio-political shift of emphasis towards the eastern parts of southern Sweden occurred in the late thirteenth century, the areas around Lake Mälaren becoming a dominant region.[6] Several towns were founded here in the thirteenth century of which Stockholm became the most important. This region will from now on stand out as the centre of the Swedish realm. Characteristic of the countryside in the east was settlement of villages and hamlets organised in a highly regulated system of land division.[7]

The western parts of southern Sweden differed significantly from the eastern region. The urbanisation of the high Middle Ages was not as extensive as in the east, the towns being small and in some areas notably instable in their spatial structure.[8] In the countryside, the settlement lacked the regulated structure that characterised the eastern parts of the country.[9]

Northern Sweden differed significantly from the other parts. Towns, landowning nobility and a social system of tenants were practically absent in the north. The population was dominated by freeholders with duties only to the royal kingship. However, there are indications of a socially stratified society in northern Sweden in the Viking Age and the early Middle Ages, such as big barrows with prestigious objects and manifest stone churches. Thus, a transition from an elitist society to an egalitarian one must have characterised the medieval development in parts of northern Sweden. The underlying causes of this process are still not fully understood, neither its possible connections with the late-medieval crisis.[10]

Formulating an archaeological approach to the late-medieval crisis, some decisive questions have to be raised. Firstly, how did the crisis affect the physical realities of the late-medieval society at the middle of the fourteenth century in terms of decline and stagnation? Here, problems concerning desertion of settlement and changes of the building of houses and churches will be included.

Secondly, how did the late-medieval society respond to the crisis? What did the people surviving the plagues of the 1350s and 1360s actually do in the new societal situation, the population being reduced by as much as 50%. How were they forced to change their everyday life in a material respect, searching for new strategies of survival?

A third question concerns regional variations. Did specific characteristics of a region affect the choice of survival strategies or were people acting in a similar way to withstand crisis and decline?

Searching for answers to these questions, an extensive, archaeological source material is available, including the traditional material categories of medieval archaeology, i.e. excavated structures as well as extant monuments. In this text it is used in two different ways. The first part of the analysis will work broadly, searching for the "good examples" all over the country, aiming for a synthesising overview.

The second part will change focus, working with a few settlement units. Studying three single farmsteads in different parts of the country, the aim will be to try to identify survival strategies in the time of the crisis in different regional contexts.

The primary area of investigation for the studies is Sweden with its present boundaries but some comparative outlooks towards other parts of the Nordic countries will complete the analyses. In a geographical sense, medieval Sweden was not the same as Sweden of today, several of its present provinces in the south and in the west belonging to Denmark

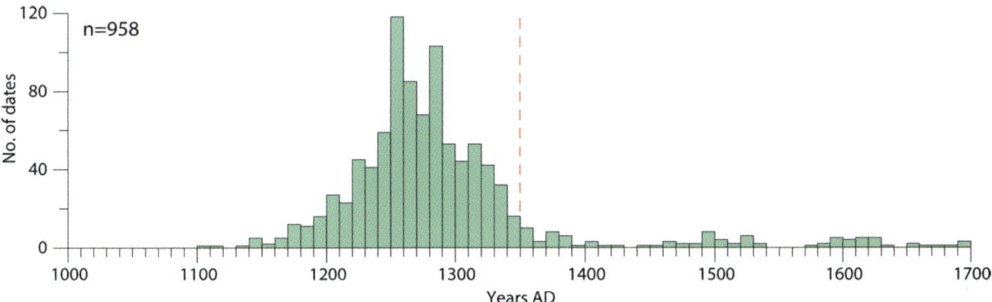

Fig. 20. All the dendrochronological dates (felling years) from medieval towns in the province of Östergötland performed by the National Laboratory for Wood Anatomy and Dendrochronology at Lund University. Bars show the number of dates per 10-year time slices. Dates later than 1700 are not included. The year 1350 is indicated by a dashed line

and Norway. On the other hand, the territory of today's Finland was part of the Swedish realm in the Middle Ages.

However, the political boundaries are of a secondary importance for this investigation. Moreover, the geopolitical situation of the Nordic countries was a very complicated one in the time of the crisis. For example, the political dominion of the province of Scania in the south alternated between Sweden and Denmark during parts of the fourteenth century. From the 1390s up to the beginning of the sixteenth century the three countries Sweden, Denmark and Norway were formally united in a political union with one common regent.

Investigating medieval settlement and its development, a conventional outline of the archaeological record will be followed, using the two primary categories *town* and *countryside* and the subcategories *profane settlement*, *churches and monasteries* and *castles*. A specific category has been denominated *proto-industrial settlement*. Using this outline has been motivated primarily by the fact that most research on the late Middle Ages so far has followed such a structuring of the source material. In addition to archaeology, a new compilation of dendrochronological data will be presented.

Late-medieval Sweden in the shadow of the crisis – an archaeological overview

Urban settlement

The extensive urban expansion of the High Middle Ages in Scandinavia came to an end in the beginning of the fourteenth century and during the remainder of this century very few towns were founded in the Scandinavian countries. Only in Sweden, including Finland, were new urban places founded during the latter part of the fourteenth century and in the beginning of the fifteenth.[11] Several of these had played a role as central places in their regions before they acquired formal status as towns, for example as market places or places of pilgrimage. In Denmark, urban expansion did not start until in the fifteenth century, while in Norway very few towns were founded in the late Middle Ages.

There are significant differences between the newly founded towns of the late Middle Ages and the places of older origin.[12] The former were mainly small units of settlement compared to the latter. They did not possess the developed institutional structure of the older towns, thus lacking buildings like monasteries, hospitals, sanctuaries etc. Usually a single church was the only institution. A famous exception of this pattern was the late-medieval town of Vadstena, the centre of the cult of Saint Bridget, where several institutional buildings were present.

Concerning urban decline at the time of the crisis, there are distinctive traces of desertion of settlement in some towns. In Uppsala a discontinuity of settlement has been observed in two places in the northern outskirts of the medieval town.[13] A rapid expansion in the later part of thirteenth century and in the beginning of the fourteenth century was followed by an abandonment of settlement in this area. At the end of the fifteenth century it was resettled by highly specialised craftsmen, indicating a new expansion of settlement during the recovery phase of the crisis.

In the town of Örebro, desertion of settlement took place in the late Middle Ages but unlike Uppsala in a central part of the town.[14] Also, in Danish towns there are indications of desertion.[15] In the town of Lund, an area in the northern outskirts, where craft buildings were located in the High Middle Ages, was abandoned after the year 1350 and was not resettled until the sixteenth century.[16]

In the town of Linköping the impact of the crisis was discernable not as desertion but as an almost total stop of construction works during the first decades after 1350.[17] This lacuna is clearly discernible in the new dendrochronological material from the towns of Östergötland where the number of dates decreases significantly after the year 1350 (Fig. 20).

A critical remark concerning the dendrochronological dates from towns is necessary. A lot of them originate from a smaller number of large-scale excavations in medieval and post-medieval towns like Söderköping in Östergötland and Jönköping and Kalmar in Småland. Excavations in the former town have generated a large amount of dates from the thirteenth century and in the latter two towns from the seventeenth century. This means that these periods will be overrepresented in the material when using it for studies of long-term development.

Totally deserted towns seem to have been less common in the late Middle Ages. Probably some urban places in medieval Denmark were wiped out, like Herrested on the island of Funen.[18] In medieval Sweden two places may most likely be considered as examples of urban desertion. One of them is the place Folklandstingstad in Lunda parish of the province of Uppland. The place was obviously an urban structure in the thirteenth and fourteenth centuries but lacking a formal status as a town.[19] According to some written evidence Folklandstingstad was located in the neighbourhood of a local thing stead at the church of Lunda. Finds of cultural layers of the High Middle Ages has given further support to this localisation. Folklandstingstad was counteracted by the Swedish kingship, deciding in 1350 that the inhabitants had to move away to the nearby town of Sigtuna. In 1385 the place seems to have been totally abandoned.

A since long accepted explanation is that solely the acting of the king caused the disappearance of Folklandstingstad. However, the fact that there is a chronological coincidence between this disappearance and the outbreaks of the bubonic plague in the 1350s and 1360s makes it reasonable to suppose that the latter highly contributed to the rapid desertion of this urban society.

Our second example of urban desertion is a place called Gamla Köpstad at the west coast of Sweden, located around 5 km south of the town of Varberg. This place is less well understood than Folklandstingstad and our knowledge of it is solely based on the results of some minor excavations of the last decades.[20] Remains of houses, cultural layers, ceramics and coins indicate some sort of coastal trading place with a principal dating to the twelfth, thirteenth and fourteenth centuries. Probably Gamla Köpstad was finally abandoned in the fifteenth century. However, a thorough discussion on the connections between the abandonment and the societal crisis must be postponed at the moment, waiting for further and hopefully more substantial results concerning the function and chronology of the place.

Urban changes, indicating a reaction to the crisis, can already be seen in some towns in the later part of the fourteenth century. In Uppsala the character of the town settlement west of the river Fyrisån seems to have changed significantly at the middle of the fourteenth century. An older, agglomerated settlement of wooden houses was replaced by a residential settlement of stone houses surrounded by open garden areas.[21] An ecclesiastical district was materialised around the cathedral. Contrasting to this was the profane settlement east of the river – the area of merchants and craftsmen – their yards filling the blocks with a coherent settlement of wooden houses. Extensive finds of bronze casting in a central part of the east riverside, indicating a specialised, large scale workshop established at the end of the fourteenth century, may be seen as an example of this new social structure of the town.[22] Furthermore, another expression of this process was the establishment of a new square in the 1380s.[23]

A decisive change seems to have happened also in the episcopal town of Linköping in the late Middle Ages. In the 1380s, only a few decades after the outbreak of the plague in 1350, new signs of expansion and restructuring became visible in the settlement. A densification and a regulation of the town plots took place and the first stone houses were built. This new expansion is absent in the dendrochronological material, a fact that may be explained by bad preservation conditions of wood in the cultural layers of the late Middle Ages.

These changes of settlement reflect, according to Tagesson, the establishment of the residential town and the building of clerical estates.[24] Thus, a differentiation of the town settlement similar to the one observed in Uppsala seems to have taken place in Linköping in the late Middle Ages.

In the episcopal town of Turku (Åbo) in the southwest of Finland a period of expansion began already in the 1360s and no signs at all of decline or stagnation are discernable.[25]

> the town grew in every direction with new buildings and the expansion of the street network. At this phase, the population of the town has increased remarkably and new technologies and innovations were also presented.[26]

So, the archaeological experience of Turku surprisingly well supports the earlier picture, obtained in Uppsala and Linköping, of the last decades of the fourteenth century as an expansive and dynamic, urban period.

Explaining this urban dynamics in the initial, severe phase of the crisis may seem rather difficult. However, there was a significant increase of gifts and donations to the clerical institutions in connection to the outbreaks of the plague in the later part of the fourteenth century, meaning a concentration of resources to the dioceses.[27] This phenomenon may probably be looked upon as a possible clue to the dynamics of the mentioned episcopal towns.

However, concerning late-medieval development, one episcopal town differs a lot from the above-mentioned places that is the town of Skara in the west of Sweden. After an expansive period in the thirteenth century and in the beginning of the fourteenth century Skara was struck by decline and desertion after the middle of the fourteenth century.[28] The dynamics, observed in Uppsala, Linköping and Turku in the late Middle Ages, seems to be lacking in Skara. On the contrary, this place together with other towns in the west were characterised by a sort of "de-urbanisation" in the fourteenth century when some administrative functions were moved from the towns to the royal castles in the countryside.[29]

The decrease of thickness in the formation of cultural layers in the later part of the fourteenth century has been a highly debated topic since the 1980s, the phenomenon being observed in urban contexts all over Scandinavia.[30] Several explanations have been presented but a connection between the change of the formation of layers and societal crisis has not been explicitly discussed.

Because of the general decrease in population the towns had to care for their own supply of foodstuff to a much higher degree than before, meaning an extension and a more rational use of their own surrounding cropland. Thus, the urban refuse was used as manure in the fields outside the towns, enforcing a new management of the garbage inside the towns.[31]

Town churches

In some cases the on-going construction of urban churches in the fourteenth and fifteenth centuries, especially the cathedrals, can be looked upon as a sort of condensed reflection of societal crisis. As mentioned above, all construction works ceased in the settlement of Linköping after the year 1350 and so did the works at the cathedral in the town. Not until in the first decades of the fifteenth century they were resumed.[32]

In the cathedral of Uppsala no stop of the construction works can be observed during the latter part of the fourteenth century. However, the walls of the southern parts of the nave, which were erected during this period, show a more deficient craftsmanship than earlier walls.[33] In the building works of the fifteenth century a higher quality of masonry is visible anew. These qualitative differences have been explained by a lack of qualified masons, caused by the general decrease of the population at the end of the fourteenth century.[34]

The cathedral of Turku shows no signs of decline in the time of the crisis but rather expansion. Extensive construction works were carried out on this building in the second half of the fourteenth century.[35] A new chancel was built together with several chapels. Furthermore the sacristy was enlarged. Thus, these changes of the cathedral harmonise well with the above-described expansion of the town settlement of Turku.

An interesting comparison has been made between the cathedral of Trondheim in Norway and the cathedral of Odense in Denmark.[36] At the former the construction of a new nave started in the thirteenth century, the work staying unfinished when the plague hit Norway in the middle of the fourteenth century. Thereafter the building had to wait for its completion until the nineteenth century.

In Odense the building of a new cathedral began around 1300 but the work was still going on at the time of the Black Death. During the later part of the fourteenth century, there was a stop of building activities, being resumed not until the beginning of the fifteenth century. At the end of the century the cathedral was finally completed.

While the Danish church reminds us a lot of the development of the cathedral of Linköping, its counterpart in Trondheim reflects something much more severe. Not only did lack of economic resources prevent the completion of the cathedral but there was also a total extinction of the knowledge of working in stone caused by a dramatic decrease of population. This was not seen in any other parts of Scandinavia, thus reflecting a much greater impact of the crisis in Norway.[37]

Rural settlement

Large-scale archaeological investigations of agrarian settlement in connection with the late-medieval crisis have been few in number, so far, and are mainly from the southern part of the country. Usually dealing with desertion of single farmsteads or villages, this phenomenon has been studied not as a primary topic but just as a phase among others of the history of the farmstead or the village. However, several deserted medieval farmsteads have been archaeologically investigated in different parts of Sweden. Often the investigations have been carried out in woodland areas where abandoned settlement is well preserved.

The impact of the late-medieval crisis in different regions has been a matter of debate in recent years. According to an earlier opinion the agrarian central areas of medieval Sweden withstood the effects of the crisis better than the marginal woodland of the north, mostly because of more favourable conditions for agriculture in the former areas.[38] This idea has been criticised by a group of archaeologists working with settlement in the woodland regions.[39] Their opinion is that such areas could cope better with decline than the central regions thanks to a multifaceted economy with several additional activities besides crop cultivation. Thus a natural flexibility should have been inherent in this kind of peasant economy, which made a rapid shift of production possible in times of agricultural decline.

A typical example of a woodland farmstead is a place called Högahylte in the southern part of the province of Småland, which was excavated in 2007.[40] The settlement was established in the thirteenth century and included buildings, crop land and places for ironworking. The economy of the farmstead was a mixed one, characteristic of a woodland area, with ironworking as an important, additional activity besides farming. The farmstead was built in a typical colonisation area but was abandoned in less than 200 years at the end of the fourteenth century. Thereafter its farmland was used for cultivation by neighbouring farmsteads. It has been assumed that the late-medieval crisis was the utmost reason for the abandonment but why this particular farmstead was abandoned is more obscure. An extremely marginal location in relation to other farmsteads in the region has been discussed as a reasonable explanation for abandonment.[41]

Deserted medieval settlement has been investigated at several places in the province of Jämtland in northern Sweden.[42] Because the farmland of deserted medieval farmsteads often were used as hay meadows or for summer pasture by nearby villages the locations of many abandoned medieval farmsteads have long been known.

A place called Eisåsen reminds of the above described in Småland. Here a farmstead was established in the thirteenth century and abandoned before 1450. Thereafter, its farmland was used for summer pasture up to the nineteenth century. However, quite a different narrative, compared to the one of the farmstead in Småland, has been presented for Eisåsen. The abandonment of this farmstead is not comprehended as the end of a phase of colonisation, but as a part of a cyclical course of events where expansion alternated with stagnation.[43] The flexibility of the agrarian society of Jämtland enabled an adaptation to the new economic realities of the late Middle Ages. Desertion was not a sign of a societal catastrophe, rather a part of dynamic change.

In other parts of Sweden where the geographical and cultural conditions were different, for example the fertile plains of Scania, a partial desertion has been observed, meaning an abandonment of only one or a few farmsteads of a village or a hamlet but not the disappearance of the entire settlement. In some places only parts of a single farmstead may have been abandoned. This type of desertion is no doubt difficult to discern in a written source material and most likely also problematic to identify archaeologically without large-scale excavations including a multitude of farmsteads.[44] However, in the province of Scania there are some good examples of partial desertion.

In the village of Kyrkheddinge outside the town of Lund a single farmstead was followed archaeologically from the end of the tenth century up to modern times. Desertion is evident during the second half of the fifteenth century when a major dwelling of three room units and a connecting barn were reduced to a minor building of only two room units.[45]

In the western part of Örja village, investigated in 2010, some kilometres east of the town of Landskrona the development of settlement could be followed from the phase of establishment in the eleventh century up to modern times.[46] The excavation area included four different farmsteads, known from the oldest maps of the village originating from the seventeenth century. A reduction of the farmsteads took place after 1400 when only two of them were in use.

The examples of medieval settlement, discussed above, represent scattered evidence of desertion from different parts of Sweden. It is of course not possible to draw some conclusions of the relative extent of desertion on the basis of these examples. Investigations showing more obvious trends of desertion usually require interdisciplinary methods.[47]

One of the most noticed of such investigations is the one by Thomas Bartholin, already presented in the introductory chapter, including dendrochronological dating of still standing log houses from the middle and north of Sweden.[48] With a dramatic clarity Bartholin's results expose a rapid impact of the crisis around 1350 and a continuous absence of building activities up to the 1450s when a new expansion seems to have started. During this period of nearly one hundred years no houses were built, which probably means that the need for new buildings then was covered by an abundance of abandoned houses available because of the demographic decline (Fig. 21a).

The new compilations of dendrochronological dates, from the provinces of Småland and Östergötland in southern Sweden, confirm in general Bartholin's results concerning a rapid impact of the crisis on the building of houses around 1350 (Fig. 21b). However, there are no total absences of dates from the later part of the fourteenth century and the first half of the fifteenth century in the southern provinces. Furthermore they do not show any clear expansion in the second half of the fifteenth century. Such an expansion is not discernible until in the seventeenth century and then only in the province of Småland.

So far discussion has centred on late-medieval settlement in terms of desertion. It is also necessary to look upon it from a perspective of long-term change. At some places in southern Sweden a lasting structural stability seems to have characterised the agrarian settlement. Excavations in the hamlet of Stora Ullevi in the province of Östergötland have revealed an adaption of the high medieval settlement to a plot system, similar to the one that is visible on the oldest maps of the eighteenth century.[49] This adaption was discernible around 1200, the settlement thereafter having stayed fixed in the plot system up to modern times, unaffected by the long late-medieval crisis. A similar structural continuity has been observed in the above-mentioned village of Örja in the province of Scania where the structural change of settlement was dated to the twelfth century.

The province of Halland in western Sweden shows quite a different kind of development of medieval agrarian settlement.[50] Unlike the eastern parts it had a distinct mobile character and the locations of settlement units were changed during the Middle Ages. An important change, occurring in the late Middle Ages, meant that settlement was moved to new locations at the border between infields and outlands. Probably this change should be seen in the light of the general restructuring of the agrarian economy during the late-medieval crisis, meaning an orientation of the production towards animal husbandry.[51] Thus, an increase of outland pasture and a more rational use of the infields caused the moving of the settlement.

Whether this development of settlement was a characteristic only of Halland is still obscure. In other parts of Sweden the picture of agrarian settlement is more complex and elusive. In the Mälaren valley, excavated remains of settlement often do not coincide with

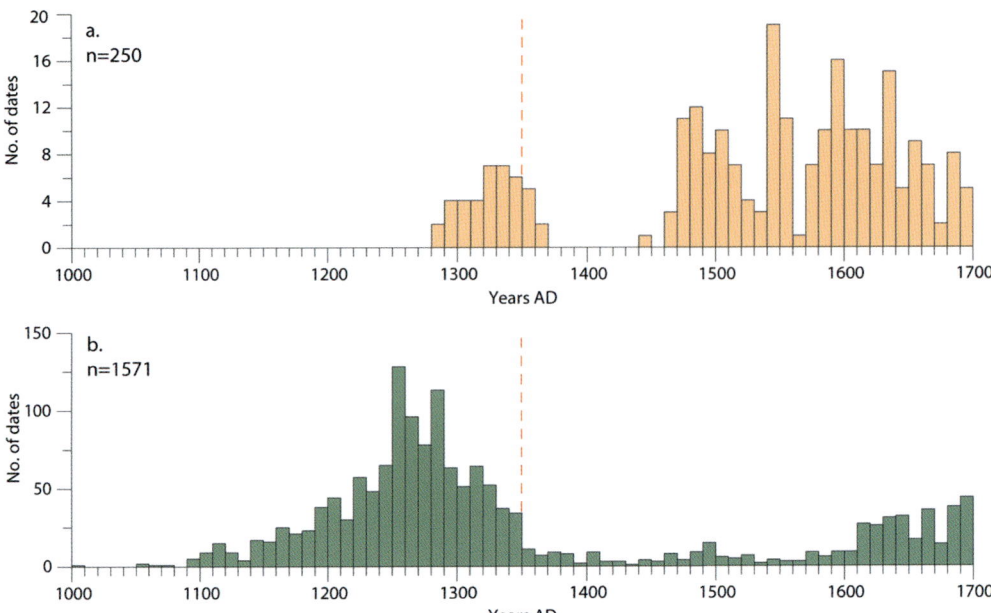

Fig. 21. Dendrochronological dates (felling years) from five Swedish provinces, AD 1000–1700. Bars show the number of dates per 10-year time slices. Dates later than 1700 are not included. The year 1350 is indicated by a dashed line. a. The provinces of Dalarna, Jämtland and Härjedalen (based on Bartholin 1989a); b. The provinces of Småland and Östergötland. Datings by the National Laboratory for Wood Anatomy and Dendrochronology at Lund University

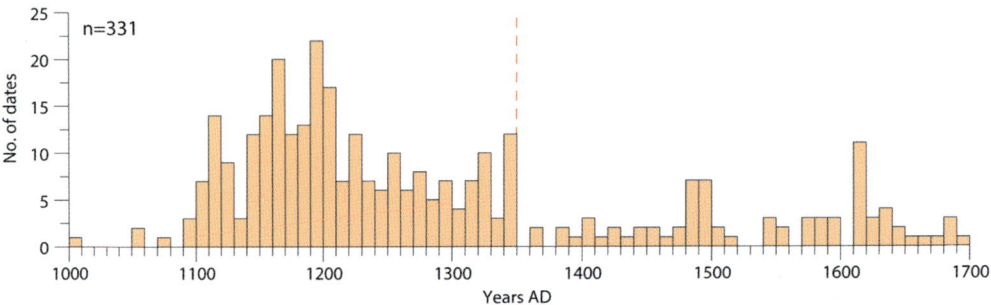

Fig. 22. Dendrochronological dates (felling years) from medieval churches in the provinces of Småland and Östergötland performed by the National Laboratory for Wood Anatomy and Dendrochronology at Lund University. Bars show the number of dates per 10-years time slices. Dates later than 1700 are not included. The year 1350 is indicated by a dashed line

locations of villages and farmsteads on the oldest maps and probably the late-medieval settlement may have had a partially mobile character.[52] However, the investigated remains are usually fragmentary and difficult to interpret, which causes great problems in identifying a late-medieval context.

Rural churches and monasteries

The building of churches in the countryside of medieval Sweden peaked in the twelfth and thirteenth centuries. Many churches, of stone as well as of wood, were erected, especially in the southern part of the country. Successively, building in stone became dominating and stone churches replaced several early wooden churches. This expansive period came to an end in the first half of the fourteenth century and during the remainder of the Middle Ages relatively few churches were built in the countryside. Instead, the late Middle Ages were characterised by extensions and reconstructions of already existing churches.

The decades following the year 1350 meant an almost immediate cessation of building activities in churches, the same pattern that was seen in the towns being repeated in the countryside. This observation is supported by the dendrochronological dates from the provinces of Östergötland and Småland (Fig. 22).[53] In some regions the stop seems to have lasted for about four or five decades. Dendrochronological dates from a number of churches in Scania show that the building activities there were resumed in the beginning of the fifteenth century.[54] However, this pattern is not valid for all regions. In the provinces of Småland and Östergötland dendrochronological dates show an increase of the building activities not until the second part of the fifteenth century.

A critical comment on the chronological distribution of the dates must be added. The purpose of dendrochronological analyses has often been to date the oldest phase of the church. Hence later phases, such as the rebuilding activities of the late Middle Ages, may be underrepresented in the material. Probably, this will be the case for the churches of Östergötland where a lot of reconstruction work, mostly vaulting, is not reflected in the dendrochronological dates from the late Middle Ages.

The extensions of the churches in the late Middle Ages included building of towers, chapels, sacristies and porches. A decisive change of the interior of the churches was the construction of brick vaults in the later part of the fifteenth century and in the beginning of the sixteenth, reflecting an agrarian surplus in the time of societal recovery being invested in new constructions. Initially cross vaults were dominating but in the course of the fifteenth century stellar vaults became common.

In searching for the aim of the vaulting, symbolic as well as functional explanations have been presented.[55] The vault may have been looked upon as a symbol of the heaven and the unearthly world and at the same time have served as a protection of fire in the church.

The geographical distribution of late-medieval vaulting shows some interesting variations, being inconceivable from a purely economic perspective. Most remarkable is the difference between the west and the east of Sweden. In the east the majority of stone churches became vaulted in the late Middle Ages, especially in the provinces of Uppland and Östergötland (Fig. 23).

In extensive parts of the western provinces, Västergötland, Bohuslän, Halland and Värmland, very few churches were vaulted in the late Middle Ages. Concerning this remarkable difference between the east and the west of Sweden, administrative as well as economic reasons have been discussed.[56] However, none of them seems convincing. If economic resources had been the decisive factor, the fertile areas of, for example, Västergötland would have had many vaulted churches. Probably an explanation is to be found in cultural differences, which are discussed below.

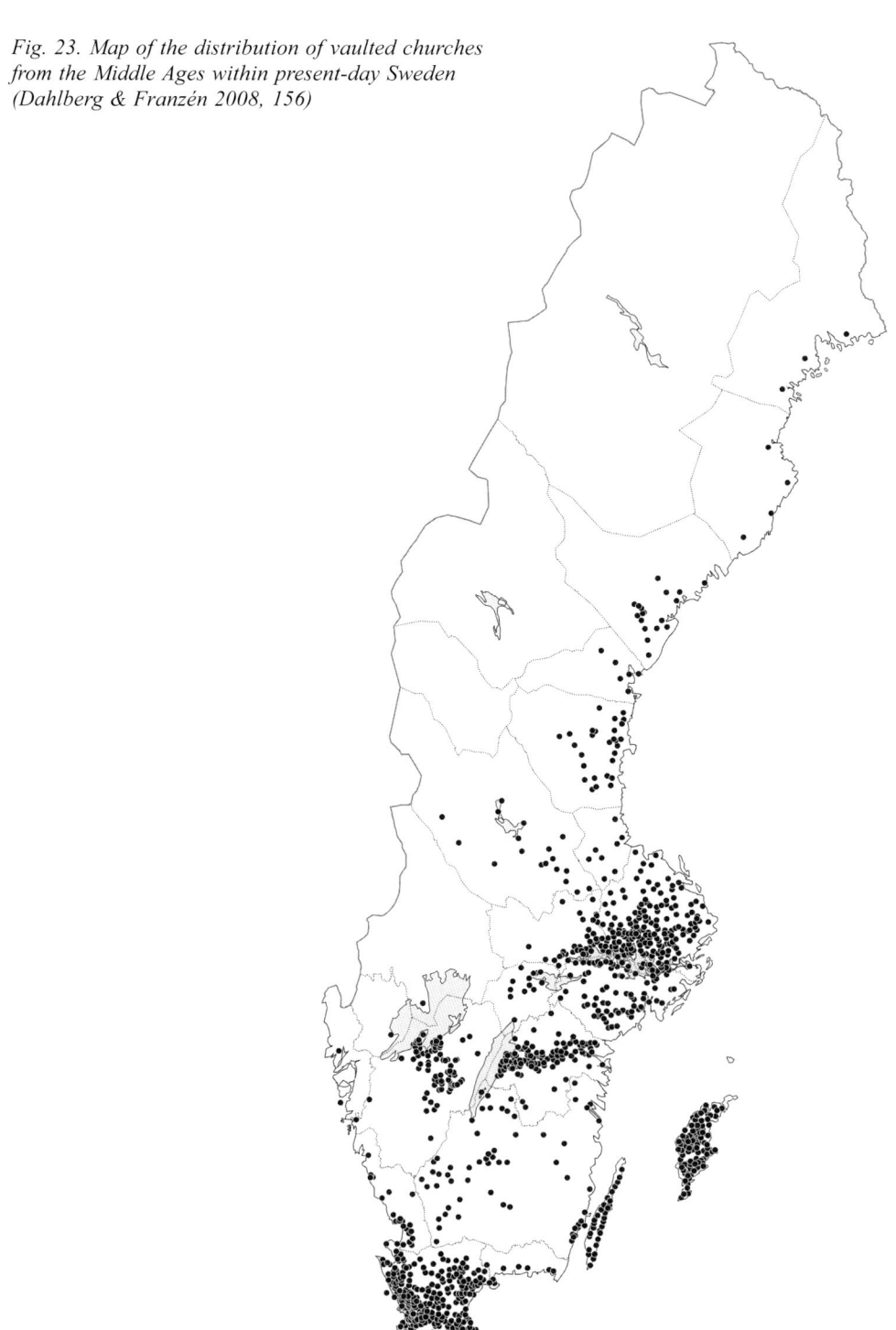

Fig. 23. Map of the distribution of vaulted churches from the Middle Ages within present-day Sweden (Dahlberg & Franzén 2008, 156)

Using the medieval monasteries in the countryside for a study of the late-medieval crisis raises some problems. Modern investigations of high archaeological quality are few and the existing source materials seldom offer opportunities for a detailed study of the late-medieval development. However, a modern investigation of the Cistercian monastery of Alvastra in the province of Östergötland, based on rich archaeological material, has provided some interesting results.[57]

A thorough analysis of the material culture of the monastery, buildings, small objects and graves, revealed a period of changes in the fourteenth century, reflecting a new approach to the world outside the monastery.[58] This change was interpreted as an expression of a greater openness to the secular world and of increased contacts with an urban culture. Nevertheless a close connection between the changes of the monastery and the late-medieval crisis has been questioned.[59]

However, it is possible to launch a hypothetical connection. A considerable part of the workforce of the monastery being wiped out by the plagues, its agrarian economy would have been severely disturbed. Being more dependent of supply from the world outside, a survival strategy may have been trade with neighbouring towns, probably also promoting an increase of urban cultural contacts. Furthermore, the monastery was not short of economic resources, being richly provided with gifts and donations in the harsh times of the plagues.

Castles

The building of castles in the late Middle Ages has been regarded as one of the most obvious material manifestations of the crisis, particularly of the "*dysfunctional reaction*" of the societal elite in the second half of the fourteenth century.[60] Developing a plunder economy when the crisis threatened to undermine its status, the nobility could use the castle as a highly effective, repressive tool. So, when all constructions of other kind were interrupted after 1350 the building of castles took another direction. A multitude of royal and aristocratic strongholds were constructed, making the second half of the fourteenth century the extreme peak of the building of medieval castles in Sweden (Fig. 24). A great number of castles were built by the royal power in the inland as well along the coasts of Sweden, several of them being located in western Sweden and in the province of Småland.[61] The castles of the nobility seem to have been more evenly distributed over the country.[62]

Many of the castles constructed in the second half of the fourteenth century became short-lived phenomena, being closed down during the first decades of the fifteenth century. Many were destroyed in connection with peasant revolts in the 1430s. Castles surviving the fifteenth century, above all castles belonging to the royal power, were often located at the coast or at strategically important watercourses, many of them in connection with towns like Stockholm, Nyköping and Kalmar.[63]

According to Janken Myrdal's interpretation of the castles built in the later part of the fourteenth century, many of them functioned primarily as centres of military repression. However, some constructions had a more complex function, detectable only by the use of archaeology. Magnus Stibeus has analysed extensive finds material of a royal castle, Piksborg, located in the southwest of the province of Småland and in use in the later part of the fourteenth century and in the beginning of the fifteenth.[64] This material, consisting among other things of a huge amount of coins, had an unmistakably urban character, indicating not only military and administrative functions but also mercantile ones.

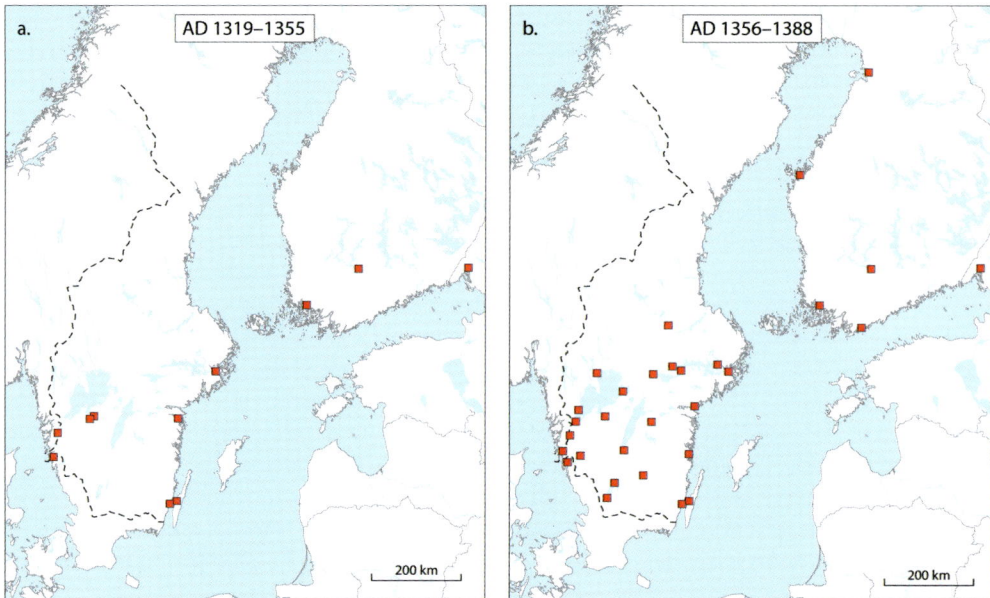

Fig. 24. Map of the distribution of Swedish royal castles of the fourteenth century. The dashed line mark the national border of medieval Sweden (based on Lovén 1996, 194–195). a. Royal castles in use 1319–1355; b. Royal castles in use 1356–1388

Thus, we may look upon Piksborg as an expression of a suppressive strategy of the royal power in an utterly severe period of the crisis, gaining a harder control not only over tax collection but also over other urban functions. For this purpose the *"urban fortress"* was a more efficient solution than the ordinary town. Hence Stibeus' results concerning Piksborg fit well with the experience of late-medieval Skara, losing some of its urban functions in the time of the crisis.

The contemporary castles of northern Sweden have also been discussed from the same perspective.[65]

Proto-industrial settlement

Here a specific kind of place, connected with iron working and fishery, will be discussed, being defined as *proto-industrial* settlement. The term *proto-industry* has been much debated within economic history, often being used to define an initial stage of industry.[66] Here a proto-industrial settlement will mean a place of a large-scale production oriented to consumption outside the actor's own home district. The work was carried out by peasants combining a specialised surplus production with ordinary agricultural supply.[67]

Medieval metalworking in Sweden and its great importance for societal development has long been well known thanks to a large amount of historical research as well as archaeology. At present, research within the latter discipline is mostly work in progress.[68]

In an area of southern Sweden, including parts of Halland, Småland and Scania, medieval iron working has been studied in a long-term perspective.[69] Here, a number of iron working sites were established in connection with colonisation of the area in the twelfth and thirteenth centuries. The iron production was organised within the context of the single farm, being oriented to a consumption of iron on this particular farm or in its closest hinterland.

In the later part of the fourteenth century the area seems to have been struck hard by the plagues and societal decline and it was not until the end of the Middle Ages that a new landscape of production was taking shape. In the recolonised area iron working was a dominant element. Although an older technique – bloomery production – was still in use, the activities had changed, both quantitatively and structurally. Bo Strömberg has interpreted late-medieval iron working in the area as a sort of *proto-industry*.[70] Its main characteristics were a volume of production much larger than before, a deliberate localisation of the working sites close to the raw material and the energy, that is the waterpower, and finally differentiated settlement at the production sites. Production was oriented to distribution outside the region, being governed by subordinate political actors.

A mining district called Näveberg in the province of Sörmland has been studied by the archaeologist Eva Skyllberg.[71] Here mining activities began in the later part of the fourteenth century, a fact discussed by Skyllberg in connection with the late-medieval crisis. She considers the establishment of mining as a strategy to cope with the consequences of the crisis. Mining provided new revenues for the nobility when the rents of agriculture tended to decrease dramatically.

A characteristic of the activities at Näveberg was an organisation of labour where tenants were the primary actors in the mining process but subordinated to a manor estate. According to Skyllberg such an organisation of metal working was a unique phenomenon in medieval Sweden.[72]

Iron working in the districts north of Lake Mälaren differed considerably from the place described above. A thorough archaeological investigation at the site of Lapphyttan has shed light on the emergence of activities at the end of the twelfth century, as well as on the introduction of the blast furnace technique in medieval Sweden – the great technological innovation of medieval metal working – enabling volumes of production never seen before.[73]

Being subject to great interest by the nobility, these activities must most likely have functioned within a manorial system from the outset, at the end of the twelfth century up to the 1350s, meaning that iron working was organised and governed by a nearby manor. Operating a number of foundries, the manor needed a considerable workforce, consisting of subordinated crofters and tenants dependent of supply from the manor when working at the foundries.

Starting in the second half of the fourteenth century, a major abandonment of blast furnaces, (around 30%) took place.[74] The closed constructions were so-called 'outland furnaces' with no spatial connection to settlement, thus reflecting the old manorial organisation of iron working. The demographic decline of the societal crisis brought this system to an end, enabling a new system of smaller, self-sufficient farms of peasant miners.[75] The latter were freeholders, dealing with iron production beside the agricultural activities. They were living in villages, the single village forming a collective enterprise with an iron foundry in the centre, surrounded by farms.[76]

This system of collaborating farms underwent a continuing streamlining and improvement of iron working during the recovery phase in the late Middle Ages. A co-location of the blast furnaces and hammer mills, beginning at the end of the epoch, was of great importance for the expansion of the activities in the hey days of the sixteenth and seventeenth centuries.[77]

The peasant miners acting as an influential group in the peasant rebellions of the 1430s; this social transformation of the mining activities must have already occurred in the end of the fourteenth century or in the beginning of the fifteenth century.

So, the late Middle Ages appear as a breaking point in the development of metal working, the crisis being a considerable causal element of this development. It was not a question of introducing new techniques – bloomery and blast furnaces were known long before. Rather it was a question of a new social organisation as well as of a specialisation and streamlining of the activities.

Concerning fishery, no desertion of production sites similar to the above-described situation in the mining districts is to be seen in the late Middle ages. There are some radiocarbon analyses of coastal settlement along the Kalmarsund strait showing a slow-down of fishing activities in the fourteenth century, probably caused by general, societal decline in the second half of this century.[78] At the major fishing sites of the Öresund strait and the southern Baltic, there was no such decline. Rather, restructuring and specialisation characterise these places in the late Middle ages.

In Skanör, one of the most important places at Öresund, the large market area was closed down in the later part of the fourteenth century. At the same time the first settlement of the late-medieval fishing camp was established, located on an island west of the town of Skanör.[79] Not until this time did the fishing camp become spatially defined, which was one of the primary conditions for the development of fishing as a large-scale activity. In Skanör and in the nearby Falsterbo, fishing became highly specialised in the late Middle Ages, the catching as well as the further processing of the fish being restricted many regulations.

Proto-industrial fishing, but of another character, was carried out along the Baltic coast of northern Sweden, starting in the fifteenth century. Burghers from the towns of the Mälaren valley organised this long distance activity as annual, seasonal expeditions to the northern archipelagos. Thus, this fishing was of a primary mercantile character but was not concentrated in big fishing camps as in the southern Baltic.

Apparently, large-scale fishing of a proto-industrial character was confined to the southern and eastern parts of Sweden, such activities entirely lacking in the western parts in the late Middle Ages.

Summing up the overview

Summing up this overview, some preliminary answers to the decisive questions, formulated in the introduction, will be presented.

Firstly, focusing on desertion and decline, it can be noted that there is abundant archaeological evidence all over the country, enhancing the picture of the crisis as a general 'wave of decline' raging everywhere. By all accounts towns as well as countryside were engulfed. However, no reliable quantification of the extent of the decline, on the basis of the archaeological material, is possible so far.

According to dendrochronological results the crisis seems to have had a very rapid impact on society in the middle of the fourteenth century, causing an immediate stop to building activities. The recovery of the fifteenth century shows, following the same results, a more prolonged course characterised by certain regional variations.

Considering significant human responses to the crisis, some towns, surprisingly soon after the first catastrophic decades, experienced a phase of restructuring and expansion. The towns in question were well-established, episcopal centres like Linköping and Turku. In newly founded towns of the late fourteenth century and first half of the fifteenth, except for the pilgrimage centre of Vadstena, there are no such signs of 'positive' development.

Concerning the countryside, the archaeological picture is more obscure, showing both continuity and discontinuity. A structural stability of settlement throughout the Middle Ages, characterising regions like Östergötland and Scania, stands out as rather different from the flexible and mobile pattern of Halland. A particular kind of change in the late-medieval countryside was the transformation of outland occupations like iron working and fishing to large scale, highly specialised activities.

Focusing on regional variations, a fragmented pattern of late-medieval development is appearing. Regional differences are discernable in almost all aspects. Signs of urban dynamics in the later part of the fourteenth century were only seen in towns in the east of Sweden and in Finland. An opposite trend was visible in the western towns, showing decline and "demi-urbanisation".

Also, agrarian settlement was characterised by great regional variation. Showing a high degree of continuity and stability in the east, the opposite was seen in the west, i.e. mobility and instability. A relocation of agrarian settlement in late-medieval Halland is the most obvious expression of this structural mobility.

Concerning churches and castles in the countryside, a great number of the former were reconstructed in the east and south, mostly employing vaulting. In the west, churches showed very little sign of such activities, most of them remaining not vaulted in the late Middle Ages. No distinct, regional differences in the building of castles are discernable except for the royal castles showing a certain concentration to the western part of the country.

Large scale activities of proto industrial character were established in the east of Sweden in the late Middle Ages, for example in the mining districts. Something similar was not to be seen in the west except for the iron working in the south of Halland.

Concluding this summarising picture of the late-medieval development it may be described in general as a complex process including elements both of decline and dynamic change as well as of great regional contrasts. With this in mind we will now continue with the second part of the investigation, studying the late-medieval crisis on a local level.

Three case studies

The previous section was an attempt to outline a late-medieval development from the perspective of the societal crisis, synthesising archaeological results of different kinds and from different contexts. Some crucial problems were discussed, however on a rather general level.

This section will approach the late-medieval crisis from a somewhat different point of view. Earlier research has often focused on the negative aspects of the crisis, for example the degree of mortality and the process of desertion of settlement. Of course the crisis caused severe and pervasive disturbances of late-medieval society but, after all, this society endured. How did people, surviving the ravages of the plague, cope with the harsh realities

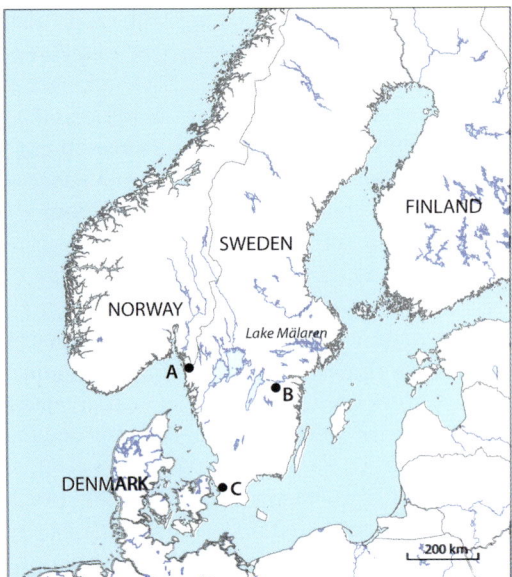

Fig. 25. Map of Scandinavia showing the locations of the three farmsteads: A. Vålle; B. Stora Ullevi; C. Örja

of the late fourteenth and fifteenth centuries in their everyday life? What strategies did they develop to withstand decline and collapse?

Hence, this study will focus primarily on survival rather than decline.[80] It will take a point of departure at a social level most essential to a majority of the population, that is the level of the single farmstead. Thus, it will concentrate interest not on deserted settlement but on settlement that survived during the long era of late-medieval decline. How did the crisis affect the people on the single farmstead? In what way were the inhabitants of the farmsteads forced to change their way of living during this severe and transformative period?

Concerning survival strategies in the time of the crisis, abandonment of the farmstead and moving to a more favourable place may of course have been a deliberate choice to avoid complete extinction, i.e. a kind of survival strategy.[81] However, to determine whether a farmstead has been deliberately abandoned or if it has been deserted because of the death of its users will hardly be possible within an archaeological context. Therefore, this section will focus on settlement remaining in use as discernible units in the time of the crisis in the places where it once was established.

The source material of the following case studies will include the archaeological results of three late-medieval farmsteads in the southern part of Sweden, all of them excavated during the last 15 years (Fig. 25). The scientific approach is a comparative one, based on farmsteads from different regional contexts. A main problem discussed in the following will be if unique regional characteristics have been of decisive importance for the choice of survival strategy of the single farmstead.

Sweden includes a large part of the Scandinavian Peninsula where the regional variations concerning topography, vegetation, climate and soils are great. Vast areas of woodland and mountains in the northern part of the country were sparsely settled in the Middle Ages. In the south the geography is more varying, with fertile plain areas alternating with woodland. Characteristic of the territory of Sweden was further an extremely long coastal zone (2400 km), giving access to maritime resources.

An optimal choice of farmsteads for the following case studies would have included examples from all the different regions of medieval Sweden. However, investigations of agrarian settlement, which almost exclusively originate from rescue excavations, are not evenly distributed over the country. In general, good examples of large-scale excavations are rare and moreover mainly to be found in the south, where modern development has been greatest. Thus, the selection of farmsteads has been restricted to this part of the country.

A point of departure for the comparative study of the farmsteads is the cultural regionalisation of Sweden, described in the introduction of this chapter, starting in the thirteenth century. With a turning point around 1250, regional characteristics were developed of which the western and eastern parts of the country respectively were paid most attention to. In several aspects these two regions differed significantly from each other.

The three places fulfil the following criteria. First, being established in the early Middle Ages, they endured the era of the crisis from the middle of the fourteenth century up to the beginning of the sixteenth century. Secondly, they represent three different regional contexts of medieval Sweden. Thirdly, the chosen farmsteads represent three different environmental contexts.

One of the three farmsteads was located in the west of Sweden, in the northern part of the province of Bohuslän. It can be characterised as a typical woodland farmstead with small lots of crop land surrounded by forests and mountains, its agrarian economy primarily being oriented to animal husbandry. In these respects the farmstead has great similarities with the agrarian settlement of northern Sweden.

The other two farmsteads were located in fertile plain areas, one in the province of Scania in the southernmost part of Sweden, the other in the province of Östergötland in the eastern part. The former was a typical coastal settlement near the strait of Öresund, a highly urbanised region of great mercantile importance in the Middle Ages. The latter was an inland settlement located in the neighbourhood of the bishop's town of Linköping. The agrarian economy of these two farmsteads was oriented primarily towards crop cultivation.

The question must be raised whether these three places may be considered as representative for their regions. Does their development show anything typical in the time of the crisis or were they just exceptions? Of course it is hardly possible to answer such a question properly. The extent and quality of the existing, archaeological source material is still too limited. However, this may not prevent us from using these examples in a discussion of survival strategies in the time of the crisis. Exposing well-discernable, human action in the late Middle Ages, they are good examples.

The farmstead Vålle in the province of Bohuslän

The analysis of each farmstead begins with a brief characterisation of the historical and topographical context followed by an overview of the development of settlement. Finally the development of the farmstead in a wider historical context during the era of the crisis, 1350–1530, will be especially discussed. The Swedish National Heritage Board investigated all the three farmsteads during the last 15 years.

The farmstead called Vålle was located in Lur parish in the northern part of the province of Bohuslän. A sparsely settled landscape, characterised by minor rift valleys alternating with mountains and woodlands, surrounded the farmstead in the Middle Ages. The settlement of the region consisted primarily of single farmsteads and minor hamlets. No manors seem to have dominated the landscape but in the written source material of the fifteenth century Vålle is mentioned as a tenant farm. On the oldest maps of the nineteenth century Vålle is denominated as a single farm but divided into several households. The investigation of the farmstead that took place in 2007 included the southern part of the settlement (Fig. 26).[82]

According to the archaeological results, the earliest settlement was established in the early Middle Ages (1000–1100), consisting of a major building probably with both residential and economic functions (Fig. 27). In the fourteenth and fifteenth centuries a significant expansion of the farmstead took place. Another large building was erected north of the existing one. The presence of a kitchen in this construction indicates a function of the building as a dwelling house. Between the two larger houses a minor agricultural building was erected.

In the fourteenth century a smithy was built just northwest of the above-mentioned buildings. How long it existed was not possible to determine but according to the radiocarbon datings the activities of the smithy peaked in the period 1350–1450.[83] The results of metallurgical analysis indicate a multifaceted working process including cleaning of iron lumps as well as forging of objects.[84]

The described structure of the farmstead remained intact up to early modern times (sixteenth and seventeenth centuries) except for the oldest building. In the eighteenth centuries all buildings were torn down and replaced with new ones.

***

There are no signs of discontinuity or desertion of the farmstead during the era of the late-medieval crisis. However, northern Bohuslän was struck hard by the crisis. Current research has estimated the desertion frequency of farmsteads in this region to be as high as 50% in the late Middle Ages.[85]

Probably the crisis caused extensive desertion in the surroundings of the investigated farmstead. However, this settlement does not reflect decline, rather dynamics through the creation of new constructions. Furthermore, one of these was the place of specialised forging, apparently a new activity in the region. An iron production site of the same date as the smithy at Vålle has been excavated further north in the province.[86]

In the less feudalised and less regulated area of northern Bohuslän the access to the vast, forested and mountainous outlands most likely was less controlled. Probably the outlands had been used, for instance for wood pasture, long before the late-medieval crisis in this area. So, when the exploitation of the outland resources, wood and iron ore, for specialised ironworking started in the fourteenth century a cultural adjustment to these areas was already long-established.

A crucial question is for what purpose were the completed iron objects produced – for sale, as items for taxation or only for use in the household of the farmstead? The activity of the smithy was of an advanced, specialised character, which probably means that forging was not intended exclusively for the household but for a wider distribution. This might have brought other revenues to the farmstead than what was possible through agriculture.

The late-medieval crisis has likely contributed to the development of a multifaceted peasant economy in the province of Bohuslän. Such an economy with additional activities besides agriculture characterised the region in early modern times and might have had its origins in the changes of the late Middle Ages. One expression for such a diversified economy was a maritime peasant trade going on since the sixteenth century up to the nineteenth century along the coasts of western Sweden.[87] Peasants from Bohuslän and other parts were also sailing tradesmen engaged in long distance trade with cargos like lime and timber to seaports in the northwest of Europe.

The archaeological find material from Vålle included some indications of this mercantile activity. Although most of the finds were of an ordinary character some of the ceramics, fragments of imported vessels from the Netherlands and Flanders, reflected external contacts less typical for an agrarian settlement.[88] Such vessels originate from the seventeenth century, i.e. rather long after the era of the crisis. However, it seems reasonable to assume that these finds reflect a long-distance trade of much earlier origin in the northern part of Bohuslän.

The farmstead at Stora Ullevi in the province of Östergötland

Stora Ullevi is a hamlet in the province of Östergötland located on a low ridge between the town of Linköping and Lake Roxen. Its hinterland is a plain area, during the Middle Ages characterised by large meadows and pastures. On the oldest map from 1764 Stora Ullevi is a geometrically regulated hamlet (Fig. 28). At the end of the Middle Ages there were 11 homesteads in the hamlet of which all but one were used by tenants under the monasteries of Askeby and Vadstena and also the diocese of Linköping. Stora Ullevi belonged to the parish of St Lars, which also included parts of the town of Linköping.

Archaeological excavations in 1998 and 2003 included three building plots of the hamlet.[89] The excavations showed that the earliest settlement here was built during the later Iron Age. The site was then continuously inhabited up to the Middle Ages. New construction elements like sills and fireplaces were introduced in the houses of the eleventh and twelfth centuries.

In the following period, the thirteenth and fourteenth centuries, the most important changes took place (Fig. 29). Of the three investigated building plots only one, plot Λ, was settled during this period. Here, four minor one-room buildings were erected, one dwelling house, one smithy and two agricultural buildings. It is obvious that this building activity was simultaneous with a regulation of the settlement in the beginning of the thirteenth century. The new houses were then adjusted to a geometrical plot system, which corresponds to a system still detectable on the oldest maps of the eighteenth century.[90]

In the fourteenth century these houses were replaced by one single building consisting of two rooms, a bigger dwelling room with a fireplace and a smaller chamber. A new expansion started in the following period, the sixteenth and the seventeenth centuries, when all the investigated plots were settled. On plot A, showing continuity of the settlement, the house of the late Middle Ages was replaced by a so called double cottage, functioning as a dwelling house.

***

There are no immediate signs of desertion or decline in the late-medieval settlement of Stora Ullevi. However, the settlement underwent a great and pervasive change during the fourteenth and fifteenth centuries.

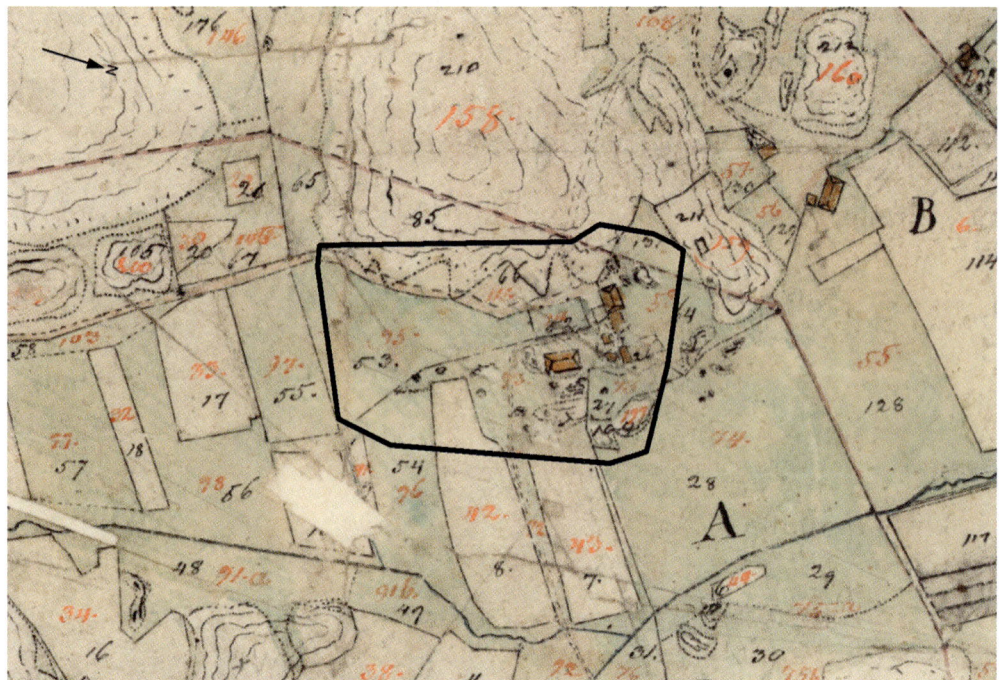

Fig. 26. Cadastral map of Vålle from 1825 showing the settlement (brown squares) and its surroundings.
Black line marks the excavation area

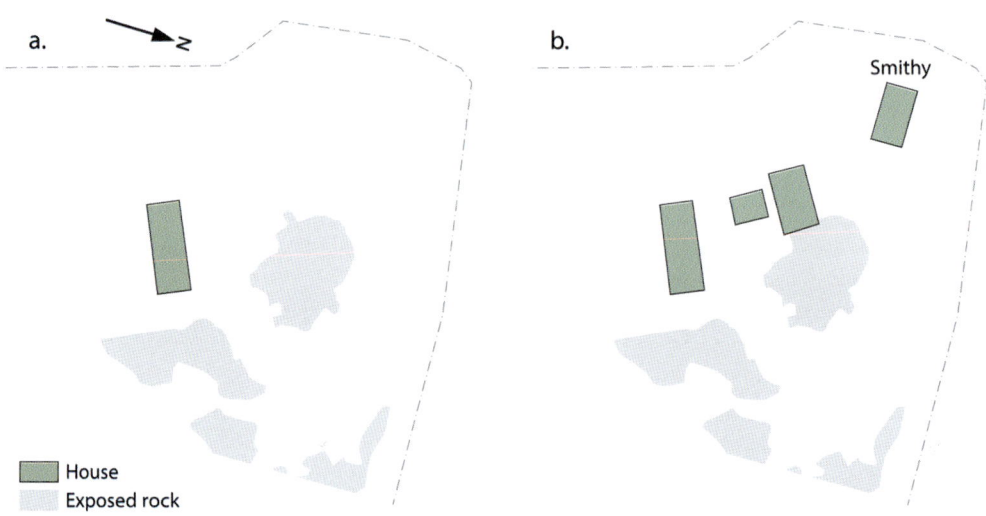

Fig. 27. Change of settlement at Vålle AD 1000–1500. Settlement dated to a. 1000–1300 and b.
1300–1500, respectively

Neither are there any signs of economic specialisation in the late Middle Ages of the kind seen at the site in Bohuslän. The smithy that was present in the thirteenth century disappeared after 1350 together with the other buildings of the early Middle Ages. Only one large building, a dwelling house, replaced them in the late Middle Ages.

However, some finds of an unmistakable exclusive character from this building give a clue to the understanding of the late-medieval Stora Ullevi. The finds consist of some book clasps, a polished rock crystal and some mountings, one with a picture of a heraldic lion (Fig. 30). Such finds are not typical of an ordinary agrarian settlement, rather of urban and ecclesiastical contexts. Similar objects have been found in residences in the town of Linköping and in the nearby monastery of Vreta.[91] These finds raise questions on the social structure in Stora Ullevi in the fourteenth and fifteenth centuries. Do they reflect the presence of some high status people and thus a major social change in the village during these centuries?

The nearby town of Linköping was an important religious centre already in the early Middle Ages, long before it got its legal status as an episcopal town at the end of the thirteenth century.[92] Most likely there must have been a close cultural connection between the town and the neighbouring villages and hamlets because of the special role Linköping played in this part of Östergötland. The fact that the hamlet of Stora Ullevi was included in one of the urban parishes might have been an expression of such a connection. Thus it seems rather logical that the formation of a survival strategy of the hamlet in the time of the crisis was highly influenced by the development of the neighbouring town.

The late-medieval crisis seems to have caused an immediate interruption of the building activities in the town of Linköping already around 1350, which lasted some decades.[93] After 1380 these activities started anew. In the last decades of the fourteenth century Linköping underwent a dynamic development characterised by expansion and densification of the urban settlement.[94] The growth of the diocese town combined with an extensive building of stone houses was no doubt of importance in this development.

Probably the town's hinterland was affected by the urban dynamics and the finds from Stora Ullevi could be a material expression of this connection. Such an assumption is further supported by the analysis of animal bones from Stora Ullevi, which indicates an economic integration between the hamlet and the neighbouring town of Linköping in the late Middle Ages.[95] A decreased consumption of beef in the hamlet can be explained by an increased distribution of cattle to the town. This trend is corresponded by an increasing consumption of mutton in the hamlet during the same period.

Thus the development of Stora Ullevi in the late Middle Ages can be comprehended as reflecting an increased integration – social, economic and cultural – between town and hinterland. The animal husbandry became more oriented to satisfy the needs of foodstuff in the nearby town. The material culture reflects a new social context in the hamlet with a non-agrarian connection.

Hence, the hamlet was in a way 'urbanised'. The ecclesiastical character of the finds indicates a link to the expanding diocese in the town, and possibly people belonging to this institution inhabited the farmstead in the late Middle Ages.

The development of the hamlet of Stora Ullevi after the Middle Ages is somewhat more obscure. The era of Reformation meant a setback for the episcopal town of Linköping, the properties of the catholic church being withdrawn to the Swedish state, possibly affecting not only the town but also the surrounding countryside.[96] However, nothing of this is

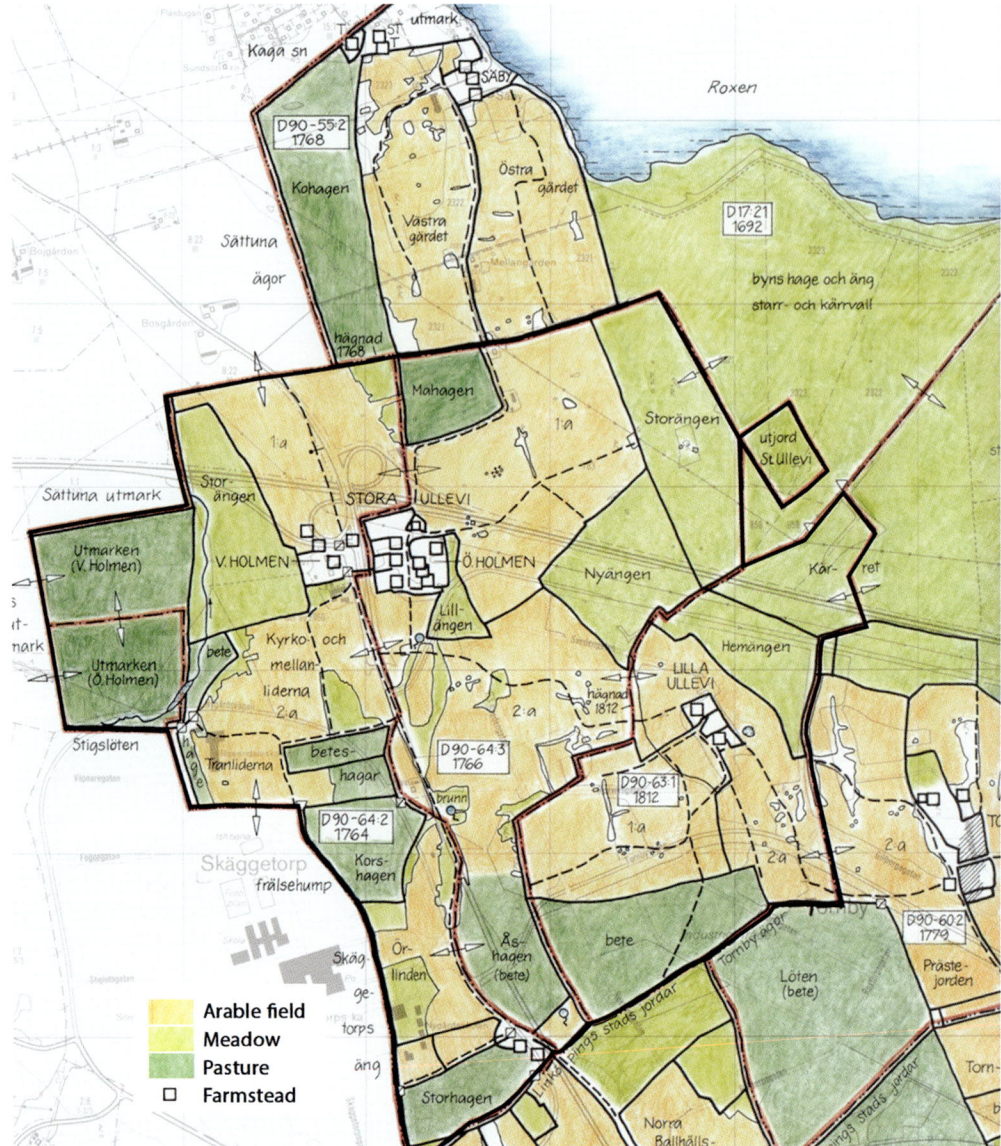

Fig. 28. Cadastral map of Stora Ullevi from the 1760s

archaeologically discernible at Stora Ullevi where the sixteenth and seventeenth centuries were characterised by expansion.

The farmstead at Örja in the province of Scania

The village of Örja is located in the western part of Scania some kilometres east of the town of Landskrona. The surroundings of the village are a fertile plain area where crop farming

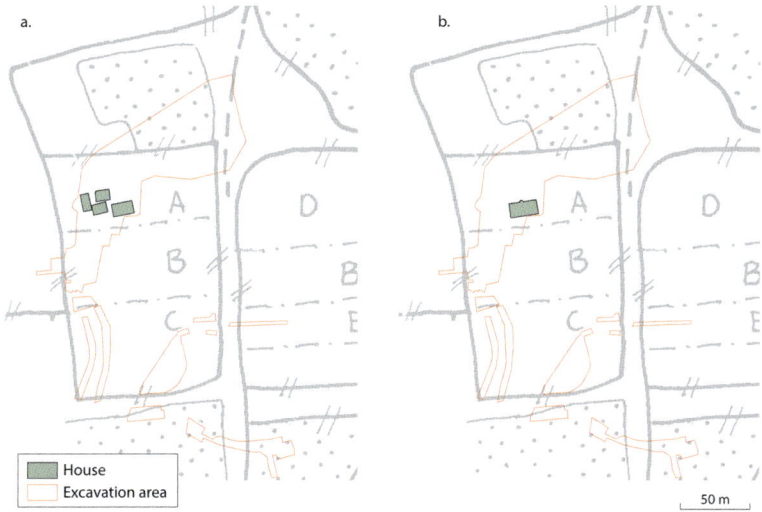

Fig. 29. Change of settlement at Stora Ullevi AD 1200-1500. Settlement dated to a. 1200–1350 and b. 1350–1500, respectively. Grey lines show the building plots from the cadastral map

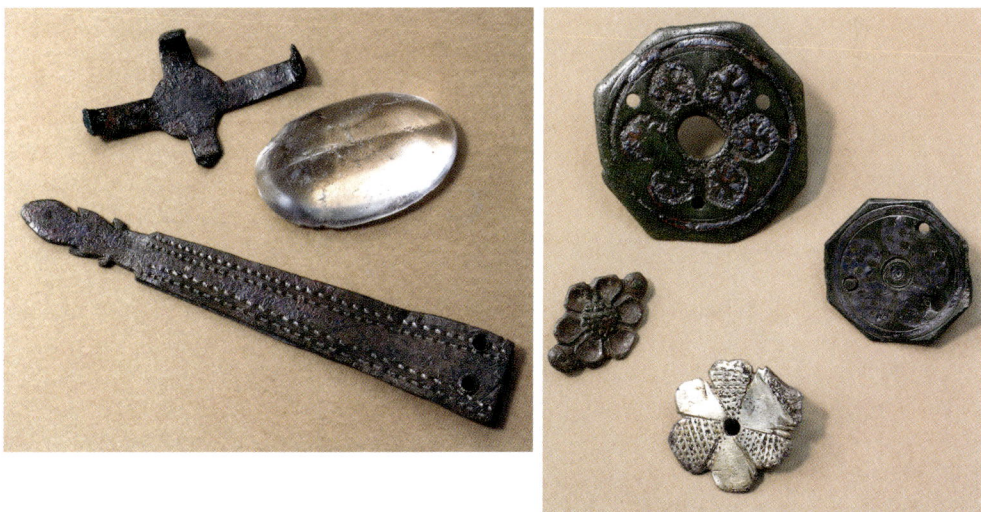

Fig. 30. Finds from the late medieval house at Stora Ullevi: a. book clasp with rock crystal and strap-end mounting; b. bronze mountings (photo: G. Billeson)

has been dominant. Örja was the church village of Örja parish, which also included the hamlet of Tullstorp. The oldest map of 1761 depicts 18 homesteads in Örja, which means a relatively large village (Fig. 31). A very scarce written source material gives no support to the assumption that this was the medieval extent of the village. All the homesteads of the village seem to have been tenant farms.

Originally the farmsteads were located around a large open area where the medieval parish church was erected at the turn of the century 1200. Possibly, there was an older church and also an early-medieval manor in the eastern part of the village.[97]

In the year 2010 the western part of Örja was excavated. Settlement remains of prehistoric as well as of historic origin were investigated. In the eleventh century a settlement, divided in four clusters of houses, was established, which coincided with the locations of the eighteenth century farmsteads. Two of the settlement units, denominated farmsteads 1 and 12 on the maps, had continuity all through the Middle Ages. One of the other two units, denominated 20 on the maps, was abandoned around 1400. The last unit, denominated 16 on the maps, existed only during the early Middle Ages and was resettled not until in the sixteenth century. Of these four units, I will focus on farmstead 12.

The four units of the eleventh century have been interpreted as a contemporary, large-scale establishment.[98] Whether they were four independent farmsteads or parts of a big manor estate is still obscure. Farmstead 12 included during this early-medieval period a big multifunctional house with three naves, probably serving both residential and economic purposes. Furthermore a long barn and three minor agricultural buildings belonged to this settlement. Outside the multifunctional building a smoke oven was found and so a cultural layer with indications of fish processing.

In the twelfth century the settlement seems to have been incorporated into to a regulated structure. A system of ditches enclosed the settlement and this system remained unchanged up to the time of the oldest maps of the eighteenth century. The farmstead now included a dwelling house in the north, a barn in the west and another two agricultural buildings in the south and in the east. Also in this phase there were strong indications of fish processing.

Small changes of the settlement happened in the thirteenth century. The agricultural buildings were the same as in the previous phase. The dwelling house in the north burned down in the beginning of the century and was replaced by a new construction. Gradually this building was used for smoking fish. A significant development of this activity seems to have happened during this period.

In the fourteenth and fifteenth centuries some important changes of the farmstead took place. There was an obvious reduction of the settled area and the farmstead now included only three buildings. The house in the north was still present but considerably changed and adjusted to the fish processing, which developed to a specialised, large-scale activity (Fig. 32).

Apparently the residential functions disappeared in this period and from now on the farmstead seems to have been used exclusively for fish processing.[99] The big barn in the west also disappeared indicating that even the animal husbandry was phased out in the late Middle Ages. In addition to the building in the north only two smaller buildings were present. Probably they served as drying houses where firewood needed for the fish smoking was dried.

The highly specialised fish processing came to an end in the later part of the fifteenth century. The smaller buildings may still have existed in the beginning of the sixteenth century but in the remainder of the century there was no settlement in the place of farmstead 12.

***

No more than a reduced building area indicates decline on farmstead 12 in the late Middle Ages. Of course, this decrease of settlement was directly linked with the changes of functions in the farmstead. However, within the excavation area as a whole there are very obvious signs of partial desertion in the fifteenth century. Only farmsteads 1 and 12 survived during this period. What happened to the farmsteads of the village outside the excavation area is of course quite obscure and the very scarce written source material gives no clues.

The change of farmstead 12 in the fourteenth and fifteenth centuries, when the economic structure of the farmstead was turned upside down, appears as a rather unexpected phenomenon in its historical context. An originally secondary occupation – fish processing – expanded and became the only activity of the farmstead. However, the large-scale expansion of this activity in the fourteenth century indicates that its aim was not only to cover the needs of the village.

The fish processing was not a new additional activity in the fourteenth century but can be traced back to the early Middle Ages. From the very beginning it is visible only on one farmstead, no. 12, which indicates some sort of allocation of specialised functions on the farmsteads of the village. On the adjacent farmstead no. 1 there were no traces of fish processing, but on the other hand there were indications of another additional activity, namely beer brewing.[100] Hypothetically, such a functional variation of the farmsteads of Örja reflects the structure of a large, early-medieval demesne farm comprising a multitude of activities. Each farmstead might have represented a specialised part of these activities, which were governed from a manorial farm in the village.[101]

It has been generally accepted that fishery was a well-integrated part of the economy of the peasants along the coasts of the strait of Öresund in the Middle Ages. Fishery was part of a common *seamanship*, which included all sorts of maritime work.[102] *The sailing peasant* will be an appropriate expression to characterise this connection between land and sea in the cultural world of the coastal population. Thus the inhabitants of Örja developed their survival strategy during the harsh years of the crisis within a cultural context that was clearly defined for centuries. Probably they could expand the processing of fish without difficulty within an economy where the agricultural and maritime activities were closely intertwined.

A connection between the fish processing in the village of Örja and the great medieval herring fishery at the strait of Öresund lies close at hand. Moreover, it seems reasonable to look upon the change towards a specialised, large scale fish processing in Örja in the fourteenth century in the light of the development of the Scanian markets, being transformed to a highly specialised fish market in the late Middle Ages. Thus, the fish processing at Örja seems to have been deliberately adjusted to trade, probably resulting in new revenues to Örja in the era of the crisis when the village was struck by a considerable decline. The absence of residential functions at farmstead 12 gives a reason to look upon the fish processing as a collective business in the late Middle Ages, inhabitants of all the farmsteads of the village taking part in the activities.

The development in Örja implies that the big herring fishery affected also this ordinary agricultural village near the coast and that the economy of the village became closer linked to a mercantile maritime context in the late Middle Ages. This conclusion is furthermore supported by the analysis of the animal bones from Örja showing a dominance of herring but also a significant presence of species like cod and flounder fish.[103]

The fish processing came to an end in the latter part of the fifteenth century and thereafter farmstead 12 stayed deserted until the seventeenth century. In this way the farmstead did not follow the development of the Scanian markets, which were still flourishing in the fifteenth century. Not until hundred years later, their final decline started.

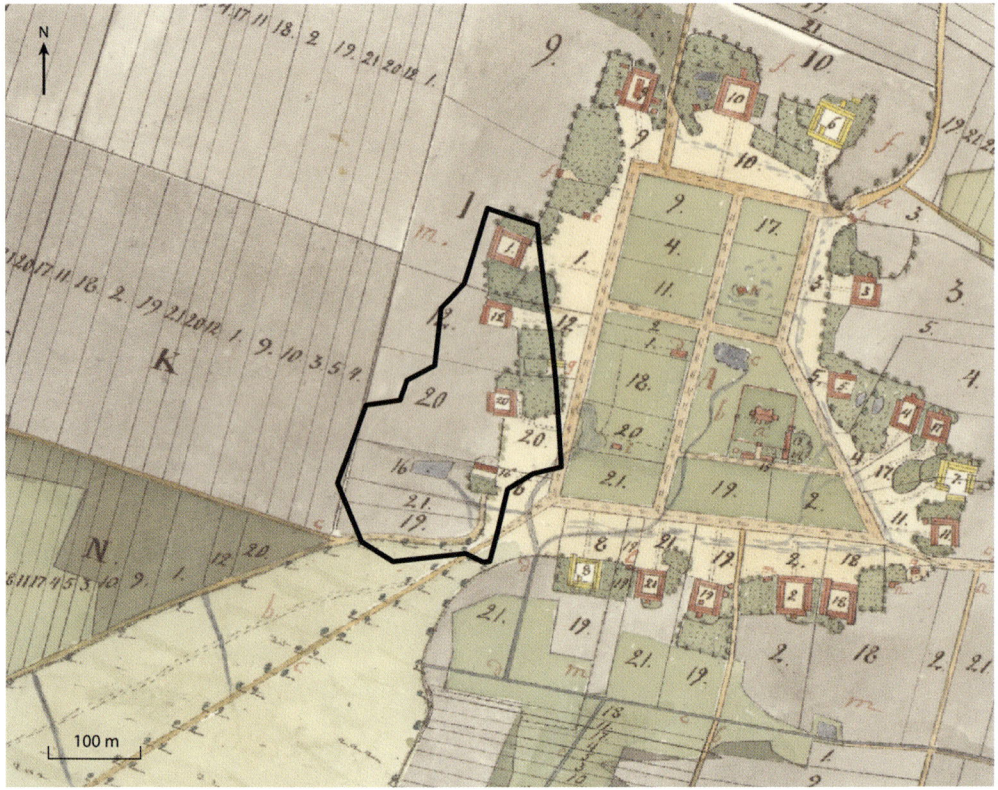

Fig. 31. Cadastral map of Örja from 1759 showing the village with its 18 homesteads (red squares). Black line marks the excavation area

Maybe the closing of the fish processing at Örja can be seen in the light of a general recovery of society and the beginning of a new agrarian expansion at the end of the Middle Ages. When agriculture expanded anew in the village the need for a large scale, additional activity may have diminished.

The expansion also meant decisive structural changes of the agrarian society. In the sixteenth century fishery was organised in a new way in this part of southern Scandinavia, from now on being performed by professional fishermen living in the towns or in permanently inhabited fishing villages by the coasts.[104] The old medieval diversity of the villages was replaced by a new specialised structure where fishermen and peasants were different social and cultural categories. The old village now became a more streamlined, agrarian unit.

The farmsteads in a comparative perspective – a brief summing-up
Despite regional characteristics, it is possible to discern some very significant resemblances in the development of the three farmsteads. It seems quite obvious that something decisive happened at all the places in the fourteenth century. The settlement of the farmsteads was fundamentally changed, either as an expansion of buildings, like in Vålle, or a reduction,

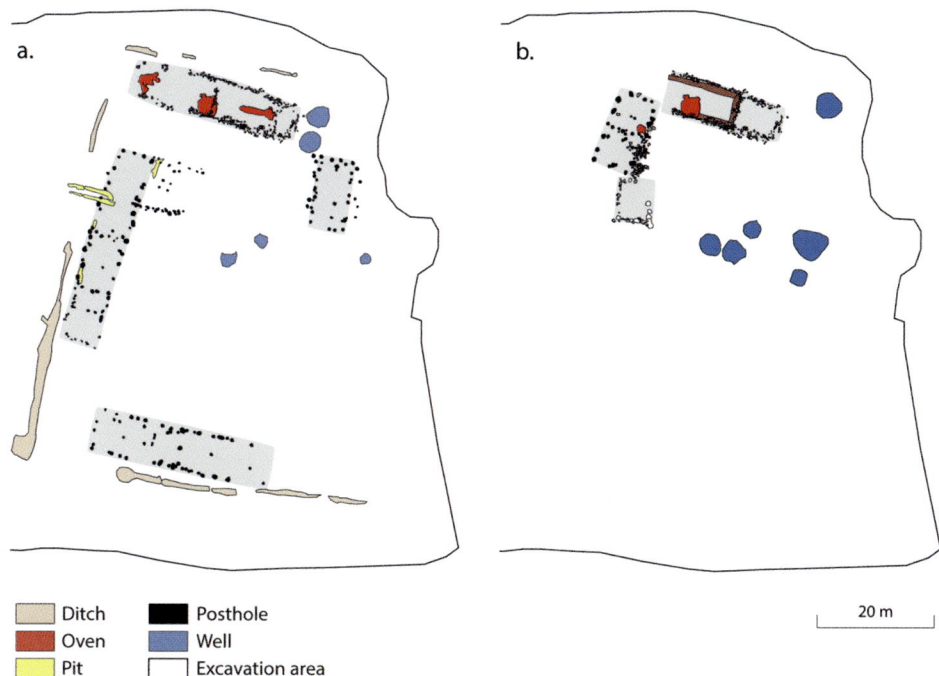

Fig. 32. Change of settlement at Örja AD 1200–1500. Settlement dated to a. 1100–1350 and b. 1350–1500, respectively

like in Stora Ullevi and Örja. This occurred in connection with major functional changes of the farmsteads. Concerning the character of the change there are some differences between the three places. A new activity, forging, was added to the agrarian settlement of Vålle. At Örja an earlier, secondary occupation was transformed to a large-scale, proto industrial activity, being the primary function of the farmstead. Stora Ullevi was characterised by a general orientation towards the nearby town of Linköping, affecting the social as well as the economic structure of the farmstead. At all the places it was a matter of specialised activities, directed to a distribution outside the own village or hamlet.

A chronological emphasis of the mentioned activities was observable at Örja as well at Vålle, to the period 1350–1450, making a connection to the initial, most severe phase of the crisis probable. At Stora Ullevi it was not possible to pinpoint the changes more precisely than to the fourteenth and fifteenth centuries.

The changes of the farmsteads were discussed in their regional contexts respectively. In the following section they will be looked upon in a wider societal connection.

General conclusions

This concluding section will use the results of the two previous investigations in one synthesising discussion on the impact of the late-medieval crisis, connecting to the initial issues. The first issue concerned desertion and decline. Different archaeological results have indicated a rapid, negative impact on society in the middle of the fourteenth century, causing an immediate stop to activities like building of houses. It supports the idea of dramatic, profound consequences of the plagues, severely disturbing important societal functions.

Regarding desertion of settlement, evidence was found everywhere, indicating a devastating movement that did not spare any remote corner of the country. Apparently, desertion was a prolonged process, as in Örja, where it occurred not until in the fifteenth century.

Of course, it will not be possible to quantify the extent of the desertion or to find out whether some regions were hit harder than others. However, the problems of partial desertion must be highlighted, being evident in Örja and probably typical of fertile areas like the plains of western Scania. As mentioned in the previous section, this kind of desertion may have been considerable in such areas, still being obscured in the source materials, the written as well as the archaeological. Challenging a general conclusion made by earlier research that such areas remained relatively unaffected by the crisis, the question must be raised as to whether that desertion was as extensive here as anywhere else.[105]

The second issue concerned the human response to the crisis. How did people act in the societal situation of the late fourteenth century and further on? We have seen the dysfunctional reaction of the nobility being materialised in an abundance of new castles in the decades following the year 1350, thus confirming Myrdal's model of development.

However, this was not the only reaction. Our investigation of the three farmsteads has shown us responses on a local level in different parts of the country, reflecting significant economic changes. Surrounded by desertion, the farmsteads seem to have responded rapidly to the crisis in the later part of the fourteenth century, developing additional, specialised activities. The changes at Stora Ullevi implied an increased orientation of social as well as economic character towards the nearby town, being a sort of specialisation, too.

What was the meaning of these changes? Apparently, parts of the production of the farmsteads became oriented towards a market to a greater extent than before. We have identified this market as the nearby town, regarding Stora Ullevi in Östergötland, or, regarding Örja, the urban, mercantile network of the Scanian markets. Thus, this meant a greater interaction between town and countryside but probably also a greater degree of collaboration between the farmsteads of the village or hamlet. At Örja, for example, the fish processing being a matter of a single farm in the High Middle Ages, it became a collective business of the entire village in the later part of the fourteenth century. The agrarian production being severely disturbed by a dramatic decrease of population, the development of an already established, additional activity like fish processing might have been a profitable enterprise for the village in a time of increasing demand for preserved foodstuff.

The traces of restructuring and expansion, discernible in some towns in the later part of the fourteenth century, are most likely to be seen in the light of such a an interacting between town and countryside, creating the basis of a new, urban development and a social emancipation of the towns.[106]

Also collaboration of farmsteads, being a consequence of the response to the crisis, is to be found at other places, for example in the mining districts north of the Lake Mälaren. Here, peasants dealt with iron working using the blast furnace technique at least since the end of the twelfth century. In the later part of the fourteenth century the activity was transformed into a new, specialised structure of collaborating farmsteads, the village of the peasant miners, replacing the old manorial system. Thus, it seems to have been a close connection between the development of specialised activities and the rise of new modes of social interaction.

How shall we look upon these creative responses to the crisis in the later part of the fourteenth century, when society was at its absolute nadir in a time of profound social and economic imbalance? Apparently, the archaeological evidence does not harmonise perfectly with Myrdal's model of the development of the crisis. The results reflect flexibility and creative change in the initial traumatic decades of the crisis rather than decline, stagnation and suppression. Is it possible to interpret this fragmented picture of the crisis in a satisfactory manner?

Probably we are dealing with reactions to the crisis on different levels of society. The "dysfunctional" acting of the nobility reflects a general survival strategy of a social class, which obviously had a paralysing effect on a socio-political level. But this may not have hampered creative solutions on a local level, where the single farm in the context of a village or a hamlet was able to form its own survival strategy.

However, the changes of the farmsteads may also be discussed in relation to the general social process transforming the agrarian society in the thirteenth and fourteenth centuries. The manorial system of the High Middle Ages, characterised by manors surrounded by subordinated crofters providing workforce to the manor, began to dissolve and was replaced by a system of larger manors functioning as fiscal centres for a number of tenant farms.[107] This process started most likely in the thirteenth century but was not completed at the time of the plagues in the middle of the fourteenth century. However, it may be assumed that the societal crisis and the demographic decline hastened the process, contributing to its completion in the later part of the fourteenth century.

The new situation around 1350 – the old manorial system being in dissolution and old social bonds between landowners and peasants breaking up – may have provided the latter a greater freedom to act on the local level. Probably we should look upon the rapid development of survival strategies at the farmsteads in the light of this new freedom. Thus the essential, societal conditions for an independent acting of the peasants were already in place in the middle of the fourteenth century. Developing their strategies, they could respond immediately to the crisis, which further hastened the social process. Of course, this development must not be looked at as being totally separated from a wider social structure, even if the initiatives to the new strategies were taken in the villages and hamlets. The peasants of our farmsteads being tenants, they most likely must have acted in a state of consensus with their landowners when developing their strategies.

So, an overall strategy seems to have been an increased interaction between town and countryside, parts of the production being specialised and orientated to an urban sphere. Still, this was not the case everywhere. In some regions people acted in a somewhat different way. I will discuss this problem here, taking a point of departure in the regional differences between the east and the west of Sweden.

At the farmstead in the west a rapid response to the crisis in the later part of the fourteenth century was observed, its economy being changed as its counterparts in the east and the south. However, signs of urban dynamics and expansion were not to be seen in the west. The towns being founded in the late Middle Ages all remained small and rather unimportant. In the western counterpart to Uppsala and Linköping, the episcopal town of Skara, there was only decline and "de-urbanisation" in this period.

Hence, not much of interaction between town and countryside was to be seen in the west. Presumably, the towns meant little for the surrounding countryside, remaining only as small, fiscal strongholds for the authorities.[108] As Christina Rosén has pointed out, an ordinary town in the west was more of a big village than of an urban centre.[109]

Then, how shall we characterise the action of people in the west in the time of the crisis? We have seen countryside, less regulated and less controlled than in the east, showing a high degree of flexibility. The latter enabled the moving of settlement in the province of Halland, adjusting it to the change of the agrarian economy in the late Middle Ages, as well as an increased exploitation of the outland in the northern part of Bohuslän. However, the specialised forging of the late fourteenth century, forming a new strategy of the farmstead at Vålle, was of a different kind compared to the corresponding activity at Örja in the south. It seems to have been a small-scale enterprise, being performed within the context of the single farm.

Thus, we may here discern an important characteristic of the west in the time of the crisis. Acting as independent units, the farmsteads of the west did not develop any large scale, collaborative projects characterising for example the villages of Scania or the villages of the peasant miners north of Lake Mälaren. Nevertheless, the peasants of northern Bohuslän were able to develop a multifaceted economy, starting in the later part of the fourteenth century. Using the natural resources of the region, such as timber, lime and iron, they developed a trade covering a far-reaching network, acting independent of regional urban intermediators. This trade of which there are abundant evidence from Early Modern times, written as well as archaeological, became an essential part of the cultural identity of the coastal regions of western Sweden.

Having identified some of the differences between the east and the west of Sweden in the time of the crisis, the relation between town and countryside stands out as a decisive element. An example from the recovery phase of the crisis in the late fifteenth century will furthermore highlight a cultural aspect of these regional differences. An absence of vaulting of the churches in extensive parts of western Sweden in the end of the Middle Ages has been commented on. Probably, the cultural incentives of late-medieval vaulting originated from an urban context, a fact that may explain the multitude of vaulted churches of the highly urbanised regions in the east and the south. The towns in the west did not interact with the countryside in the same way as in the east, thus never being able to function as transmitters of cultural influences.

The western and eastern parts of Sweden appear as two different and well discernible cultural entities in the late Middle Ages. This cultural regionalisation was not a result only of the crisis, but started long before 1350. However, in the late-medieval society of the crisis, the cultural differences became further explicit, appearing in a more clear light than before. Hence, the crisis had a deep impact on the cultural process, contributing strongly to a strengthening of the regional cultural differences.

Thus the late-medieval crisis has to be considered in the light of the two movements discussed above, the one of cultural regionalisation, the other of social emancipation. Emphasising the complex relation between these two movements will be a primary contribution of archaeology to the study of the crisis.

Notes

1   Cf. Gissel *et al.* 1981; Österberg 1981b
2   Berglund 1991
3   Andersson & Anglert 1989
4   Andrén 1985, 102ff
5   Myrdal 2012a
6   Lindkvist 2010, 34
7   Ericsson 2012, 338f
8   Andersson 1982
9   Winberg 2000, 113
10 Myrdal 2012a, 209
11 Broberg 1992, 56f
12 Broberg 1992, 62f
13 Ersgård 1986, 91
14 Ljung 1991, 120
15 Andrén 1985, 102
16 Christophersen 1978
17 Tagesson 2002, 157f
18 Tagesson 2002, 1
19 Beronius Jörpeland & Bäck 2003, 185f
20 Connelid & Zedig 2007
21 Ersgård 1986, 94
22 Anund *et al.* 1992, 227
23 Uppsala. Medeltidsstaden 3. 1976, 15
24 Tagesson 2002, 159ff
25 Seppänen in press, 6f
26 Seppänen in press, 6f
27 Myrdal 1999, 116f
28 Vretemark 1997, 13
29 Carlsson 2007, 163
30 Andrén 1986; Beronius Jörpeland 1992
31 Andrén 1985, 101; 1986, 265
32 Tagesson 2002, 157f, 281f
33 Malm 1984, 58
34 Malm 1984, 60f
35 Pihlman & Kostet 1986, 123
36 Nyborg 2009, 188–193
37 A similar loss of knowledge concerning the art of healing, caused by the decrease of population in the late Middle Ages, has recently been discussed by Johanna Bergqvist (Bergqvist 2013, 333–337)
38 Cf. Österberg 1981b
39 Berglund *et al.* 2009; Svensson *et al.* 2013
40 Åstrand 2007
41 Åstrand 2007, 77
42 Hansson *et al.* 2005; Olausson 1989; Gauffin 1989
43 Hansson *et al.* 2005, 162
44 C.f. Karsvall 2011
45 Schmidt Sabo 2001, 74f
46 Schmidt Sabo (ed.) 2013

47   See Chap. 4
48   Bartholin 1989a
49   Lindeblad & Tagesson 2005. In this article the terms *village* and *hamlet* are used to classify the
     local contexts of the medieval, agrarian settlement (cf. Jones 2010, 13–16). 'Village' is used for
     a cluster of cooperating farmsteads that have had some central functions in the parish, usually
     through the presence of the parish church. Thus 'hamlet' will be used for clustered settlements
     with no such functions. The term 'single farm' concerns a farmstead that does not cooperate
     agriculturally with other farms
50   Connelid & Rosén 1997; Connelid & Mascher 2003
51   Connelid & Mascher 2003, 105
52   Beronius Jörpeland 2010
53   See also Chap. 4 for a discussion on the Småland datings
54   Bartholin 1989b
55   Wienberg 1993, 44ff
56   Bonnier 2008, 164
57   Regner 2005
58   Regner 2005, 229
59   Regner 2005, 238
60   Myrdal 2012a, 230f
61   Lovén 1996, 195
62   Lovén 1996, 348
63   Lovén 1996, 197
64   Stibeus 1986
65   Grundberg 2001
66   Cf. Magnusson & Isacson 1988
67   These characteristics are in accordance with Bo Strömberg's definition of proto industry (Strömberg
     2008, 28–31, 53–54)
68   Cf. papers in *Med hammare och fackla* 51 (2010)
69   Strömberg 2008
70   Strömberg 2008, 28ff
71   Skyllberg 2003
72   Skyllberg 2003, 65
73   Magnusson 1985
74   Pettersson Jensen 2012, 251
75   Pettersson Jensen 2012
76   Pettersson Jensen 2012, 56ff, 213ff
77   Magnusson 2010, 114ff
78   Norman 1993, 61, 181
79   Ersgård 1988, 95
80   Such an approach on the late-medieval crisis has already been paid attention to within recent
     archaeological research in Sweden. Cf. Svensson *et al.* 2012
81   Myrdal 2012a, 225
82   Rosén 2009; Rosén 2013
83   Rosén 2009, 54f
84   Grandin *et al.* 2008
85   Framme 1985, 174–175
86   Lindman *et al.* 2004, 119
87   Sandklef 1973
88   Rosén 2009, 44–46

89   Carlsson *et al.* 2001; Lindeblad & Tagesson 2004; Lindeblad & Tagesson 2005
90   Lindeblad & Tagesson 2005, 250
91   Feldt & Tagesson 1997, 114
92   Tagesson 2002, 234ff
93   Tagesson 2002, 157ff
94   Tagesson 2002, 159ff
95   Lindeblad & Tagesson 2004, annex 1
96   Tagesson 2002, 260f; Lindeblad & Tagesson 2005, 278
97   Schmidt Sabo (ed.) 2013, 30
98   Schmidt Sabo (ed.) 2013, 230
99   Bolander 2014, 192
100 Bolander 2014, 193
101 Cf. Myrdal 2012a, 208
102 Stoklund 2000, 199
103 Stoklund 2000, 197
104 Ersgård 2001, 103
105 Cf. Österberg 1981b; Skansjö 1983
106 Cf. Andrén 1985, 100ff
107 Myrdal 2012a, 209; Ericsson 2012, 43–54
108 Andersson 1985
109 Rosén in press

6.

Living conditions in times of plague

Caroline Arcini, T. Douglas Price, Maria Cinthio,
Leena Drenzel, Mats Andersson, Bodil Persson,
Hanna Menander, Maria Vretemark, Anna Kjellström,
Rickard Hedvall & Göran Tagesson

Introduction

The Black Death shook society in its foundations. Contemporary chroniclers describe the rampage of the plague and the immediate shock for society. But there were also long-lasting effects of the population drop, which may have affected the living conditions not only for the survivors of the plague but also for following generations for centuries. This chapter will use skeletons from medieval churchyards to investigate living conditions before, during and after the crisis. Burial customs and what they tell us about social customs and religious beliefs in the times of plague will be discussed.

When the Black Death struck in the mid-fourteenth century, Sweden like much of Europe had experienced a marked increase in population size over the centuries. Several different factors had contributed to agricultural expansion and population growth. Technological innovations in agriculture and iron production played an important role, together with changes in the social organisation and household conditions. Decline in household size, freedom of slaves and new opportunities for the poor to marry and found families favoured population growth.[1] However, this period of expansion came to a definitive end with the Black Death, which hit Sweden in 1350. It was the first of a long series of plague outbreaks, which lasted all the way up to the early eighteenth century. During the Middle Ages, in particular the outbreaks of 1350 (the Black Death), 1359–60 and 1368–69 appear to have been particularly devastating.[2]

The plague obviously caused death and suffering, broken families and abandoned farms. In addition to these direct effects, there were social effects in the wake of the plague that added to the misery. Increased oppression and plundering by the landowning elite resulted in peasant resistance and revolts, and much of the late fourteenth century was characterised by social unrest and conflicts.[3] It is easily understood that living conditions must have been hard, at least during the initial phase of the crisis. However, in a longer time perspective the picture gets more complex. Even though plague continued to haunt the population there were social changes during the fifteenth century that appear to have had positive effects on everyday life for many people. The peasant revolts eventually turned successful and together with the urgent shortage of labour they resulted in lower rents and higher wages. As a consequence, living standards of the large number of common people may have improved and consumption increased. Also the average agricultural production per head increased, because the smaller population after the Black Death concentrated to fertile areas, leaving less productive holdings to abandonment.[4]

For the above reasons several authors have concluded that living conditions improved distinctly after the Black Death,[5] but mortality was still high and it was not until the late fifteenth century or the early sixteenth century that population numbers started to increase again.[6] Also the changes in living conditions may have affected social classes differently and there may also have been regional variation. Furthermore, improved living conditions due to population drop may have been confined to regions that suffered from high population density before the crisis. Hence, the picture is complicated and still very little is known about short-term and long-term effects of the crisis on the standard of living for common people.

Living conditions in general are reflected in stature, and because archaeological excavations of medieval cemeteries all over Europe have resulted in the recovery of thousands of skeletons from different periods of the Middle Ages, there should be great possibilities to study living conditions before and after the Black Death. However, the numbers of Black Death cemeteries, used specifically for plague victims, are still very few and few studies have focused on health and living conditions before and after the Black Death. The most used material for this purpose is from the Black Death cemetery at East Smithfield in London.[7] Other examples are the mass graves at Hereford, England, and Heiligen Geist, Germany.[8] This study takes a closer look at the medieval skeleton material from Sweden. Medieval burial customs are examined and – based on a combination of cemeteries of different age and a chronological distinction within one specific cemetery – stature estimates from a large number of skeletons are used to investigate possible changes in health and living standards.[9]

In addition to improved living conditions in general there may have been specific changes in diet that affected health and stature. Written sources together with pollen records indicate that the population drop was followed by changes in the agricultural system, in particular by an increase in the relative importance of animal husbandry.[10] When there were fewer people left to cultivate the land, former fields were turned to meadows and pastures, and the production of meat and milk products in relation to cereals increased. A plausible consequence would be a change not only in production but also in consumption, with a larger intake of meat and dairy products.[11] To test this hypothesis, stable-isotope composition of carbon (C) and nitrogen (N) in teeth from medieval skeletons was examined. The material used comes from the Trintitatis cemetery in Lund, which spans 990–1536 and enables a comparison of different periods of the Middle Ages.[12]

Another question that may be reflected in stable-isotope composition is the migration of people. Strontium-isotope analyses of medieval skeletons from the Trinitatis cemetery have been used in an attempt to trace possible migration into Lund in the wake of the plague. Written documents indicate that trade and craftsmanship flourished during the late-medieval crisis and even though the plague probably hit the town populations hard, newcomers may have filled vacancies.

The written sources from Sweden concerning the period of the Black Death are few, but from the last plague of 1710–1713 sources are richer. The last section of this chapter leaves the osteological source material and takes a closer look at the church books from this last plague epidemic. The aim is to gain some clues on plague's epidemic behaviour, how it spread from parish to parish, how it affected lowlands and uplands, and how long it took for population to recover.

Where are the victims of the Black Death buried?

When the Black Death swept through Europe people died in unprecedented numbers. Chroniclers from the time emphasise the high mortality, and modern historians who base their conclusions on a wide range of historical records give the same picture.[13] Although opinions differ on the exact amount of the population decrease – estimates on a European level usually range between one-third and two-thirds – it is believed to have been the most significant population drop in Europe's history.[14] The Black Death – the first strike of the plague – was followed by several recurring outbreaks during the late fourteenth century and throughout the fifteenth century.[15] Increased mortality was connected to all of them, but in most parts of Europe the first event appears to have been the most devastating.[16] It ravaged Europe in 1347–51, but on a local scale the visit by the plague in any particular region or town usually lasted only a few months or weeks.[17] These months must have been characterised by shock and sorrow but also by the practical problems of taking care of the dead.

It is easy to imagine that the super mortality of the Black Death called for extraordinary measures, and in the popular mind the plague is much associated with mass graves – 'plague pits.' The historical records provide some glimpses of such measures. For instance, Pope Clement VI, who resided in Avignon, bought a piece of land near Our Lady of Miracles and inaugurated it as a cemetery for plague victims. And more drastically, he consecrated the River Rhone so that the dead bodies could be safely thrown into the river.[18] In the ports of Spain dead bodies were thrown directly into the sea.[19]

From Boccaccio's *Decameron* – the most frequently cited eyewitness account on the Black Death – a vivid picture is obtained of how the high mortality of the plague affected the funeral customs of the city of Florence:[20]

> It had once been customary, as it is again nowadays, for the women relatives and neighbours of a dead man to assemble in his house in order to mourn in the company of the women who had been closest to him; moreover his kinsfolk would forgather in front of his house along with his neighbours and various other citizens, and there would be a contingent of priests, whose number varied according to the quality of the deceased; his body would be taken thence to the church in which he had wanted to be buried … But as the ferocity of the plague began to mount, this practice all but disappeared entirely and was replaced by different customs … it was rare for the bodies of the dead to be accompanied by more than ten or twelve neighbours to the church, nor were they borne on the shoulders of worthy and honest citizens, but by a kind of grave digging fraternity, …
>
> As for the common people and a large proportion of the bourgeoisie, they presented a much more pathetic spectacle, … they fell ill daily in their thousands, and since they had no one to assist them or attend to their needs, they inevitably perished almost without exceptions. Many dropped dead in the open streets, both by day and by night, …

Whenever people died, their neighbours nearly always followed a single, set routine, ... Either on their own, or with the assistance of bearers whenever these were to be had, they extracted the bodies of the dead from their houses and left them lying outside their front doors, where anyone going about the streets, especially in the early morning, could have observed countless numbers of them. Funeral biers would then be sent for, upon which the dead were taken away, though there were some who, for lack of biers, were carried off on plain boards. It was by no means rare for more than one of these biers to be seen with two or three bodies upon it at a time; on the contrary, many were seen to contain a husband and wife, two or three brothers and sisters, a father and son, or some other pair of close relatives. And times without number it happened that two priests would be on their way to bury someone, holding a cross before them, only to find that bearers carrying three or four additional biers would fall in behind them; so that whereas the priests had thought they had only one burial to attend to, they in fact had six or seven, and sometimes more ...

Such was the multitude of corpses (of which further consignments were arriving every day and almost by the hour at each of the churches), that there was not sufficient consecrated ground for them to be buried in, especially if each was to have its own plot in accordance with long-established custom. So when all the graves were full, huge trenches were excavated in the churchyards, into which new arrivals were placed in their hundreds, stowed tier upon tier like ships' cargo, each layer of corpses being covered over with a thin layer of soil till the trench was filled to the top.

Boccaccio was upset by the unchristian and unworthy dissolution of traditions and moral values, and his colourful testimony brings us the horror and despair. But looking at it in hindsight, the degree to which funeral practices actually prevailed during these hard times is perhaps even more stunning. In spite of the high mortality, people were still buried in coffins, and funeral processions lead by priests were held whenever possible. The dead were buried on cemeteries, although not always the particular graveyard wished by the diseased.[21]

When looking for the physical remains of the plague victims, it may be concluded that some may be lost forever, for instance if thrown in the river or the sea, whereas others may be found on cemeteries. Although surprisingly few, in the light of the disaster, some Black Death cemeteries have been identified and archaeologically investigated. The most well-published and thoroughly studied is the plague cemetery of East Smithfield in London.[22] It has been estimated that a total of 2400 plague victims were buried in the cemetery, of which the skeletons of 759 individuals have been archaeologically documented. In the cemetery there were both single graves and mass burials. The latter were obviously necessitated by the high mortality and by the need to bury many dead in a short time. However, the phrase 'mass grave' may give a false impression. The bodies at East Smithfield were not carelessly just thrown into a pit. The mass graves constituted long trenches in which the dead bodies were placed side by side in an orderly manner. Even though they were densely packed, they were carefully placed beside each other, oriented in east–west direction as was customary (Fig. 33). There were up to five layers of bodies buried in the trenches and small children were put between the adults. Of the bodies in the trenches, 13% had coffins. Apart from the long trenches, there were also smaller multiple graves that contained only a few bodies buried together.[23]

The long trenches with orderly placed bodies documented at East Smithfield fit well with the description from Florence by Boccaccio. Similar mass graves have also been documented elsewhere, for instance at St Bartholomew's Hospital,[24] Charterhouse Square,[25] Blackfriars and Guildford Friary in London,[26] and at Hereford, England.[27] Other examples are from Lübeck, Germany,[28] Grossmünster in Zurich, Switzerland,[29] and Barcelona, Spain.[30] In Scandinavia there is one possible Black Death mass grave reported from the Church of Our Lady (Vor Frue Kirke) in Randers, Denmark.[31] The grave is from the Middle Ages (*c.* 1100–1550), but it lacks a more precise dating and it has not been osteologically analysed. From Sweden there is one possible example from outside the St Nicolaus cemetery in Lund.[32] It was a partly excavated trench with twenty individuals that appeared to have been buried more or less at the same time. However, the skeletons are not available anymore, and similar to the Danish grave it was only broadly dated to the Middle Ages.

Hence, identified mass graves from the Black Death are still few but they seem to give a rather unanimous picture. In spite of the many dead that had to be buried in a short time, plague victims from the Black Death were taken care of in a relatively dignified manner, given the circumstances. When mass graves were necessary, these were well-ordered trenches with east–west oriented bodies. This picture stands in contrast to some plague pits from later outbreaks, which show no signs of dignity or of any attempts to follow traditional, religious customs. One example is the plague pit belonging to Lazzaretto Vecchio on Quarantine Island in Venice, from a plague outbreak in 1485 (Fig. 34). The pit contained 1500 individuals buried out of order and some of them placed in prone position. Similar plague pits have been found in Martigues, north of Marseille, France, dated to 1720–21.[33] These mass graves from later plague epidemics give a completely different impression than for instance the Black Death cemetery at East Smithfield.

Extraordinary measures were sometimes also taken in connection with the Black Death, for instance those of Pope Clement VI mentioned above, but these may have been spectacular exceptions that caught the attention of chroniclers. The well-ordered mass graves at East Smithfield, where there were also single and small multiple graves, together with the description from Florence by Boccaccio, give another impression and indicate that Black Death burials may not necessarily be very different from ordinary burials. Could this be a reason why identified Black Death graves are still surprisingly few? Have we overlooked the most obvious place to search for them – in the ordinary medieval cemeteries?

People at the time of the Black Death seems to have stuck to traditional burial customs as far as possible, and mass graves were dug only when necessary. The need for mass graves would have depended on the number of dead in a given time and the number of people left to bury them. In Sweden there are no detailed records from the Black Death of the number of dead in any particular area, which otherwise could have indicated the possible need for mass burials. However, on a national level, the average population drop in Sweden during the late fourteenth century has been tentatively estimated to about 40–50%.[34] This population drop was probably due not only to the Black Death in 1350, but also to the two severe outbreaks that followed in 1359–60 and 1368–69.[35]

The area covered by present-day Sweden had a population of approximately 1.1 million before the Black Death.[36] If two assumptions are made that (1) the total population drop from the first three plague outbreaks was 50% and (2) that the first outbreak was the most devastating, a simple estimate suggests a 40% drop in 1350 (from 1,100,000 to 660,000), a 10% drop in 1359–60 (from 660,000 to 594,000), and then another 10% drop in 1368–69 (594,000 to 534,600). The increased mortality during each of these three different outbreaks may then be divided by the number of cemeteries in Sweden, which has been estimated to approximately 2350.[37] It gives us an average estimate of the number of extra burials per

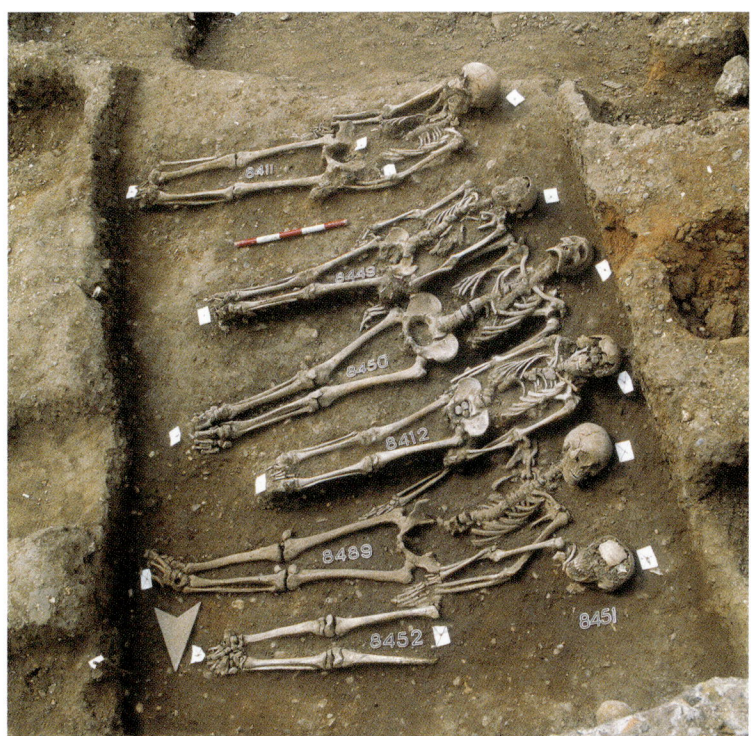

Fig. 33. Part of a burial trench investigated at the Black Death cemetery East Smithfield in London (photo courtesy of Museum of London Archaeology Service)

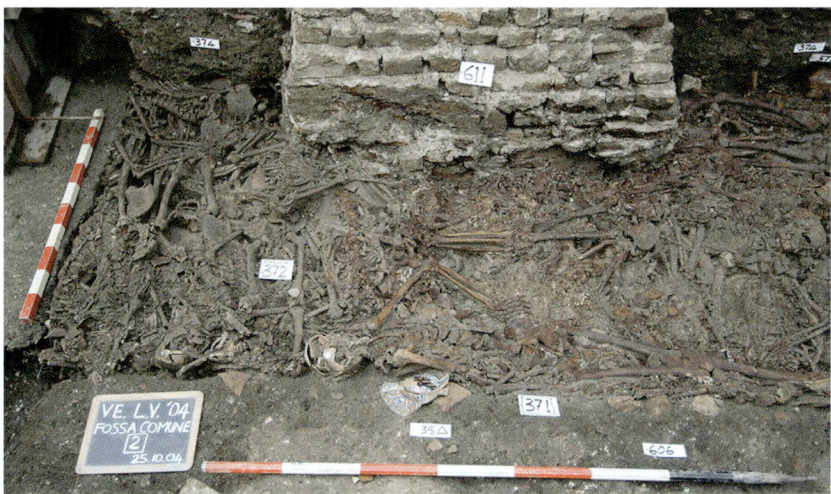

Fig. 34. Mass grave with plague victims from 1485 on the Island of Lazaretto Vecchio, the Venetian Lagoon, Italy (photo used under the licence of Italian Republic, Ministry for Culture, Soprintendenza per i Beni Archeologici del Veneto, Copyright reserved)

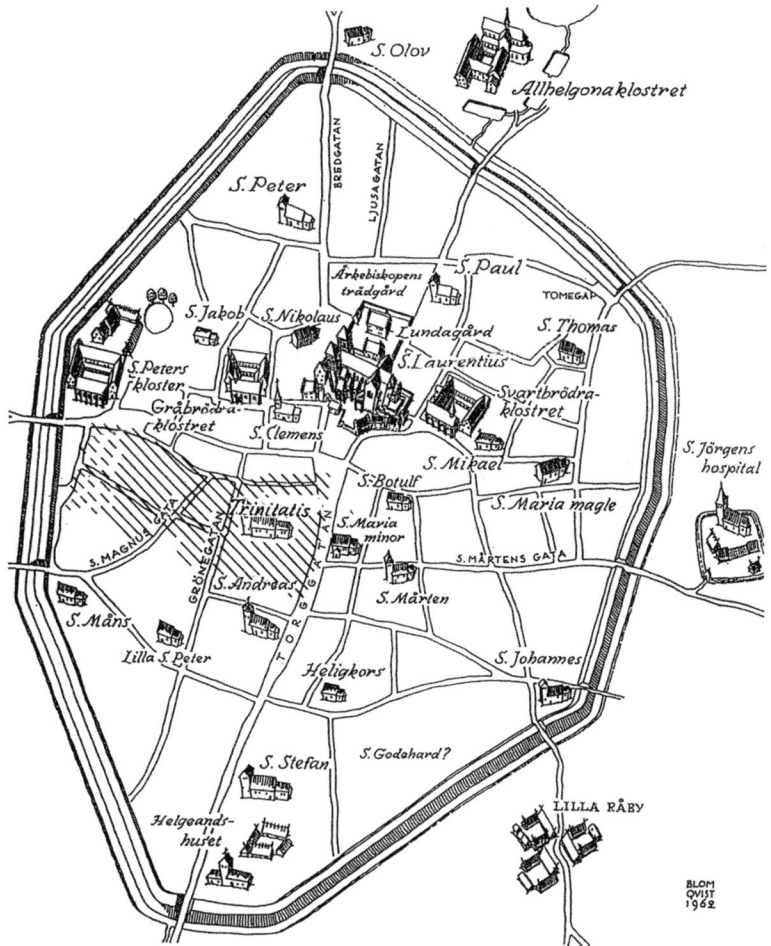

Fig. 35. Map of Lund in 1536 with churches. The hatched area marks Trinitatis parish (original drawing by Ragnar Blomqvist 1962, with some later additions)

cemetery during the plague years. During the first wave, i.e. the Black Death, there were on average 187 more burials per cemetery than in a normal year, in the second wave there were 28, and in the third 25 more than normal. Whether the cemeteries could accommodate this amount of additional bodies depends on how large the cemeteries were and how many died at the same time – 187 more dead than normal in a year or in a month would be very different.

From these hypothetical numbers on a national level we may now look closer at the most thoroughly studied medieval cemetery in present-day Sweden, the Trinitatis Cemetery in Lund (Fig. 35). The cemetery spans the period 990–1536 and 2953 graves have been osteologically investigated.[38] The total number of graves at Trinitatis, which was the largest cemetery in medieval Lund, has been estimated to approximately 5700 graves. Based on stratigraphy, dendrochronology and radiocarbon dates in combination with time-characteristic arm positions of the buried individuals, the graves have been divided into chronological groups.[39] The group tentatively dated to the late fourteenth century is characterised by increased burial activity in general (Fig. 36a, b), and also by the occurrence of several double and triple graves (Fig. 36c). This concentration of graves is interpreted here as reflecting victims of the Black Death together with the two subsequent outbreaks. Layers with increased numbers of graves containing two, three, four and occasionally five individuals have been identified also at other medieval cemeteries in Sweden, for instance in Åhus,[40] Skänninge,[41] Linköping,[42] Stockholm[43] and Westerhus (Fig. 37).[44] They may represent plague victims, but in the absence of detailed chronological studies this remains a hypothesis. Although Lund has particularly good dating and preservation conditions, our study indicates that it may be fruitful for future studies to return also to several of these other excavated materials to try to make refined chronological distinctions.

Based on the chronological grouping at Trinitatis, the average number of burials per year in the excavated part of the cemetery has been estimated at 4–5 individuals in the centuries before the Black Death. The accumulation of burials in the late fourteenth century consists of 270 individuals. If they represent the three epidemics 1350, 1359–60 and 1368–69, then 90 normal burials may be expected during this 20-year period (4–5 per year), which leaves us with 180 burials that may be plague victims. Divided by three, it equals 60 extra burials per plague epidemic on this cemetery.

Lund at the time had 26 cemeteries.[45] They were of different size and some of them, in particular those of the monasteries and convents, where mainly for the higher social strata. Still a rough extrapolation from Trinitatis can be made based on the different sizes of the cemeteries. The number of 180 extra burials at Trinitatis would then represent approximately 1500 extra burials in Lund. The population of Lund during the High and Late Middle Ages has been estimated to 3000–4500 people.[46] Even though this figure has not been specified, 1500 extra burials would represent a population drop of 30–50%, provided that the moving of people in or out of the town is negligible. This figure is of course very tentative, given all the uncertain parameters of the calculation. However, the most important conclusion is that a population drop of this size would not necessary call for mass graves. The increased mortality could be handled with single burials in combination with smaller multiple burials in the ordinary cemeteries.

Lund was a small town in an international perspective and much higher numbers of dead have been suggested for several larger European towns. For instance, in Parma, 40,000 victims of the Black Death were buried in 6 months, on average more than 220 per day, and in Avignon the death toll reached an incredible 150,000, of whom 1800 died during the first 3 days.[47] Also, London was a large town, estimated to have had 45,000–80,000 inhabitants.[48] From this population, 30–50% (15,000–40,000 people) died from the Black Death. London at the time had more than 100 cemeteries,[49] but still there was need to establish at least two emergency plague cemeteries – the East Smithfield, discussed above, and the neighbouring West Smithfield/Charterhouse Square.[50] These two cemeteries had mass graves but also single burials and small multiple burials similar to the ones at Trinitatis.

It may be concluded that the need for mass graves differed greatly between towns and between regions, and that the lack of safely identified mass graves from the Black Death

a.

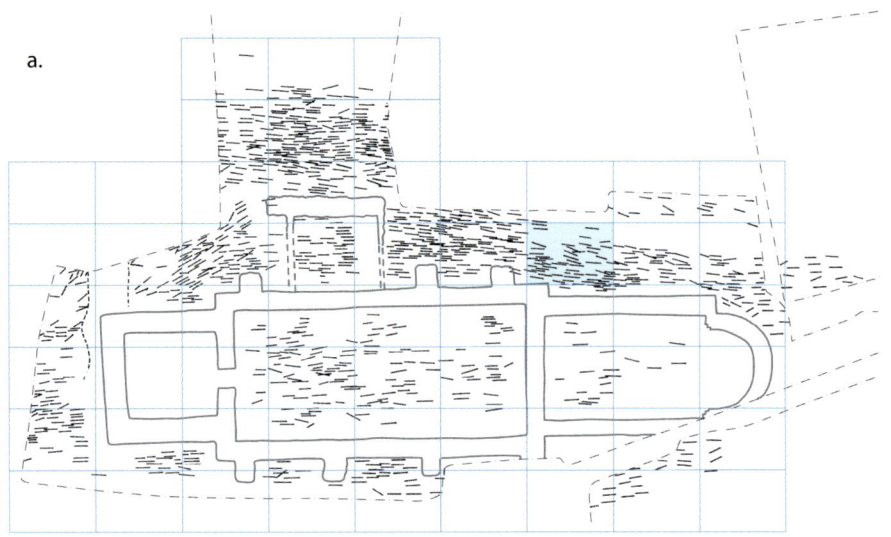

b.

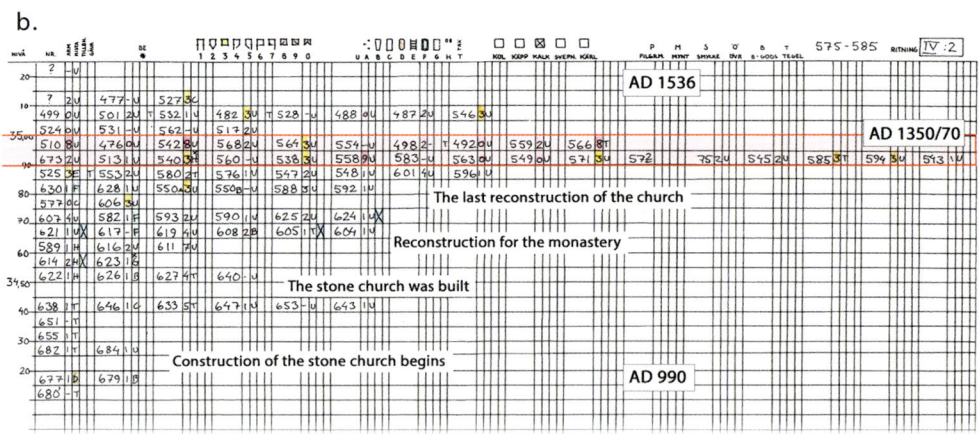

c.

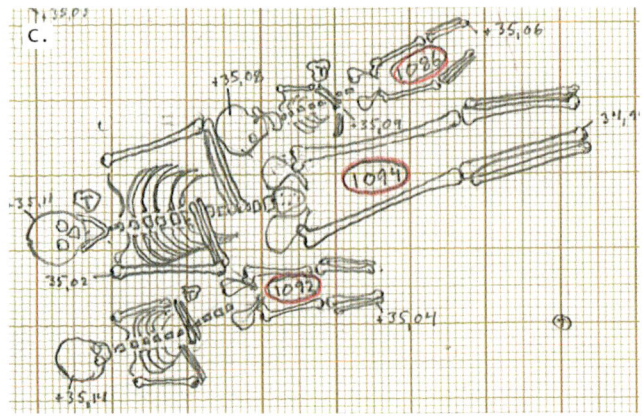

Fig. 36. (opposite page) Archaoelogical documentataion of the Trinitatis Cemetery in Lund; a. plan of the Trinitatis church with cemetery, 1300–1536. Blue grid indicates the 5 × 7 m squares used for archaeological documentation (drawing by Maria Cinthio); b. the dating and chronological grouping of graves from Trinitatis were made using relationship diagrams and grave levels for each of the 5 × 7 m squares. The picture shows the documentation from one such square (light blue in a), with the number of buried individuals at each level. Vertical axis represents height above sea level (the graves here range 34.10–35.25 m a.s.l.). In the period c. 990–1536 the ground level was gradually raised due to the accumulation of building layers from the construction and renovation of the stone church together with the numerous buried. Burial customs (arms position, type of coffin) is listed with symbols at each grave number. Grave levels were based on the measured levels of the skulls. The relationship diagram provides a picture of the changes in funeral customs and grave digging intensity at different levels; c. original drawing of one of the triple graves from Trinitatis

in Scandinavia indicates that the plague victims could probably be handled in ordinary cemeteries. This is true also for later plague epidemics from which we have written records. For instance, in the small village Sørby-Magle Kirkerup in Denmark, the church book from 1656 describes the burial of plague victims in the cemetery. Sometimes the burials could not be paid for, since also the relatives had died, and in some cases siblings were buried together in the same coffin. In one occasion it is mentioned that one person was buried just as he was, without a coffin. Obviously all customs could not be followed but they were still buried at the cemetery.[51]

In Sweden, there are good records on the last plague of 1710–13. During this epidemic approximately 200,000 died, which represent almost 15% of the population. In November 1710, royal authorities proclaimed that plague victims should be buried in other places than in the ordinary cemeteries.[52] One example of a town where the new regulation was followed is Linköping, which lost about one-third of its population. In the initial phase of the epidemic, plague victims were buried in the Cathedral Cemetery, in a part of the cemetery normally used for thc poor.[53] Following the regulation, a specific plague cemetery was established at a nearby military training camp.

The only plague cemetery in Sweden that has been archaeologically documented was also the result of the new regulation of November 1710. It was situated in the village of Holje, Blekinge, in southeastern Sweden. From this cemetery 90 graves containing 115 individuals were excavated (Fig. 38), whereas the total number of graves was estimated to 300–350.[54] All the burials had coffins and the majority of them were single graves. There were some double graves and a few graves with three individuals (Fig. 39), but no mass graves. There was also one grave where two children were put in the same coffin. All the graves were put neatly in line with no intercutting or disturbance.[55] The burials seem to have followed the authorities' regulation that the plague victims should not to be washed and wrapped. They were apparently buried in the clothes they wore when they died, as indicated by preserved buttons, hooks and eyes from the cloths, and by the absence of the needles normally used when wrapping the diseased. They also had necklaces, scissors, knives, metal toothpicks and ear-spoons, the latter usually carried in a leather strap or thin chain around the neck. The body of young girl still had a thimble on its finger. Another sign of hurry is that the graves were shallow dug. According to the regulations, graves should be at least 1.8 m deep, but the ones in Holje reached a depth of only 0.8–1.2 m. Apart from this, the establishment of

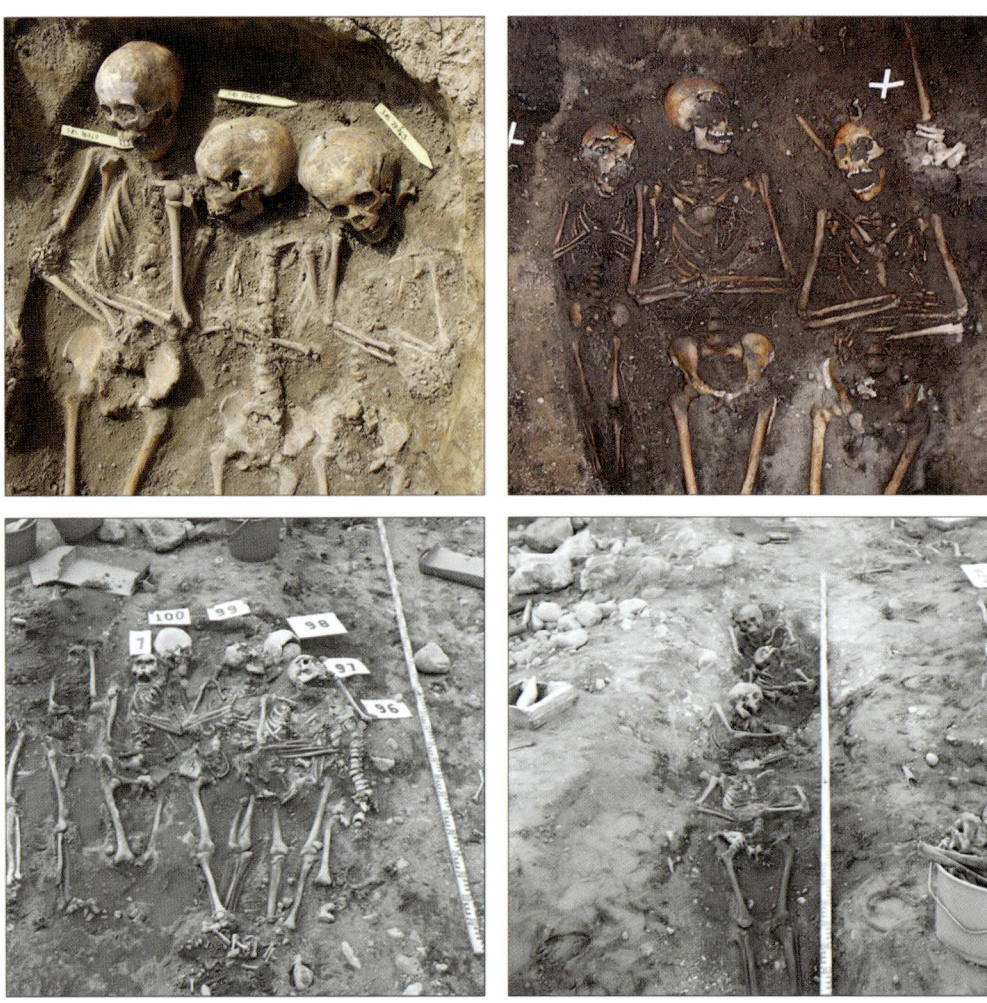

Fig. 37. Photos from medieval cemeteries in Sweden: a. three children buried close together in the cemetery of the Black Friar convent in Skänninge, Östergötland, c. 1237–1536 (photo: Swedish National Heritage Board, UV Öst); b. Triple grave with two adults and one child from the cemetery of the cathedral of Linköping, Östergötland, dated to the Late Middle Ages (photo: Swedish National Heritage Board, UV Öst); c. Several adult individuals buried very close together at the cemetery of the Sanctuary at Helgeandsholmen, Stockholm, dated to c. 1320–1531 (photo Stefan Kriig); d. Several adult individuals buried in a long row, like in a ditch, at the cemetery of the Sanctuary at Helgeandsholmen, Stockholm, c. 1320–1531 (photo Annika Olson)

a special plague cemetery and the burial procedures in Holje seem to have followed the regulations. However, this went not without protests. According to the priest's diary he was threaten by his parishioners and at some occasions even violently forced to bury plague victims in the ordinary cemetery.[56] The deeply rooted customs of cemetery burials were not easily thrown overboard.

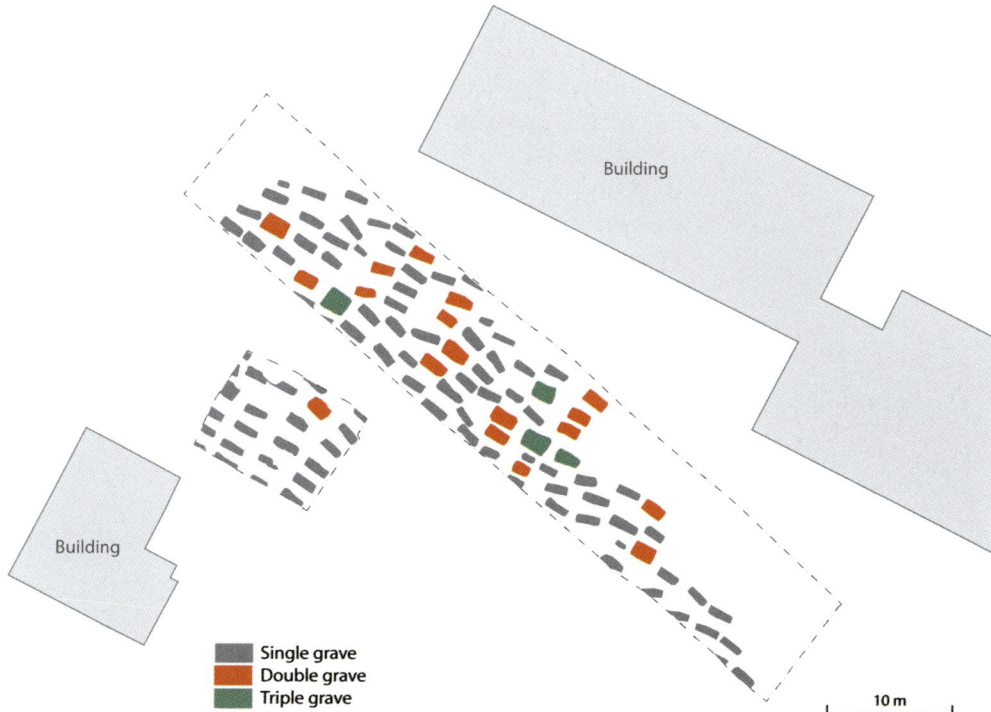

Fig. 38. Excavation plan showing the distribution of single, double and triple graves at the plague cemetery Holje, Jämshög village, in the province of Blekinge, from 1710

In conclusion, most victims of the Black Death as well as of later plague epidemics were probably buried in ordinary cemeteries. In large and densely populated towns of Europe, special plague cemeteries were established, which contained single graves, multiple graves and mass graves. However, the only safely identified plague cemetery in Sweden was established in connection with the last plague epidemic of 1710–13. It followed a new national regulation, according to which the burial of plague victims on ordinary cemeteries was no longer allowed. We cannot exclude the possibility that some plague cemeteries, and even mass graves, were established in Sweden also before, for instance in connection to the Black Death. But based on present knowledge, the best place to search for the victims of the Black Death is probably in the ordinary medieval cemeteries. Indications to look for may be accumulations of single graves as well as multiple graves with two, three or more individuals. Hopefully this can be tested in the future by more thorough chronological and stratigraphic studies in combination with aDNA analysis.

Stature – a health parameter through history

Stature varies greatly among individuals and around the globe, and it has also varied

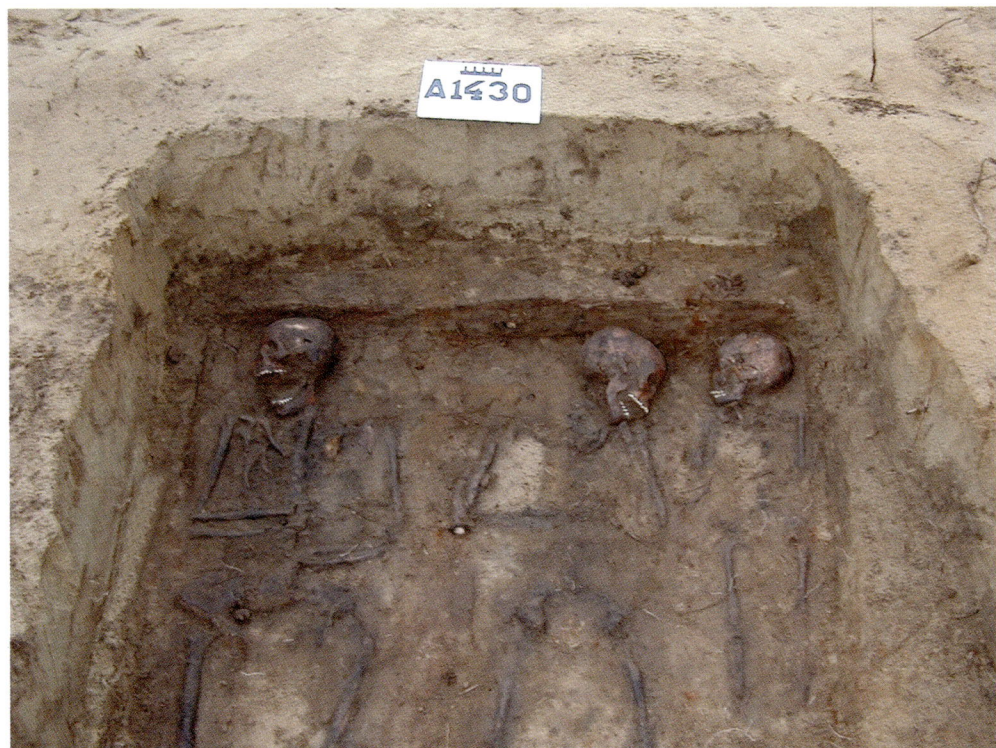

Fig. 39. Triple grave containing one adult woman, one young person (14–18 years) and one child (4–5 years). The plague cemetery in Holje, Jämshög village, Blekinge, from 1710 (photo: Bengt Jacobsson)

significantly through history. Long-term changes may be studied first of all by osteometric analysis of skeletons from different periods, while written records may also contribute with statistics for the last few centuries. In Sweden the earliest systematic records derive from the nineteenth century and the conscription of soldiers. Based on this combination of sources and methods we have a fairly clear picture of the long-term trends in stature in Scandinavia.[57]

People living in the nineteenth century were short, actually as short as the hunter-gatherers who lived in Sweden 6000 years ago. But between these two low points stature has varied considerably, and during the Roman Iron Age (first to fourth centuries AD) people were almost as tall as we are today.[58] From the Roman Iron Age to the eleventh century average stature decreased by 5 cm. During the Middle Ages there were relatively small changes (see our new results below), until stature started to decrease steadily to reach a nadir in the mid-nineteenth century. Since then, stature increased again to reach present-day values.[59] This increase was very sharp. In only 150 years, average stature of men in Europe increased by 11 cm, which is the fastest change recorded so far (Fig. 40).[60]

What are the causes behind the long-term fluctuations in stature through history? According to studies of modern living populations, stature depends on both genetic factors and on living conditions and lifestyle. Particularly important are living conditions that affect the mother during pregnancy and child during the early years of childhood.[61] Factors that

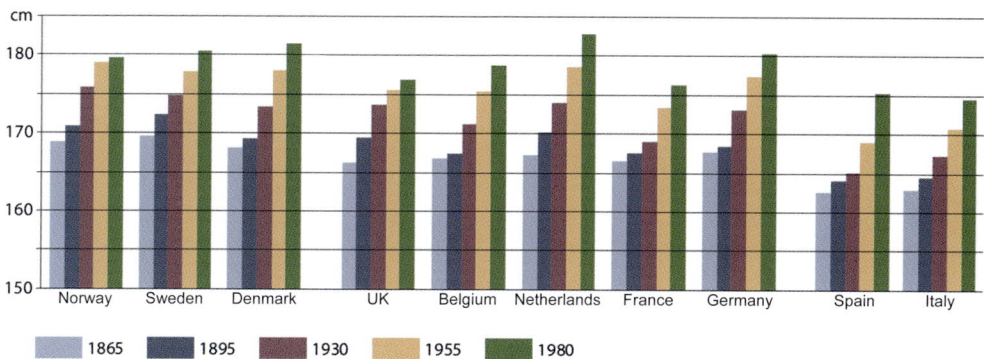

cm

Norway   Sweden   Denmark   UK   Belgium   Netherlands   France   Germany   Spain   Italy

1865   1895   1930   1955   1980

Fig. 40. Diagram showing the increased stature of men in some European countries during the last 150 years (based on data from T. J. Hatton 2013)

have been proved to influence living conditions are social class,[62] income and education,[63] environment (urban or rural) and family size,[64] which in turn can affect nutritional status and exposure to infectious diseases. Hence, stature is affected by a multitude of social factors, and may be used as a general indicator of the average living conditions in a society.[65] It is used today by WHO as a sensitive health indicator and a measure of the nutritional state within a population.[66]

Regarding the connection between stature and food intake, the nutritional composition is considered to be a more decisive factor than the amount of food. In general, there is a relationship between protein intake and stature, and particularly animal protein, fat, vitamin, essential fat and amino acids are vital substances concerning growth.[67] Studies of the population of Japan, which has undergone a marked increase in stature during the last 50 years, indicate that an important underlying cause to the observed increase in stature is a larger intake of animal protein and energy.[68] In this case it is particularly connected to an increased intake of milk products.[69] Also the marked increase in stature in Europe during the last century is considered a reflection of better living conditions, together with improved control of diseases and decreased infant mortality.[70] It has also been shown that it could not be explained by genetic evolution.[71]

In other words, the scientific community agree that changes in stature in a population are strongly linked to living conditions (lifestyle, health and welfare), and we may therefore use it as an indication also of living conditions in the past. In this section medieval stature will be discussed, and the focus will be on possible changes in living conditions in connection to the Black Death and the associated population drop.

Estimations of stature presented here are based on length measurements of femur (thigh bone) according to standard protocols.[72] Two different femur measures have been used – maximum length (M1) or physiological length (M2). To be able to compare all the materials, comparison is based on the estimated stature, not on the femur measurements.[73]

The skeleton data collected for this study derive from cemeteries in different environmental settings and from different periods of the Middle Ages (1050–1536). Some materials are older while others are younger, so that the total period covered by the study is *c.* 990–1620. From this period approximately 16,500 skeletons have been analysed and of these stature has been

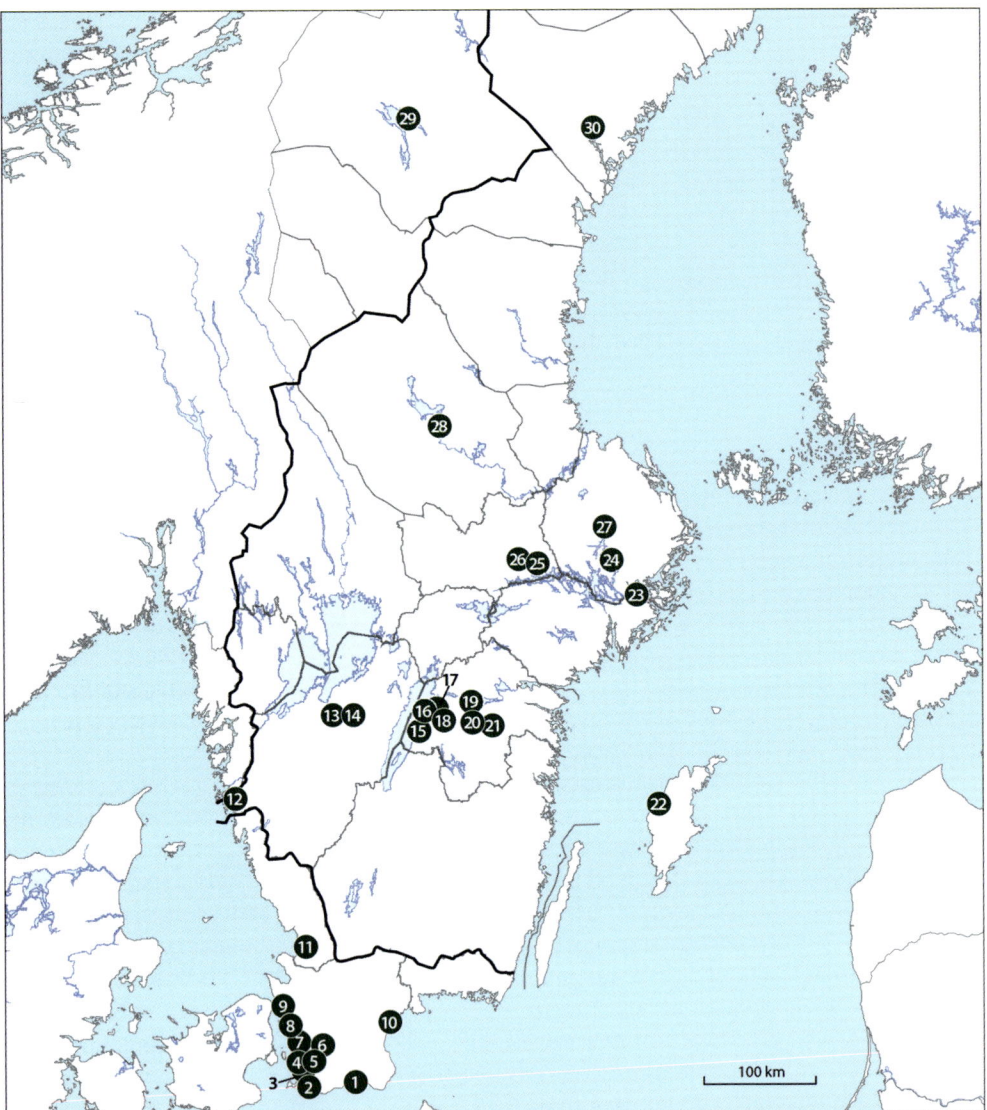

Fig. 41. Map of Sweden showing sites with osteological materials used in the present study. Numbers refer to Appendix 2.

estimated for 4876 adult individuals deriving from 65 different cemeteries. Geographically the cemeteries are distributed over a large part of present-day Sweden, from the province of Jämtland in the north to Scania in the south, and from Västergötland in the west to the Baltic island of Gotland in the east (Fig. 41). However, the majority are from Östergötland and Scania. These two provinces are today densely settled, and the high number of investigated cemeteries partly reflects the intensity of archaeological activity in connection to exploitation, but they were also the most heavily populated during the Middle Ages. All the cemeteries are from within the borders of present-day Sweden, but several of them are from provinces that belonged to Denmark during the Middle Ages (see Appendix 2 for details).

The major goal was to find materials to compare stature before and after the Black Death in 1350 and therefore chronology was essential. The different materials have been dated using different methods, such as dendrochronological dating of the coffins, radiocarbon dating, stratigraphy, the position of arms (which varies over time) and written sources. Many of the medieval cemeteries have been in use for several hundred years. For most of the cemeteries with such a long history, it has not been possible to make any fine chronological distinctions. Only at Trinitatis in Lund, which covers the time period 990–1536, have several different phases of the Middle Ages been distinguished within one and the same cemetery (see above).[74] It enables comparison between populations from the same area through time. In addition, cemeteries with a shorter history have been most valuable. Several of the medieval cemeteries were in use only before the Black Death, whereas others cover only the period *c.* 1300–1536. Very few new cemeteries were established after 1350. For the most part, the establishment of cemeteries reflects overall population development. When population numbers were drastically reduced after the Black Death there was no need to establish new cemeteries, not until a few centuries later when new towns were founded.

Hence, there are few medieval cemeteries that exclusively represent the period after 1350 and they are mainly from later periods. Some of them are from special circumstances, like the executed individuals buried at St Michael in Lund, the execution places like Slottsvången in Helsingborg and Galgberget in Vadstena, and the mass grave from the battle of Good Friday in Uppsala. There are also two ordinary cemeteries from after 1350 – St Gertrud in Visby and the Nya Lödöse cemetery.

Materials from Helgeandsholmen in Stockholm and St Jörgen in Malmö were initially regarded as post-Black Death materials based on previous publications.[75] However, the dating of the establishment of these two cemeteries is uncertain. Finds of several graves containing 2–5 individuals, which may be plague victims, indicate an establishment already by the time of the Black Death.

The material does not only represent different periods and different geographical areas, but also different social classes. Ordinary parish cemeteries can be expected to represent all social categories, whereas monasteries, convents, military mass graves, execution places, sanctuaries and hospitals reflect different parts of society (Appendix 2). In monasteries and convents many of the buried were monks or nuns, but the majority were wealthy people from outside.[76] The monastic orders represented are Dominican Black Friars and Cisterciensians. The monks and nuns of Dominican Black Friars survived through almsgiving and were not allowed to own property, while the Cisterciensians and Premonstratenser were landowners, sometimes with numerous farms and very large estates. The materials from the monasteries and convents span the whole period *c.* 1100–1536.

In the military mass graves are found professional soldiers but also peasants. Only occasionally, when they ended up in the grave wearing their armour, can professional soldiers be distinguished from other men.[77] Skeletons from execution places represent a mixture of individuals from different parts of society.[78] According to the written sources, 90% of those who were sentenced to death were convicted for murder, theft or adultery. But people who had committed suicide were also buried at the execution places. In cemeteries belonging

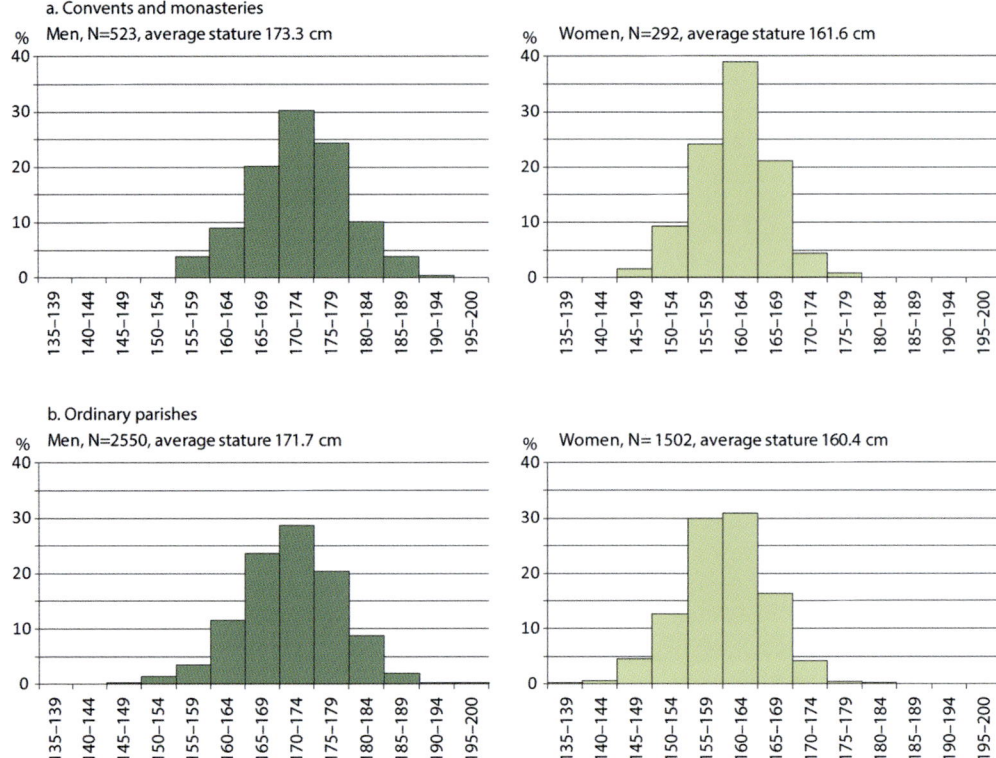

Fig. 42. Stature distribution of men and women from (a) convents and monasteries and (b) ordinary parishes

to sanctuaries and hospitals, finally, we find the sick who stayed at these institutions for medical treatment, but also elderly who used the sanctuaries as a place of retreatment.[79]

To test if different life conditions due to social status is reflected in stature, not only today but also in medieval populations, monasteries and convents were compared with ordinary parish cemeteries. It is known from written records that monastery and convent cemeteries were not only for the brothers and sisters, but particularly for people who could afford to buy a grave there. If these wealthy people had experienced better life conditions and eaten a more well-nourished diet than common people, it may be expected that they would be taller than average. The material from ordinary parishes consisted of 4052 individuals (1502 women and 2550 men) and the material from monasteries and convents of 815 individuals (292 women and 523 men). Interestingly, both women and men buried in monasteries and convents were significantly taller than those buried in the ordinary parish cemeteries. Mean values for women and men in monastery and convent cemeteries were 161.6 cm and 173.3 cm, whereas women and men in parish cemeteries measured 160.4 cm and 171.7 cm, respectively (Fig. 42; Table 1). The difference is significant for both women and men,[80] indicating that stature could be used as a parameter for social difference during the Middle Ages.

Table 1. Estimated stature for different populations and time periods

	Phase and population	n.	Min.	Max.	Mean	SD
Women	c. 1100–1536 monasteries, convents	292	141.7	178.3	161.6	5.4
Men	c. 1100–1536 monasteries, convents	523	155.2	191.1	173.3	6.1
Women	c. 990–1620 ordinary parishes	1502	181.2	138.8	160.4	6.0
Men	c. 990–1620 ordinary parishes	2550	199.9	145.1	171.7	6.8
Women	c. 980–1350 all populations	727	138.8	181.2	160.2	6.1
Men	c. 980–1350 all populations	1408	147.9	192.0	171.5	6.4
Women	c. 1350–1620 all populations	53	154.1	173.6	162,7	4.6
Men	c. 1350–1620 all populations	126	156.2	199.9	172.5	6.6
Women	c. 990–1350 Trinitatis in Lund	321	138.8	179.4	160.7	5.7
Men	c. 990–1350 Trinitatis in Lund	428	151.5	192.0	172.0	6.8
Women	c. 1350–1536 Trinitatis in Lund	31	154.1	168.3	161.2	3.7
Men	c. 1350–1536 Trinitatis in Lund	31	156.2	199.9	170.8	8.7
Men	1361 Battle of Visby	366	157.5	189.9	172.0	6.3
Men	1520 Battle of Good Friday	34	163.0	185.7	173.6	5.8

Several authors have argued that living conditions improved after the Black Death.[81] There may have been several reasons for this. One may simply be that the most poor and under-nourished died from the plague. The most common explanation, however, is that the smaller population resulted in a shortage of labour, which after a period of conflicts and resistance resulted in higher wages and lower rents and taxes. This resulted in higher popular consumption and better living conditions for the majority of ordinary people. According to another line of reasoning, the shortage of manpower and excess of land in agriculture after the population drop resulted in a gradual shift from crop growing to animal husbandry.[82] The pollen record presented in Chapter 4 indicated that such a shift actually happened, at least in marginal uplands. An expected consequence of increased animal production would be an increased consumption of meat and milk products. However, documentary sources provide very little information on the consumption of food among ordinary people in medieval Sweden.

If living conditions improved after the Black Death and if the consumption of meat and milk products increased, it may show up in stature. To test this it is important to distinguish between population from before and after the Black Death. Of the 65 cemeteries (also including execution places and military mass-graves), 24 (39%) were in use only before the Black Death and seven (11%) only after. From the first group stature has been calculated for 727 women and 1408 men, and from the second and much smaller group, for 53 women and 126 men. Based on these populations, mean stature for women was 160.2 cm before the Black Death and 162.7 cm after. For men mean stature was 171.5 cm before the Black Death and 172.5 cm after (Fig. 43; Table 1). Hence, both women and men show a slight increase in stature after the Black Death, but only for women is the change statistically significant.[83]

Apart from changes in mean stature, the frequency of really tall individuals – that is to say women taller than 170 cm and men taller than 180 cm – was also higher after the Black Death. The relative number of tall women increased from 3.9% to 9.4%, whereas the relative number of tall men increased from 8.9% to 12.7%.

It can be concluded that there was no decrease in stature after the Black Death, and therefore no indication that living conditions got worse. On the contrary, there was an

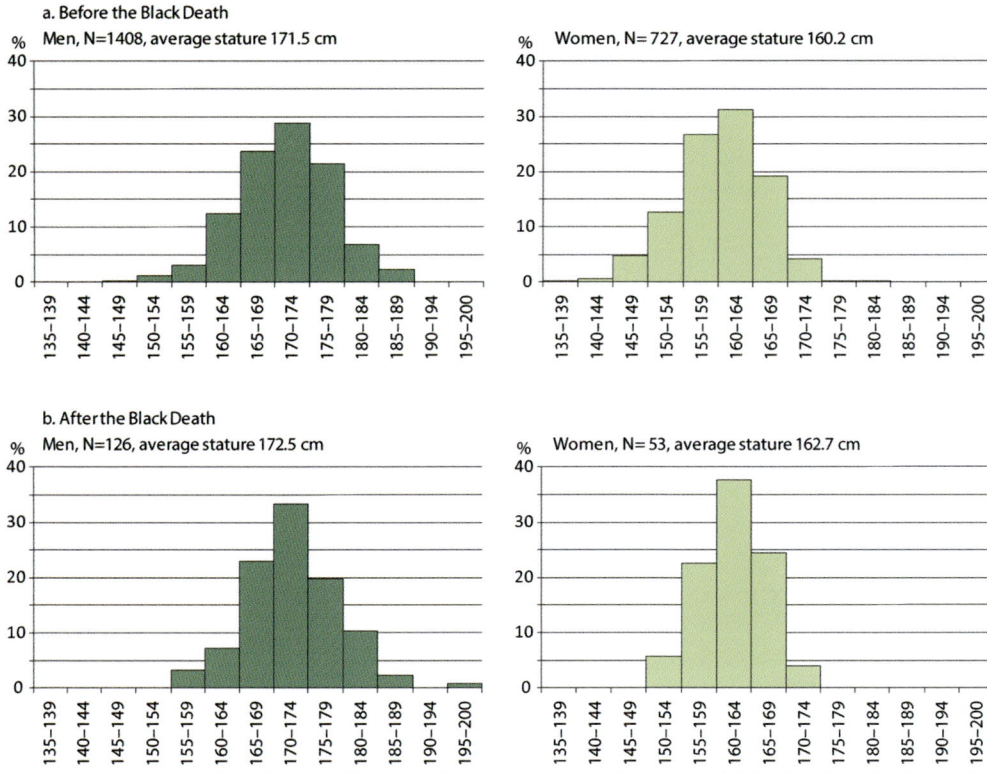

Figure 43. Stature distribution of men and women from (a) before and (b) after the Black Death

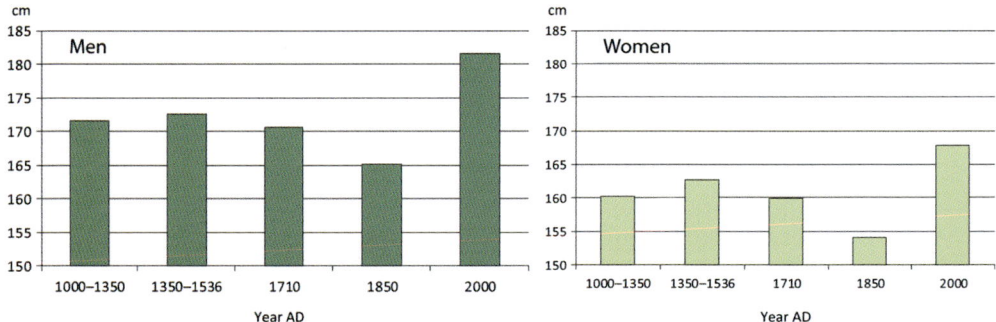

Fig. 44. Diagrams showing changes in mean stature for men and women in Sweden 1000–2000. Medieval stature before and after the Black Death is based on the present study, 1710 stature is based on a skeletal plague material published by Arcini et al. (2006), 1850 stature is based on measurements on living population (Hultkrantz 1927) and so is present-day stature (Gustafsson et al. 2007)

increase in stature indicating improved living conditions, although the change is statistically significant only for women. Also the number of very tall increased, both among women and men. A limitation is the rather small sample after the Black Death.

A similar comparison of stature was made based on only the material from Trinitatis in Lund. In this cemetery a tentative distinction has been made between graves from before and after the Black Death (see Fig. 36). According to this distinction, mean stature for women was 160.7 cm before the Black Death and 161.2 cm after, hence a small increase. However, mean stature for men decreased from 172.0 cm to 170.8 cm (Table 1). None of the changes is statistically significant.[84] When looking at the relative number of very tall people, contrary to the result from the larger study, they became fewer in the Trinitatis material after the Black Death. However, the tallest man in the entire material is one individual from after the Black Death in Trinitatis. He measured 199.9 cm.

The fact that stature seems to have increased more for women than for men – both in the total material and in the material from Lund – indicates that the height difference between the sexes was reduced after the Black Death. Possibly women in particular benefited from improved living conditions.

Two other populations that may be compared are the two military mass graves. The majority of those who died in the Battle of Visby were ordinary farmers from the island of Gotland and some were Danish soldiers. The battle took place in the summer 1361, which means that they must have been born and raised before 1350. Possibly they were stronger and better fed than average because they had obviously survived the Black Death as well as the plague of 1359–60. The Battle of Good Friday in Uppsala took place in 1521. In this case also there were both farmers and professional soldiers among the dead. They were born around the turn of the century, 1500, after the nadir of the late-medieval crisis in a time when society had slowly started to recover. These two military mass graves represent two comparable groups of men born and raised before and after the Black Death.

The mean stature for men who died in the Battle of Visby was 172.0 cm and 9% of them were taller than 180 cm (Table 1). The men who died in the Battle of Good Friday show a mean stature of 173.6 cm and 14.7% of them were taller than 180 cm. Hence, the comparison shows that the later population was slightly taller, but again the difference is not statistically significant.[85] However, this is yet another indication that there was a slight increase in stature after the Black Death.

The new results on medieval stature are put in a longer time perspective in Figure 44. As evident from the figure, the increase in stature after the Black Death was only temporary. After the end of the Middle Ages, stature started to decrease again to reach a low-point in the mid-nineteenth century, before it increased strongly during the twentieth century. The long-term development was similar for men and women.

Changes in diet?

Written sources indicate that the supply of food products may have changed after the Black Death. As mentioned above, agricultural production changed not only in quantity but also in composition and in particular animal husbandry seems to have increased in importance, at least in some regions.[86] However, written sources on food habits are restricted to monasteries, convents and the ruling classes of society. If we want to study food consumption among ordinary people and to look for possible changes in diet other methods have to be used.

During the last decades new methods have made it possible to study the palaeodiet of individuals by stable isotope analysis.

Stable isotope analysis for palaeodietary reconstruction is based on the principle that the isotope composition in body tissues of both animals and humans reflects the isotopic composition of the food they have eaten. In the present study the isotope compositions of carbon and nitrogen have been measured, which are particularly useful in this context.[87] For carbon, $\delta^{13}C$ (the ratio between ^{13}C and ^{12}C expressed in ‰) reflects the relative amount of proteins from marine food sources (marine fish, shellfish, seals, seabirds) in comparison to terrestrial. For nitrogen, $\delta^{15}N$ (the ratio between ^{15}N and ^{14}N expressed in ‰) reflects the relative amount of proteins from animal products (meat, milk products, eggs, fish, shellfish) in comparison to plant products (vegetables, cereals, beer, etc.). However, different types of plants may also result in different $\delta^{15}N$. Furthermore, when it comes to animal products, $\delta^{15}N$ is affected by the trophic level, i.e. the position in the food chain, so that food derived from higher trophic levels results in higher $\delta^{15}N$ in human tissue.[88] Other factors may also influence the isotope values.[89] When interpreted in relation to the isotopic signatures of available food sources, the combination of carbon and nitrogen isotope ratios in archaeological bone provides a proxy of the diet of an individual. It is important to note, however, that it reflects only the main protein sources and not the diet as a whole.[90]

For this study the material from the Trinitatis cemetery in Lund, dated to 990–1536, was chosen, which allows a comparison before and after the Black Death. The study is based on teeth from 99 adult individuals representing five different phases of the Middle Ages (Appendix 3).[91] In the selection of individuals for sampling, three criterions had to be fulfilled: well-preserved teeth (first molar, incisive and second molar), femur length measurements and sex identification. To also investigate the possible relationship between dietary composition and stature in the studied population, the skeletons of the longest and shortest individuals that fulfilled these three criteria were also selected for analysis. By using teeth the diet signal of the child is caught, which is important since diet during childhood affects adult stature. The results are presented for the 99 individuals (46 men and 53 women) in Appendix 3.

The stable isotope values in the whole material irrespective of time period range for $\delta^{13}C$ from -22.3‰ to -18.7‰ (average -19.9%) and for $\delta^{15}N$ values from 8.1‰ to 14.6‰ (average 11.6‰). The results indicate that nearly two-thirds of the individuals acquired a certain part of their nutrition from the sea. The distance between Lund and the coast was not far and findings of fishing gear in the oldest settlement of the town indicate that fish may have been brought to the city with fishermen who lived there.[92] Osteological analyses of fishbone from Lund show that consumed fish consisted mainly of cod, although herring dominated during some periods and also flounder was common from time to time. Freshwater or brackish-water fish, with few exceptions, was not on the menu very often, but when it did it consisted of roach, perch and pike.[93]

A closer look at the results from the different periods indicates clearly that there was a change in diet. However, this change did not happen when might be expected, i.e. in connection with the Black Death, but some centuries earlier, around 1100. As evident from the diagrams in Figure 45, there are several individuals with very low nitrogen values from the period 990–1100, but not from later periods. No less than one-third of the individuals from the early period display $\delta^{15}N$ values between 8.1‰ and 9.8‰. Depending on these low values, the average $\delta^{15}N$ value for that period is only 10.5‰. It is significantly separated from the later phases of the Middle Ages,[94] which show average δ^{15}N values between 11.9 ‰ and 12.2‰. However, the early period shows a great variety of values and one third of the individuals have relatively high nitrogen values, between 11.0 and 14.0.

How then should the different nitrogen values from Lund be interpreted in terms of diet composition and possible change in diet? The individuals with low nitrogen isotope values in the early period (990–1100) probably had a diet based primarily on cereals. A similar pattern, with unusually low nitrogen isotope values in an early phase of the town, was noted also in the medieval town of Sigtuna, in the province of Uppland. In that case also the low values were interpreted as an indication of a high relative input of cereals and vegetables.[95] A closer look at the material from Lund reveals that all the individuals with low nitrogen values were buried in a peripheral part of the cemetery, and the burial custom indicates that they had something in common as a group.[96] Because the peripheral part of the cemetery during the Middle Ages was generally reserved for the poor, the low nitrogen values probably reflect low social status. The buried individuals may have been slaves or other poor people with a lower consumption of meat than other social groups.[97] Hence, the great variety in isotope values in the earliest phase of Lund may reflect strong social stratification. The increase of mean nitrogen isotope values after 1100 reflects an average increase in the relative intake of meat or other animal products. This change was probably due to the disappearance of the very poor and may hypothetically be associated with the gradual termination of slavery.

The observed variation in diet is however not reflected in stature. In Figure 46, δ^{15}N‰ is plotted against femur length, where δ^{15}N‰ is used as a proxy for the relative amount of animal proteins in the diet and femur length as a proxy for stature. The two parameters show no correlation. This may be explained by the fact that also other living conditions than diet affects stature, and that δ^{15}N‰ does not catch all the dietary factors of importance. For instance, even though it reflects the protein composition, it says nothing about the amount of protein intake, or for that matter the amount of food.

Migration and stature

The medieval town of Lund was, like many other urban centres, a magnet that attracted people from different places. The intensity of migration has of course varied over time for various reasons. To test if observed variations in stature could be related to migration, it was decided to examine mobility as another characteristic of the population. The aim was to see if migration to the town changed over time and specifically following the Black Death when cities were likely in need of labour. Strontium isotope ratios in tooth enamel were used to investigate this question.

Isotopic ratio of strontium has been used in a number of studies for proveniencing human remains. The isotope ratio of interest is ^{87}Sr/^{86}Sr. The basic principles are straightforward. ^{87}Sr/^{86}Sr varies among different types of rock and enters the human body through the food chain as nutrients pass from bedrock through soil and water to plants and animals. Strontium substitutes for calcium in the hydroxyapatite mineral of skeletal tissue and is stored there. Human tooth enamel forms during the first years of life and remains unchanged during life

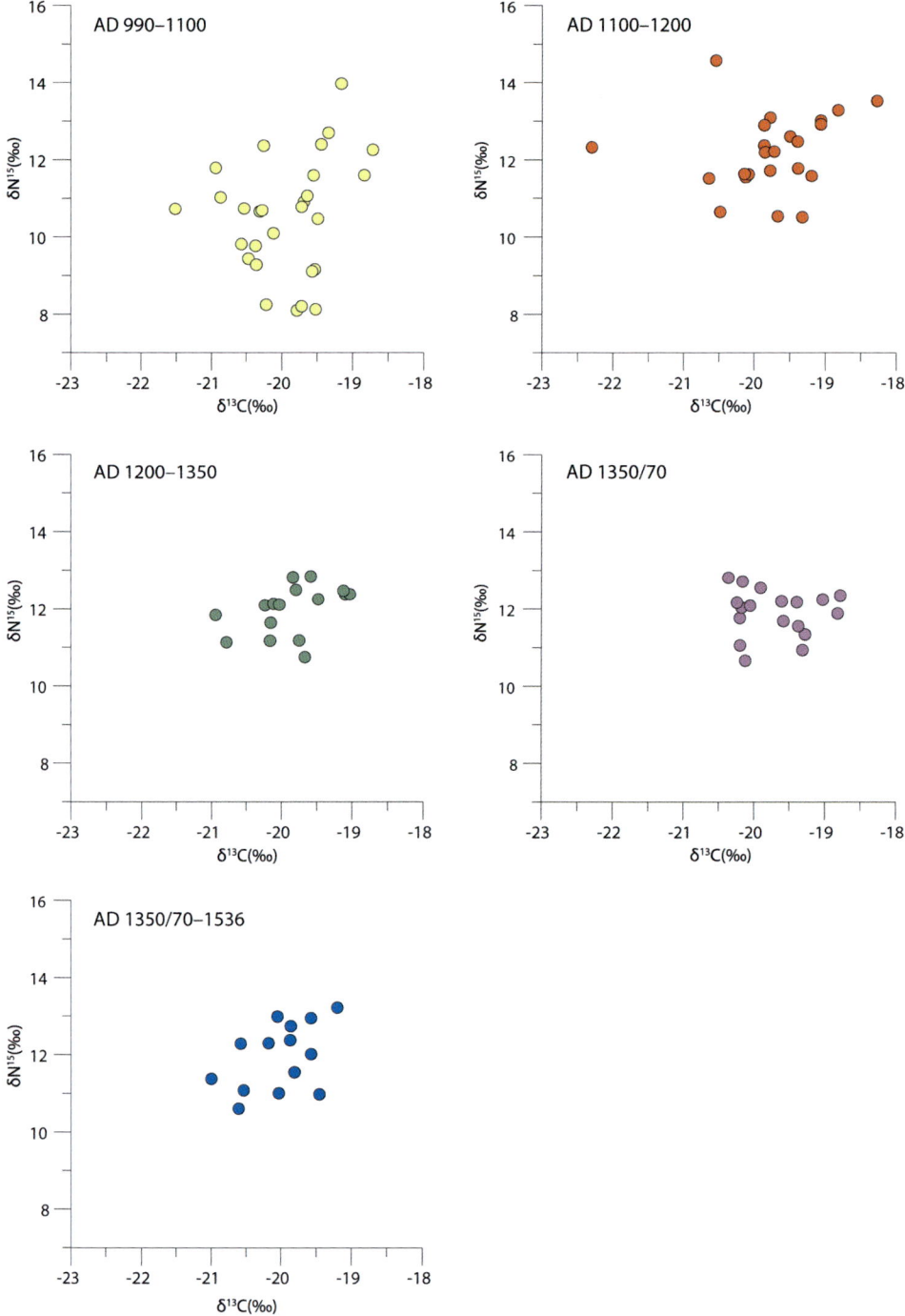

Fig. 45. Carbon and nitrogen isotopic ratios for humans in medieval Lund (Trinitatis Cemetery) during different time periods. AD 1350/70 includes possible Black Death victims

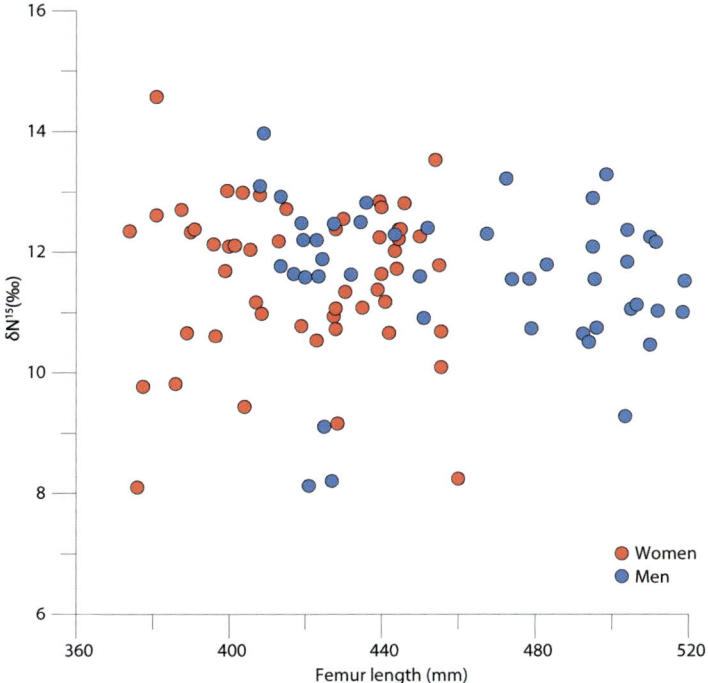

Fig. 46. Nitrogen isotopic ratios and femur length for men and women in Lund during the Middle Ages. No correlation between the two parameters was found

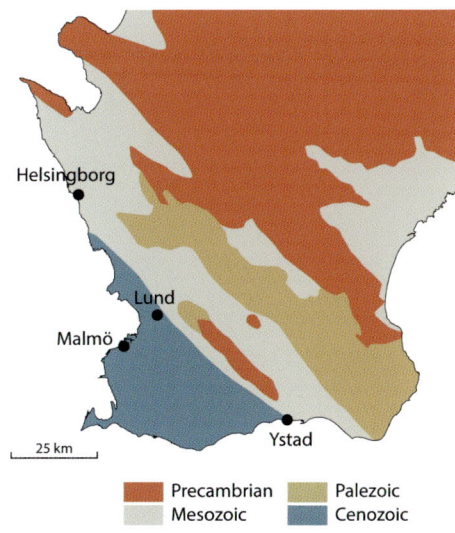

Fig. 47. Bedrock map of the province of Scania

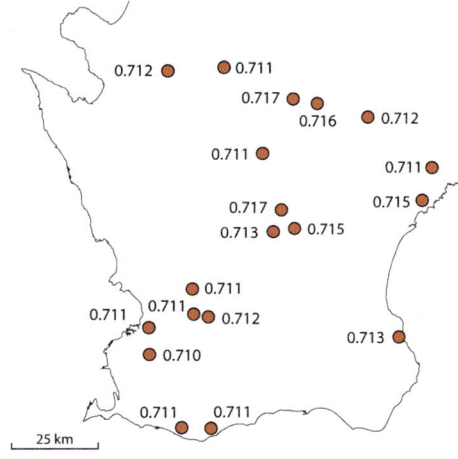

Fig. 48. Map of Scania with $^{87}Sr/^{86}Sr$ baseline values from archaeological studies. Values between 0.710 and 0.711 are mainly found in south-western Scania and values above 0.712 are rare

and often long after death. Isotopes of certain elements (strontium, lead, oxygen) vary in amounts according to geography and are deposited in tooth enamel as it forms. Thus, tooth enamel retains an isotopic signal of the place of birth. If that signal differs from the place of burial, then the individual must have moved during his/her lifetime. The application of strontium isotopes in a variety of archaeological settings has revealed significant movement in the past.[98]

[87]Sr represents approximately 7% of total strontium in nature and [86]Sr around 10%. Thus, the measured [87]Sr/[86]Sr ratio has a value in nature between approximately 0.703 and 0.750, and sometimes higher. While the range of these numbers may seem small, [87]Sr/[86]Sr ratios can be measured very accurately to the sixth decimal place and have been used by geologists for many years to characterise and date rock formations. These isotopic ratios work well for identifying non-local individuals in a population but identifying the place of origin is more difficult because similar isotopic ratios are often found in a number of locations.

Although a potential complication of strontium isotope analysis in bioarchaeology is post-burial contamination (diagenesis), tooth enamel is generally resistant to diagenesis and may be relatively well preserved even when bones are contaminated.[99] In any case, a non-local isotopic signature is always significant because 'contamination' is a local signal. Hence, diagenesis does not result in the misidentification of locals as immigrants. It is also important to note that the analysis can distinguish only first generation migrants, not their offspring. In a community occupied for several generations, only a small proportion of the individuals in a cemetery might be from the first generation.

An essential issue in strontium isotope analysis involves determination of the local strontium isotope signal for the area in which a burial is found. Measurement of these baseline values is essential for identifying non-local individuals.[100] The local bioavailable isotopic signal of the place of burial can be determined in several ways: in human bone from the individuals whose teeth are analysed, from the bones of other humans or archaeological fauna at the site, or from modern fauna, water, soil extracts or vegetation in the vicinity.[101]

The province of Scania has varied bedrock, characterised by old granites and gneisses in the north and east, and much younger bedrock primarily composed of marine sediments such as limestone and chalk in the southwest (Fig. 47). The bedrock has varied strontium composition, which is reflected in bone material from archaeological sites. Information is available from several archaeological studies of strontium isotope ratios in southern Sweden,[102] and the data from Scania are summarised in Fig. 48. In general values between 0.710 and 0.711 are found in southwestern Scania and range somewhat higher to the north and east. Values above 0.712 are rare.

Bioavailable samples from cattle and pig tooth enamel have also been examined from the nearby site of Uppåkra,[103] located about 5 km south of Lund. There are slight differences between the two species. The mean value for 14 cattle teeth was 0.7118 ± 0.0009 with a range 0.7097–0.7134. The mean value for six pigs was 0.7115 ± 0.0002 with a range 0.7113–0.7118. The very low variance for the pigs suggests that this range of values likely reflects the local value at Uppåkra. The variation among the cattle, particularly one very low and two very high values, suggests that some of these animals were imported. Finally measurements from two faunal samples from Lund itself were used – archaeological specimens of black rats – with [87]Sr/[86]Sr values of 0.7112.

In order to examine changes in mobility over time, burials were sampled from the parish cemetery of Trinitatis, presented above. Strontium isotope ratios were measured in tooth enamel from 74 adult individuals (36 male and 38 female),[104] and these values had a mean of 0.7116 (±0.002) with a range 0.7082–0.7191 (Appendix 3). The strontium isotope ratio results are presented in a rank-ordered bar graph in Figure 49. The local baseline appears quite clear in this graph and includes all the individuals with values between 0.710 and 0.712. Approximately 37% of the analysed individuals are indicated as non-locals, with 11/74 below 0.710 and 17/74 above 0.712. The variation in $^{87}Sr/^{86}Sr$ values indicates that non-local individuals came from several different places. A kernel density plot[105] clearly shows this multi-modality in the values (Fig. 50). Kernel density estimates are a data smoothing technique that reduces the problem of interval size in standard histograms.[106] The plot shows a primary mode between 0.710 and 0.712 within the local range. A slightly lower mode below 0.710 may represent individuals from elsewhere in southwestern Scania, Denmark, or northern Germany. The small modes above 0.712 reflect individuals from a variety of different places in the older geological terrain elsewhere in Sweden or northern Scandinavia.

Regarding changes in mobility over time, the highest rate of non-locals appears in the earliest period of the history of Lund, the establishment phase (Fig. 51). That greater variation in strontium isotope ratios occurred during the earliest period of the city is not surprising. Lund was founded in the late 900s during the reign of King Sven Forkbeard on a royal initiative to serve as an administrative and religious centre for eastern Denmark. It was populated by priests, administrators, soldiers, merchants, and workmen of all kinds – minters, artisans, goldsmiths, blacksmiths, comb makers, shoemakers and slaves. Burial customs like different types of coffins, charcoal, and chalk in the graves, finds of coins as well as written sources indicate that among the buried were men and women from England, Germany, the Slavic area and of course parts of present-day Denmark.[107]

Variation then declined and of particular note is the absence of non-locals during the period of the Black Death, from 1350 to 1370. A medieval town like Lund usually harboured people from both far and near. Most of them were temporary visitors who came there for trade. The strontium results indicate that this exchange with a wider surrounding broke down during the plague. At the same time we see that Lund in the period after the Black Death once again exhibited increased immigration and that the contacts with a wider world were resumed. Perhaps it indicates that the city had need for labour in the wake of the plague.

Lessons from the last plague 1710–1713

In Sweden there are few written sources from the time of the Black Death but more plentiful records from later plague epidemics. Particularly from the last plague of 1710–1713 there are detailed records that shed light on how plague spread and how the local society reacted. The most useful records are church books containing information about when the plague appeared in the parish, how many died, and sometimes also the sex and age of the diseased. They also provide data on the number of births and marriages.[108]

The last plague may tentatively be used as a reference for the Black Death. There are several reasons for this. In the early eighteenth century, when Sweden was struck by the plague for the last time, the country was not much more densely populated than at the time

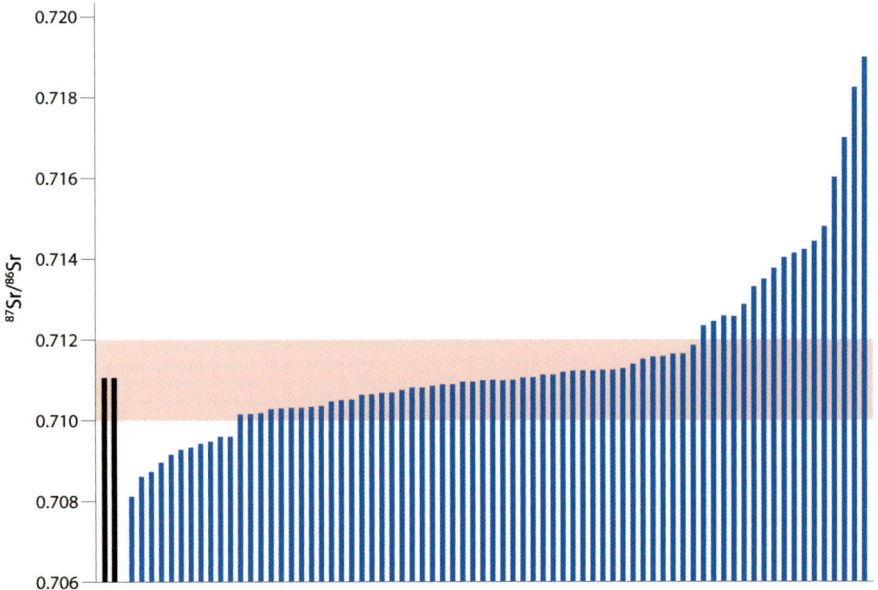

Fig. 49. Ranked $^{87}Sr/^{86}Sr$ *values of two fauna samples (black) and 77 human samples (blue) from Lund. Red band marks the estimated local baseline range at Lund. The human samples are from the Trinitatis Cemetery*

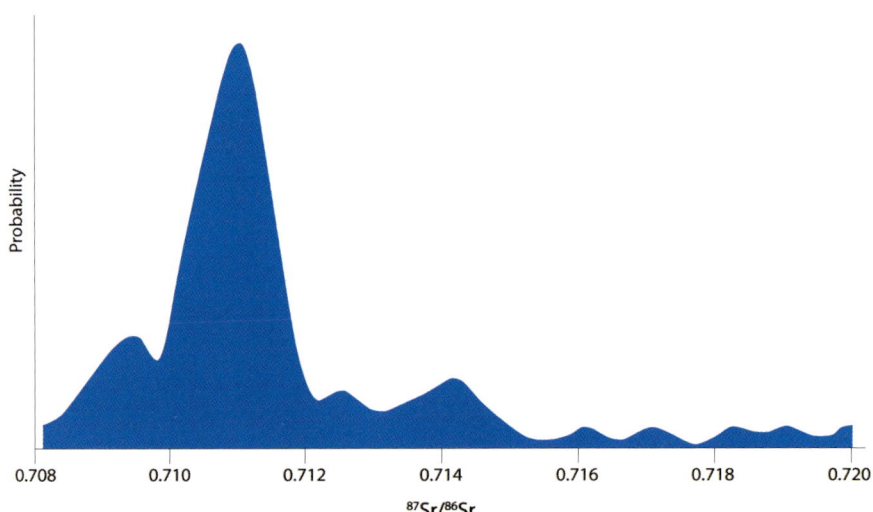

Fig. 50. The Kernel Density plot of $^{87}Sr/^{86}Sr$ *values from human tooth enamel from Lund shows a primary mode between 0.710 and 0.712 within the local range. A slightly lower mode below 0.710 may represent individuals from elsewhere in south-western Scania, Denmark, or northern Germany. The small modes above 0.712 reflect one or a few individuals from a variety of different places in the older geological terrain elsewhere in Sweden or northern Scandinavia*

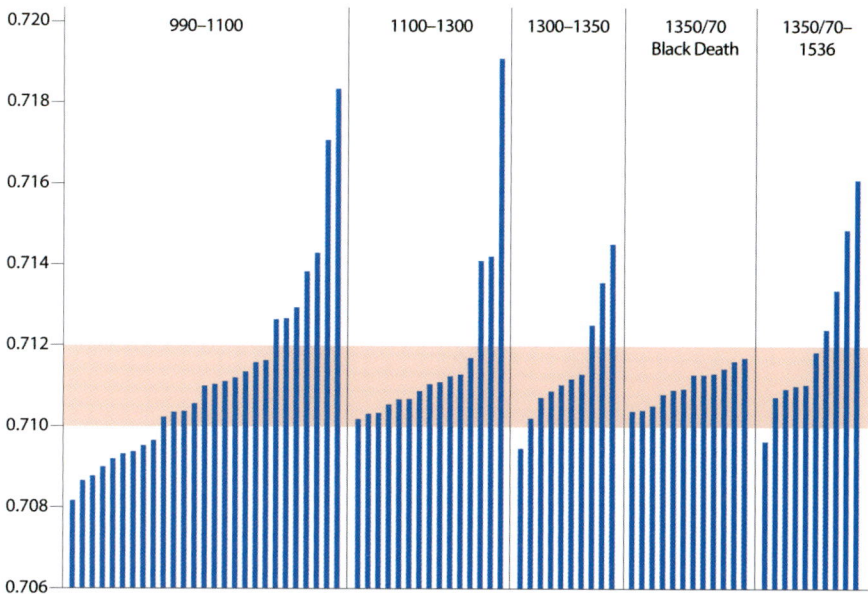

Fig. 51. Strontium isotope ratios from Lund ranked by time period. Red band marks the estimated local baseline range at Lund

of the Black Death in the middle of the fourteenth century. In the area covered by present-day Sweden, the population in the mid-fourteenth century before the Black Death and in the beginning of the eighteenth century was approximately 1.1 million and 1.4 million, respectively.[109] In the early eighteenth century the majority of the population still lived in rural areas. Furthermore, agricultural systems were not very different from the medieval ones.

The most important difference between the fourteenth century and the early eighteenth century was the very different preparedness to plague. When the Black Death struck Sweden in the fourteenth century there were only religious precautions. In letters to the dioceses in the autumn of 1349, Magnus Eriksson, king of Norway and Sweden, warned of a disease with great mortality that was approaching Sweden.[110] King Magnus dictated that all the people of Sweden, clerks and lay people, old and young, women and men should every Friday come barefoot to the church, hear the mass and on the alter sacrifice a coin (a penning) or less according to ability. Everyone should fast every Friday on bread and water, not even eat fish, lean their conscience and humbly do penance and repent of their sins. He hoped that this would make God turn the plague from them. When the last plague struck in the early eighteenth century, it was no longer seen only as a divine punishment for human sin, but as a phenomenon that could be prevented and limited by human countermeasures. Sweden had experienced several plague epidemics since the devastating Black Death and now authorities were more on guard and regulations were more developed. However, in spite of the better preparedness, 200,000 Swedish citizens died.

In southern Europe regulations intended to stop the plague were established earlier than in Sweden, in some places already in connection with the Black Death. In 1348 special health commissions were established in the Italian cities of Venice and Florence, and in Ragusa (present-day Dubrovnik) 30 days of quarantine for incoming ships was stated in 1377.[111] In 1370 the authorities of Milan and Mantua prohibited all contact with areas that were contaminated by the Black Death,[112] and from later plagues in the fifteenth and seventeenth century they imposed health passports in order to stop the rampage of the disease.[113] Sometimes these countermeasures were taken too late, when local authorities tried to deny and underplay the arrival of plague in their town.[114] In Sweden the earliest evidence of quarantine regulations are from a plague epidemic in 1577, and in 1638 the death penalty was imposed on those who broke the isolation rules.[115] In Denmark the first regulations intended to protect the population from plague came in the second half of the sixteenth century.[116]

However, in her study of the plague in Scania 1710–1713, Bodil Persson showed that despite proclamations and rules from the authorities, people continued to gather at burials and in houses where people had died of plague, to mourn the diseased and to share the belongings. Also during times of plague, people gathered not only for burials but also for other religious traditions like marriage and baptism.[117] Obviously, new regulations could not easily change deeply rooted cultural behaviour, customs and traditions. When authorities, in November 1710, declared that plague victims should no longer be buried in the ordinary cemeteries but in special places far away, people refused to accept it. Priests were threatened by their parishioners and forced to break the regulations, and in some cases relatives dug up their dead and dragged them in to the graveyards.[118] To get a decent burial on sacred ground was as important in the eighteenth century as it was during the Middle Ages.[119]

Finally, a closer look can be taken at some aspects of the last plague in the province of Östergötland. From this province more than 80% of the parishes have preserved church books that provide relatively detailed information on the plague years of 1710–11. They represent both densely populated agricultural plains and more sparsely populated woodlands. The church books reveal that the first case of plague in Östergötland was seen in the parish of Lönsås on 23 September, 1710, and already within a month the plague had reached several other parishes both far away and nearby (Fig. 52). One year later, by the end of 1711, 89% of the parishes had been affected (Fig. 53).[120] Some parishes were hit hard, others not so hard and some appear not to have been affected by the plague at all. As an estimate of how severely the plague ravaged the different parishes the Crises Mortality Ratio (CMR) has been used, which is frequently used to identify mortality crises in a population.[121] It measures the mortality in a year of crisis in proportion to the average mortality of normal years. Mortality 3× times higher than normal (CMR>3) is defined as a demographic crisis, whereas mortality more than 15× higher than normal (CMR>15) is a demographic catastrophe.[122] According to these criteria the plague resulted in a demographic crisis in 66%[123] of the parishes of Östergötland and in 3.6% of them it reached a demographic catastrophe (Fig. 54).[124]

Hence, in spite of a better preparedness, the plague of 1710–13 hit parts of Sweden hard. Plague was still a deadly disease that was very difficult to stop, partly due to the unwillingness among the general public to change deeply-rooted customs and traditions. Similar religious traditions were probably important also for the transmission and spread of the Black Death. Although devastating in some areas, the last plague did not reach all parts of Sweden and at a local scale it showed a mosaic pattern of spread. This is evident from Östergötland, where even neighbouring parishes suffered to very different degree. The local variation may be due to chance, but also to different precautions taken by the parishioners. If the Black Death also showed this spatial variation at a local scale is not known.

In Östergötland, the agricultural lowlands, characterised by relatively small and densely populated parishes, appears to have been struck harder than the forested uplands by the last plague (Figs 53 and 54). There are several exceptions – some upland parishes were affected whereas some parishes on the plains were not affected at all – but in general the central lowlands were most hardly hit. This was also the case in Scania.[125] Probably the plague could spread more easily in the lowlands, where population density was higher and the settlement pattern was characterised by hamlets and villages. However, it is important to note that also several sparsely populated parishes in the uplands, where single farms dominated, were hit by the plague.

Little is known about migration, both during the last plague and during earlier outbreaks. It is likely that all plagues resulted in social reorganisation, remarriages, etc., which involved moving to new farms and settling in new areas. For the Black Death the large-scale farm abandonment in marginal uplands may to some degree reflect such migration, when people moved to better holdings in the more fertile lowlands.[126] The last plague gives some support to such an interpretation, by indicating that the plague hit the agricultural plains somewhat harder than the uplands. However, the high mortality rates of some upland parishes show that the plague sometimes also reached remote farms in the woods.

The church books from Östergötland also give interesting insights into recovery after the plague. For 20 randomly selected parishes the annual numbers of deaths and births have been used to estimate the time it took to reach pre-plague population numbers. The calculations are based on the relationship between deaths and births only, and take no heed of the possible influence of migration, which is not known. The results show that birth rates increased soon after the arrival of the plague in 1710–11, and already in 1720, population numbers were back at pre-plague levels in 76% of the 21 parishes (Fig. 55). However, in some parishes recovery took longer. In Bjälbo the population reached pre-plague levels in 1723, in Kaga in 1728, and in Sya and Väderstad in 1730. The parish of Skänninge had almost recovered in 1734 when mortality suddenly peaked again, probably due to some other epidemic disease, and the same happened in 1743. It did not reach pre-plague population number until 1750 (Fig. 55). Even though plague did not return to Sweden after the outbreaks of 1710–13, there were several different diseases that could lead to increased mortality. The most serious ones were smallpox, typhus, measles, dysentery and whooping cough.

However, even though different diseases and other difficulties may have added to the problems and delayed the recovery, Figure 55 shows a clear relationship between Crisis Mortality Ratio and recovery time. All the parishes with a CMR lower than 3 recovered within less than 5 years, whereas the parish with the highest CMR needed the longest time to recover. During the Middle Ages, recurring outbreaks of plague together with different social factors may have delayed recovery after the Black Death, but the most important factor behind the very long time needed to recover was probably an exceptionally high mortality ratio.

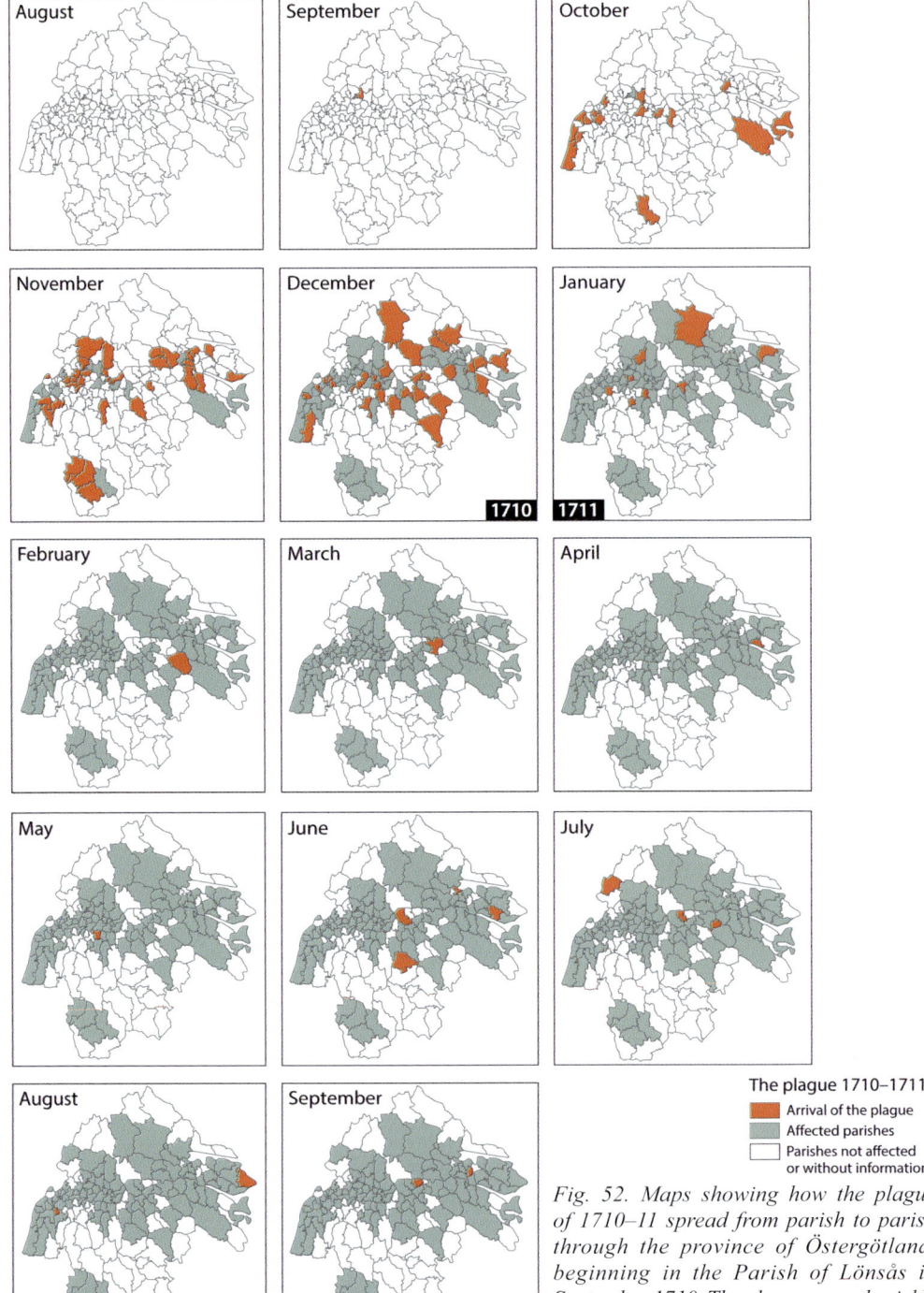

Fig. 52. Maps showing how the plague of 1710–11 spread from parish to parish through the province of Östergötland, beginning in the Parish of Lönsås in September 1710. The plague spread quickly in October, November and December

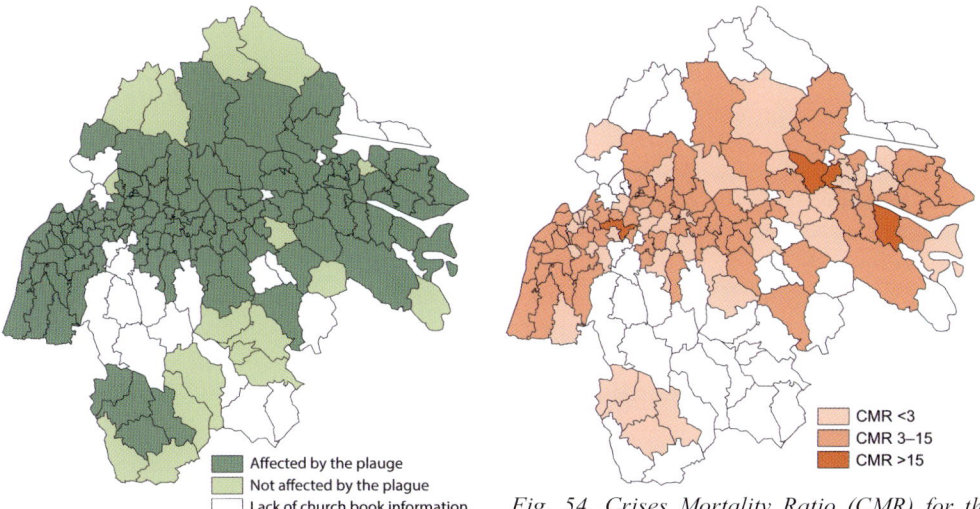

Fig. 53. Parishes affected by plague 1710–11 in the province of Östergötland

Fig. 54. Crises Mortality Ratio (CMR) for the different parishes of Östergötland in connection to the plague 1710–11

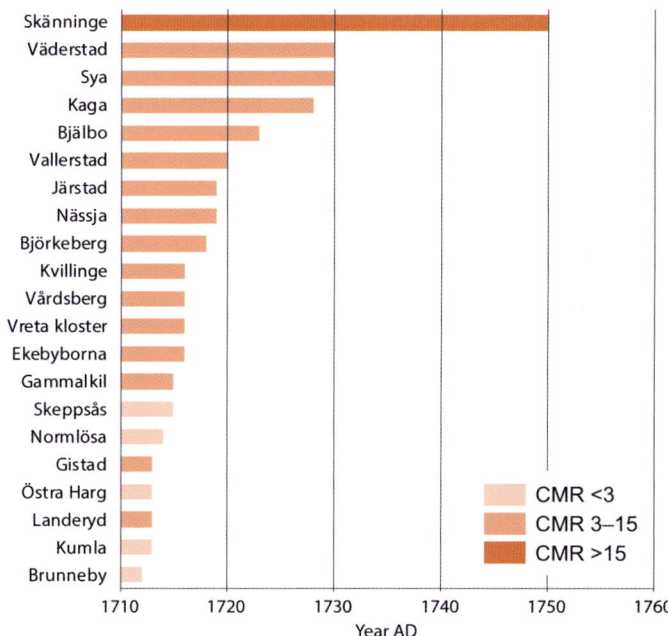

Fig. 55. Diagram showing the time needed for population recovery in some parishes of Östergötland after the plague of 1710–11. Bars show the number of years needed before population numbers were back at the same level as before the plague. By 1720 76% of the parishes had recovered and some of them already after a few years. Others took longer to recover. Skänninge, which had experienced a demographic catastrophe in connection to the plague and also was hit by other epidemics, took 40 years to recover

Conclusions

The higher density of graves and the increased numbers of multiple graves in layers from the Late Middle Ages at ordinary cemeteries are here interpreted as a reflection of the Black Death and recurring plague outbreaks in the late fourteenth century. This observation, together with the absence of any documented mass graves, indicates that the majority of the plague victims were buried in the ordinary cemeteries. If so it tells us that, even though mortality was high, the dead were taken care of according to the existing customs and practices as far as ever possible.

The hypothesis that living conditions improved after the Black Death was tested by means of changes in stature estimated from skeleton material. The results showed that people born after the Black Death were taller than earlier generations, which indicates improved living conditions. However, the change was small and only statistically significant for women.

One aspect of living conditions that may be particularly decisive for stature is diet. Stable isotope analysis of carbon and nitrogen was used to investigate the intake of animal proteins among a medieval population in Lund. The results indicated increased intake of animal proteins like meat and milk products around 1100, but no noticeable change after that. Hence, the results indicated no difference in diet before and after the Black Death in the population studied. The largely vegetarian diet of some individuals before 1100 may be associated with low social status.

Strontium isotope analysis of the Lund population indicated a high rate of non-locals in the earliest phase of the medieval town, before 1100. Variation decreased after that and of particular interest is the absence of non-locals during the brief period of the Black Death, from 1350 to 1370. It indicates that the ordinary exchange of temporary visitors paused during the plague.

Written documents from the last plague in Sweden 1710–13 were used as a reference to the Black Death. The last plague resulted in a population drop in Sweden of approximately 15% on average but in the studied province of Östergötland of as much as one-third. There was great spatial variation, both on a regional and local scale. Even neighbouring parishes were sometimes struck to a very different degree. Agricultural lowlands seem to have suffered most, but the plague reached also forested uplands. Recovery took one or a few decades in most parishes. The apparently much slower recovery after the Black Death may have been due to several reasons. Probably the initial population drop was much larger and also the recurring outbreaks of plague held population numbers down.

Notes

1   Myrdal 1999, 93–95
2   Myrdal 2006, 154
3   Myrdal 2012a, 205
4   See Chap. 2
5   Dyers 2002, 296; Benedictow 2004, 390; Myrdal 2012a, 229
6   Campbell 2012, 151; Myrdal 2012, 227
7   Grainger 2008; DeWitte 2009, 2014; DeWitte & Wood 2008; DeWitte & Huges-Morey 2012
8   Stone & Appleton-Fox 1996
9   Werdelin *et al.* (2002) made a similar study based on a smaller material
10   See Chap. 4

11 Myrdal 1999, 130, 137, 154; Campbell 2006, 186; Thomas 2007
12 The year 1536 marks the reformation and the end of the Middle Ages in Denmark. Lund is situated in the province of Scania, which belonged to Denmark at the time
13 Cf. Chap. 2 for an introduction
14 E.g. Livi Bacci 2000, 81
15 Myrdal 2012a, 223
16 Benedictow 2004, 5; also the pollen record presented in Chap. 4 indicates a sudden decline at 1350
17 Scott & Duncan 2001, 106
18 Scott & Duncan 2004, 24–25
19 Scott & Duncan 2004, 27, 31
20 Boccaccio 1353 [1995], 9–12
21 Boccaccio 1353 [1995], 10
22 Grainger *et al.* 2008
23 Grainger *et al.* 2008, 12–18
24 *Proceedings of the Society of Antiquaries* 1906–07
25 Barber & Thomas 2002, 12–14
26 Poulton & Woods 1984, 52
27 Stone *et al.* 1996, 24–25
28 Lütgert 2000, 255–265
29 Etter & Schneider 1982–83, 43–49
30 Archaeology Magazine, Barcelona's Black Death Victims. August 19, 2014
31 KHM 35/89 Fideikommisgården, Kirkegård ved Vor Frue kirke. Randers
32 Ragnar Blomkvist 14/9 1953, unpublished document, Kulturen Museum
33 Signoli *et al.* 2002, 829–854
34 Myrdal 2011, 80; 2012, 227
35 Myrdal 2006, 154; Bisgaard 2009, 97
36 Palm 2001, 28
37 Bonnier 2008, 167
38 Arcini 1999, 160
39 Cinthio 1992, 30–39 and this study
40 Lilja *et al.* 2001, 38
41 Menander & Arcini 2013, 222
42 Arcini & Tagesson 2005, 292
43 Unpublished photo from the ATA archive
44 Ranåker 2009, 26–39
45 Blomqvist 1951, 324
46 Carelli 2001, 118
47 Scott & Duncan 2004, 22, 25
48 Keene 1984, 101; 1989, 107
49 Brook & Keir 1975, 123–125; Keen 1989, 99
50 Grainger *et al.* 2008, 10; Barber & Thomas 2002, 12–14
51 Højrup & Jensen 1963
52 Royal letter dated 08-11-1710 (Stiernman 1775)
53 Ecclesiastical book Linköping 1710 containing data on deaths. Archive of Swedish church books, Linköping Domkyrkoförsamling, CI: 2
54 Jacobsson 2002, 16
55 Arcini *et al.* 2006, 16
56 Arcini *et al.* 2006, 59

57   Koepke & Baten 2005; Steckel 1995; Hatton 2014
58   Sellevold 1984, 227; Arcini 1996, 91–100
59   Hultkrantz 1927; Arcini *et al.* 2006, 80–81; Gustafsson *et al.* 2007
60   Hatton 2014
61   Tanner 1987; Bielicki *et al.* 1986
62   Kuh *et al.* 1997
63   Meyer & Selmer 1999
64   Chinn *et al.* 1989
65   Tanner 1987; Bielicki *et al.* 1986
66   WHO 1983
67   Allen & Uauy 1994; Tanner *et al.* 1982
68   Kimura 1984; Takahashi 1984; 1994
69   Tanner 1982; Takahashi1984; 1994
70   Hatton 2014
71   Hatton 2014
72   Martin & Saller 1957
73   The method is based on Sjøvold 1990
74   Cinthio 2002
75   Dahlbäck 1982, 118–119; Weises 2009, 39
76   Menander & Arcini 2013, 226
77   Thordeman 1939
78   Arcini 2008, 72
79   Dahlbäck 1982, 113
80   The result of the t-test (two-tailed P-value test) for stature of women were P = 0.0015 and for
      men P = 0.0001 and the level for significance is P<0.05
81   Dyer 2002, 296; Benedictow 2004, 390; Myrdal 2012a, 229; Campbell 2012, 124
82   Cf. Chap. 2 for further discussion
83   t-test: women P=0.0036, men P=0.0939
84   t-test: women P= 0.6327, men P=0.3531
85   t-test: P=0.155
86   The pollen record from the South-Swedish Upland indicates a relative increase of pastures and
      meadows in relation to arable land after the Black Death (see Chap. 4)
87   Fjällström 2013
88   DeNiro & Epstein 1978; 1981. According to these studies, $\delta^{15}N$ increases with 3–4‰ by each
      step up the food chain (Schoeninger *et al.* 1983, Schoeninger & DeNiro 1984), but recent studies
      suggest that 6‰ would be a more correct value (O'Connell *et al.* 2012)
89   For example, if the meat consumed were from young animals that were still suckling, the nitrogen
      value would be higher than if the meat were from adult animals. However, nothing in the kill-off
      patterns in faunal remains from Lund indicates any change through time in the consumption of
      young animals (Magnell 2006, 19–33). Regarding cereals, nitrogen isotope values are affected
      by the degree of manuring, and cereals from heavily manured crops may reach similar nitrogen
      isotope values as meat from herbivores (Bogard *et al.* 2013)
90   Schwarcz & Schoeninger 1991; Ambrose & Norr 1993, 1–37; Howland *et al.* 2003
91   Fjällström 2013
92   Cinthio 2002, 64
93   Magnell 2006, 19–33; Cardell in prep.
94   P<0.05
95   Material from the Nunnan block in Sigtuna, dated to 970–1100, showed an average nitrogen
      isotope value of 10.73% (Kjellström *et al.* 2009)

96 Cinthio 2002, 63–89
97 The use of slaves in early-medieval Sweden was mentioned for instance by Adam av Bremen in the eleventh century (1984, 207)
98 Price *et al.* 1994; 2011; 2013; Cox & Sealy 1997; Grupe *et al.* 1997
99 Price 1989; Kohn *et al.* 1999; Budd *et al.* 2000; Lee-Thorp & Sponheimer 2003
100 Price *et al.* 2002. Ratios of strontium isotopes in human tissue may vary from the actual geological background for a number of reasons (e.g. Sillen *et al.* 1998; Price *et al.* 2002; Maurer *et al.* 2012)
101 Price *et al.* 2002; Maurer *et al.* 2012
102 Sjögren *et al.* (2009) and Sjögren and Price (2013) analysed $^{87}Sr/^{86}Sr$ in human remains from megalithic burials in the Falbygden region of western Sweden along with numerous bioavailable samples from the surrounding region. Frei *et al.* (2009) recorded strontium isotope ratios in sheep wool and soil leachates from several areas in Sweden and Denmark. Arcini & Price (in press) measured strontium isotope ratios in human teeth from the Viking period and various biological materials from the Swedish island of Gotland and southern Sweden in a study of place of origin for the inhabitants of Viking Gotland
103 Larsson 2007; Hårdh & Larsson 2007; Price 2013
104 The tooth sampled is mainly from mandible but there are also some from maxilla. The majority of the sampled are incisors or first molars, however a canine tooth is used in three cases (Appendix 3)
105 Shimazaki & Shinomoto 2010
106 Wand & Jones 1995
107 Cinthio 2002
108 These records have been used for studies of different aspects of the last plague. Illmoni (1846–53) has studied the transmission routes but also the measures authorities took in the Nordic countries; Hult (1916) studied the plague's rampage in different regions in Sweden; Kellgren (1930, 76–105) showed how Gotland was hit; P. G. Vejde (Preinitz 1987) studied the plague in county of Kronoberg; Persson (2001) studied the plague in Stockholm and Scania; and Knudsen (2009) studied how it struck Zealand in Denmark
109 Andersson 2001, 28
110 Nordberg 1995, 160
111 Carmichael 1986, 110–112
112 Carmichael 1986, 110–112
113 Cipolla 1981, 19–50
114 Slack 1985, 256–257; Cipolla 1976, 47–66
115 Persson 2001, 266
116 Knudsen 2009, 115
117 Persson 2001, 423
118 Arcini *et al.* 2006, 59
119 Arcini *et al.* 2006, 56
120 Frequency based on 112 of 133 preserved church books. In some church books it is just mentioned that plague was present and in a few we have drawn the conclusions only from an increased number of deaths
121 30 parishes thave been sampled to calculate Crises Mortality Ratio (CMR) and the number of deaths for 1705–1709 and 1713–1717 used (the mortality in the two highest and two lowest years were removed). The number of individuals for each parish is not known for the year 1710, but there are estimates done by Palm for 1699 that have been used. The calculated frequency of death based on the 30 investigated parishes is 2.3%. According to Palm the mortality at that time is assumed to have been 2–3%. Based on Palms data regarding estimated number of individuals

in 1699, the number of expected deaths a normal year has been calculated in order to see how it relates to the mortality during the plague years in 1710 and 1711

122 Persson 2001, 348; Knudsen 2009, 116

123 74 of the 112 investigated parishes that have been affected by plague and where CMR could be calculated for each year

124 Four of 112 investigated parishes that have been affected by plague. For comparison, in the province of Scania a demographic catastrophe was reached in 6 of 155 (3.9%) of the investigated parishes (Persson 2001, 349)

125 Persson 2001, 355–357

126 See discussion in Chap. 4

PART III

CONCLUSIONS IN A
WIDER PERSPECTIVE

7.

Environment–society interactions

Per Lagerås

The dominating trend in the relationship between human society and the natural environment in a long-term perspective is one of increased human impact through time. This impact has affected plants and animals as well as soil, bedrock, water and the atmosphere and it has increased tremendously during the last one or two centuries. It has now become such a major factor in altering the conditions and processes on Earth, that it has been suggested that the latest part of the Holocene, from the late eighteenth century onwards, should be distinguished as a new geological epoch – the Anthropocene.[1] The technological development, including the introduction of fossil fuels, has enabled fast population growth and (for parts of the population) increased consumption *per capita*, but it has also put enormous pressure on ecosystems, resources and the natural environment. Today, much environmental concern is about anthropogenic global warming, which may be seen as the ultimate and most spectacular effect of human impact on the environment witnessed so far.[2]

However, these accelerating effects during the last few centuries should not blind us to the fact that human influence on the environment has a much longer history. Already early hunter-gatherers had great influence on ecosystems, whereas a systematic manipulation of the environment started with the first agriculture about 12,000 years ago.[3] Since then, woodland clearing, cultivation, herding and fodder collection have gradually transferred natural environments to cultural landscapes as agriculture has spread around the globe. Tightly linked to agricultural expansion is deforestation. Even though half of the world's deforestation has happened in the last 50 years (due to strong deforestation in the tropics), there has been a long-term process of deforestation from the introduction of agriculture to the present day.[4]

On the very broad temporal scale, the historical development of global population numbers and human pressure on the environment shows an exponential increase, with slow and steady expansion during prehistory and most of history, followed by a very sharp increase during the last century. However, this is a matter of scale. The incredibly strong population growth during the last century – the number of people in the world first reached 1 billion in 1825 whereas the latest 1-billion-increase (from 6 to 7 billions) took only 12 years – tends to diminish any previous variations in population numbers and to make past developments look linear, smooth and steady. By large this is a false impression. A zooming in on almost any period or specific region would reveal a much more complex development, characterised not only by gradual population growth and agricultural expansion, but also by periods of stagnation and decline.

The late-medieval crisis of Europe, which has been the topic of this book, is one such period of decline and it is far from the only one. There have been several other major social crises during the course of history. Some of them have gained much attention, like the collapses of the Western Roman Empire, the Classic Lowland Maya and the Rapa Nui on Easter Island,[5] but these are only a few grand and well-studied examples of a common phenomenon. Even though the long-term trend on a global scale is characterised by expansion and population growth, stagnation periods and crises of different magnitude and duration are part of human history. In many regions, due to recurring and alternating periods of expansion and decline, population numbers tend to show a cyclic or wavelike development superimposed on a long-term increase, rather than just exponential growth.[6] This cyclic appearance of population growth has been much discussed. In particular Thomas Malthus' view that population growth would eventually outstrip food production, leading to population check by famine, disease or warfare, has been criticised for being too deterministic.[7] However, regardless if periods of crisis and decline are direct consequences of previous expansion and population growth in a Malthusian sense, or if they are caused by other independent factors, it is an important observation that there have been recurrent periods of decline throughout history. These periods were also periods of decreased human impact on the environment.

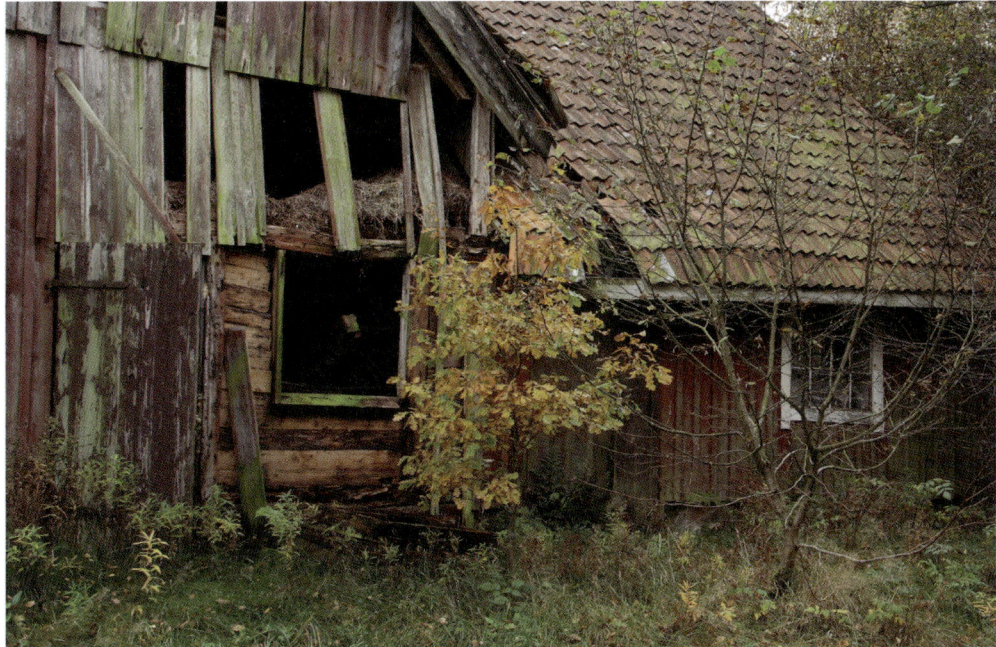

Fig. 56. A recently abandoned farm in the uplands of southern Sweden. Farm abandonment and reforestation was not restricted to the late-medieval crisis, but have happened several times during history (photo: Per Lagerås)

In Sweden, as in much of Europe, particularly two such periods of decline during the last two millennia have gained attention. One is, of course, the Black Death and the late-medieval crisis of the fourteenth and fifteenth centuries. The other is a societal crisis during the sixth century. The causes and processes behind the sixth-century crisis are unclear and several different contributing factors have been suggested. Like for the late-medieval crisis plague may have been involved also in this crisis. The so-called Justinian Plague ravished the Mediterranean and much of Europe in 541–43,[8] but it is still unclear if it reached Sweden. Also climatic deterioration has been suggested, in particular a series of unusually cold summers that started in 536, caused by volcanic dust in the atmosphere.[9] A third explanation may be political and social unrest, possibly as an indirect effect of the fall of the Western Roman Empire.[10] Probably several different factors worked in combination. When it comes to agricultural change and environmental responses, the sixth-century crisis shows great similarities with the late-medieval crisis, with settlement abandonment and woodland regrowth, in particular in marginal areas. The latter is reflected in several pollen records from northern Europe, including Sweden.[11]

Hence, the long-term history of environment-society interactions cannot be characterised simply as a one-way development of agricultural expansion and deforestation and an ever-increasing human impact on the environment – there have also been periods when the pressure from agriculture eased. Depending on the natural and climatic conditions as well as the duration of a crisis, abandonment would in most environments eventually lead to reforestation. In Europe during the last two millennia we have seen two major periods of reforestation – the sixth century and the fourteenth–fifteenth centuries – both periods connected to population decline. In many regions there has also been a third one, which started in the nineteenth century and continues today. Unlike the two earlier ones, the latest one is not a reflection of a societal crisis or a general population drop, but rather the transformation of non-profitable agricultural land to forest plantations, particularly in poor uplands (Fig. 56).[12] Parallel to this reforestation of marginal land there has been an intensification of agriculture on the most productive land.

In addition to these three major periods of farmland abandonment and reforestation, there have been several short-lasting interruptions and more local crises that affected smaller areas or regions. Some were caused by outbreaks of plague and other epidemic diseases, either among people or their livestock.[13] Others were caused by war and plundering. In Sweden, for instance the late sixteenth century was a period of warfare, which left parts of the countryside devastated.[14] In areas with poor conditions for agriculture there may also have been abandonment due to soil depletion and climate deterioration. Occasionally, also harvest failures due to poor weather may have resulted in famine and depopulation. Very little is known about these short-term and local crises and their possible environmental consequences.

Studies of the relationship between societal crisis and environmental change have focused primarily on those cases where overexploitation and mismanagement appear to have been the origin of the crisis, or where cultural maladaptation or societal rigidity prevented necessary actions and decisions to be made.[15] Less attention has been paid to environmental changes that followed upon other types of crises, like disease and warfare.[16] Such crises were not caused by environmental mismanagement, but may still have had important environmental and ecological consequences.

Urban Emanuelsson suggests that recurrent periods of decreased human impact in the history of the European cultural landscape have been beneficial for the overall biodiversity.[17] Several species of plants and animals are favoured by secondary succession and reforestation and would probably have gone extinct if there had not been interruptions in the agricultural land use. Many species are favoured by agriculture – in particular the many herbaceous plants that thrive in open grasslands – but few species would tolerate a continuous pressure from agriculture in the long run. The key to high biodiversity is the dynamic, both temporal and spatial, between well-managed agricultural land, abandoned land in different stages of secondary succession and grown-up forest. This dynamic has provided a rich variety of ecological habitats, species richness and genetic variety within species.

This is a hypothesis, and still little is known about the ecological consequences of societal crises in Europe's history. However, in the study presented here a couple of vegetation changes in Sweden in the wake of the Black Death have been identified, which may be a starting point for a discussion on the ecological consequences of this particular crisis. First of all, pollen and dendrochronological data show that some abandoned land was overgrown by woodland. These data thus confirm the generally held belief that forest cover increased during the crisis, at least in marginal uplands. The abandonment of fields in combination with decreased grazing pressure enabled the sprouting of shrubs and trees and started a process of natural woodland succession. In particular birch woodland expanded but there was also regeneration of oak and pine and to some degree spruce. Several forest plants and animals must have been favoured by this change, particularly those associated with light, early-successional woodland.

But not all abandoned farms were overgrown by forest. Even though settlements and arable fields were abandoned, many of them were used for grazing and occasionally for hay mowing, which kept the landscape open by holding back the forest. Hence, another vegetation change was associated with the turning of arable fields into pastures and meadows. When cultivation ceased, the immediate effect would have been enhanced flowering of annual weeds, but soon a grass sward would develop and a rich flora of perennial herbs typical of grazed and mowed environments would take over.

The most apparent vegetation changes after the Black Death, such as the expansion of birch woodlands, lasted for about 200 years until the sixteenth century. By the late sixteenth century, the re-establishment of arable fields, meadows and pastures had again replaced much of the secondary woodland. There may, however, also have been more long-lasting ecological effects. Dendrochronological data show that some trees, particularly of pine, that germinated in connection to abandonment in the mid-fourteenth century lasted for several hundred years. They consisted the oldest tree generation of the forest for a long time to come. Still in the early eighteenth century there were living trees that had germinated around the time of the Black Death. By that time they were about 350 years old. Such old trees are usually the home for a large number of plants and animals, like fungi, lichens and insects, and contribute significantly to the species richness of forests.[18] We may therefore conclude that the Black Death of the mid-fourteenth century still affected biodiversity more than 300 years later.

There have been no studies on changes in the fauna in Sweden in the wake of the Black Death, but such changes certainly occurred. Insects and other invertebrates, birds and also mammals were affected by the expansion of woodland and other changes in the vegetation.

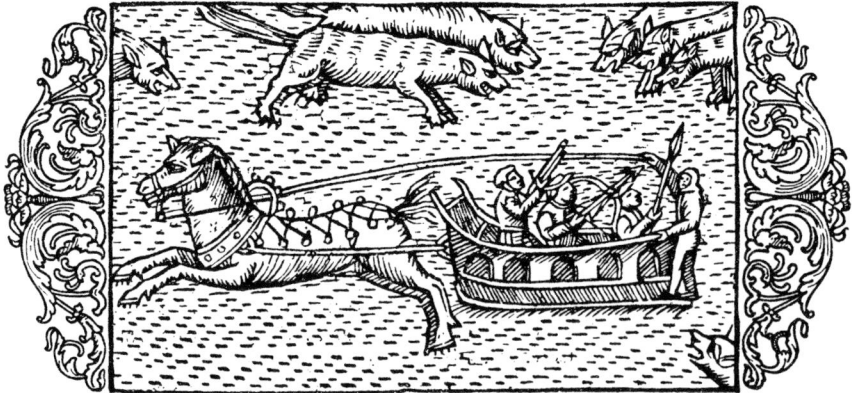

Fig. 57. Wood carving from Olaus Magnus' History of the Nordic People, published in 1555, showing wolves attacking a sledge. A letter from 1376 indicates that wolves may have increased in numbers in the wake of the Black Death

Herbivores like deer and elk could browse the new shrub vegetation on abandoned land and benefit from decreased competition by domestic animals.[19] Mammals, and particularly carnivores, may also have been more directly affected by the decrease in human population numbers, due to reduced hunting pressure. A royal letter from 1376 indicates that this was actually the case. According to the king, people complained that wolves and bears everywhere made much damage to humans and their livestock. He therefore proclaimed increased hunting and demanded one wolf skin to be delivered to the bailiffs each year by six farmers together. Janken Myrdal interpreted this as a direct effect of the population drop.[20] With a much smaller population in the wake of the plague, particularly in marginal woodlands, it was impossible to maintain hunting pressure on carnivores at the same level as before (Fig. 57). Another immediate effect of the plague may have been that there were unguarded cattle and sheep roaming the woods. Accessible prey and decreased hunting pressure gave the populations of wolves and bears, and possibly also of lynx and foxes, the opportunity to grow stronger during the crisis.

In addition to changes in vegetation and fauna, the population drop may have had wider environmental consequences. According to a hypothesis by William Ruddiman, reforestation in Europe in the wake of the Black Death, together with reforestation in the Americas in connection to the population drop of the sixteenth and seventeenth centuries, affected global climate.[21] Expanding woodlands resulted in lower levels of carbon dioxide in the atmosphere, a reduced greenhouse effect and a colder climate. Hence, the Little Ice Age may have been a consequence of the Black Death, at least to some degree. The hypothesis has been debated and climate modelling indicates that the observed changes in carbon dioxide concentrations may also be explained by natural factors.[22] According to Ruddiman the observed increase in carbon dioxide concentrations during the Late Middle Ages amounts to an average reforestation in Europe at a level of 25–45%.[23] The study presented in this book confirms that there was reforestation due to farm abandonment, at least in marginal uplands of southern Sweden, but to a lesser degree. According to the pollen-based landscape reconstruction, woodland expanded by approximately 20% in the higher parts of the uplands, whereas reforestation at lower elevations was less or insignificant. However, studies from several parts of Europe are needed to fully test the hypothesis.

The Black Death and the late-medieval crisis may also have affected marine environments. Today, nutrient leaching from modern agriculture leads to eutrophication and the spread of hypoxia (low oxygen conditions) in the bottom waters of the Baltic Sea. However, sedimentological studies show that hypoxia occurred in the Baltic Sea also during specific periods of the past. Warm climate seems to have been a driving force during most of the Holocene, but for later periods also human impact may have contributed. One such period of hypoxia corresponds to the Medieval Warm Period of AD 800–1300, which was also a period of agricultural expansion. It was followed by a period of oxic condition, 1300–1850, which roughly corresponds to the Little Ice Age, and then again hypoxia from 1850 to present. Lovisa Zillén and Daniel Conley suggest that the period of hypoxia, 800–1300 may have been caused by a combination of warm climate and increased agricultural land use in the Baltic catchment, and that the turn to more oxic conditions that followed was the combined effect of colder climate and a sudden decline in agriculture due to population drop.[24] Similar to the Ruddiman hypothesis it is difficult to separate natural factors from human impact, but taken together the two examples suggest that the environmental consequences of the late-medieval crisis may have been more far-reaching than what has been hitherto believed.

Leaving the still hypothetical impact on climate and sea aside, we can conclude that there were changes in the vegetation and fauna as direct consequences of the crisis. The next question is whether these changes had any influence back on society. Some of the changes may have had a positive effect by creating good preconditions for agricultural re-expansion. Others may have had a negative effect by making re-expansion difficult, troublesome and laborious.

Starting with the positive effects, the period of agricultural abandonment was a period of soil recovery and may be compared with long-term fallow. Before the introduction of chemical fertilisers, recurrent fallow periods were an integrated an important part of most agricultural systems. The aim of fallow was to restore some of the nutrients extracted from the soils by the crops during cultivation. However, fallow periods were usually not long enough to restore all the lost nutrients, leading to long-term declining fertility and gradually smaller yields.[25] When fields were abandoned in the wake of the plague, they were turned to grassland used for pasture or mowing, or they were overgrown with shrubs and trees and eventually turned into woodland. In either case, this unintended fallow transformed depleted arable fields to rich and fertile brown-earth soils. After the crisis, when abandoned farms were re-established and fields were put under the plough again, the new settlers could enjoy fully restored soils and high yields.

Also some other agricultural changes that were originally caused by necessity may have been beneficial for agricultural expansion after the crisis. Due to shortage of labour and excess of land, animal husbandry had gained in relative importance in comparison to crop growing during the crisis. Surviving farms had expanded their pastures and livestock by incorporating the land of abandoned farms. When population numbers started to recover and fields were put under the plough again, larger livestock provided rich access to manure to enrich the soils. In some regions, the incorporation of abandoned land may also have facilitated the introduction of crop-rotating systems that were based on systematic fallow in the infields.[26] In comparison to the older one-field system, they provided a better basis for a productive and sustainable agriculture.

It can be concluded that environmental and agricultural changes in the wake of the plague in some ways created good conditions for agricultural expansion and thereby may have facilitated societal recovery. But they had negative consequences as well. One example is the increased number of big carnivores. If reduced hunting pressure during the crisis led to expanding populations of wolf and bear, it certainly made the forests more insecure. New settlers who tried to reclaim abandoned land in forested areas had to accept a higher than normal predator pressure on their livestock. Furthermore, the responsibility to watch over the animals and to protect them from wolves and other threats was now on the shoulders of women and children. They had taken over the herding task from adult men during the crisis, probably as a consequence of labour shortage.[27]

Another environmental consequence of the crisis, which in turn may have delayed agricultural re-expansion, is the overgrowing by woodland and other vegetation on abandoned land. In general it requires more work to bring abandoned land back into use again than it takes to maintain continuous land use. Less work is needed to continue cultivation on a well-managed field than it takes to establish a new field or to re-establish an abandoned one. The same is true for hay meadows – less work is needed to continue mowing than what is needed to restore a meadow overgrown by shrubs and trees. The consequence of this would be, that if it takes a certain working force to keep a farm going, it would take a larger working force (or a harder working one) to put the same farm back into use again after abandonment. In general, the longer the interruption in cultivation, the more work is needed to re-establish full production. According to Urban Emanuelsson, who refers to this as the cultivation hypothesis, this effect of abandonment tends to prolong societal crises by keeping food production down.[28]

In the case of the late-medieval crisis, the degree of reforestation on abandoned land may have been a decisive factor. To clear abandoned and overgrown fields from trees and shrubs is a labour-intensive task. Also to restore a field turned into grassland requires more work than continuous cultivation, but it takes much more work to clear a field overgrown by woody vegetation. We may therefore expect a high degree of reforestation to raise the threshold for agricultural re-expansion. In the present study, pollen data show that there was reforestation in the wake of the Black Death, at least in the higher parts of the uplands, which probably delayed agricultural expansion in those areas. However, in other parts of the uplands the land of deserted farms was not reforested, but to a large degree kept open by grazing even when settlement and arable fields were abandoned. To turn to animal husbandry was obviously a rational strategy in a time of land excess and labour shortage. But it was strategic also in another sense. Grazing the abandoned farms and holding back the forest during the crisis facilitated future reestablishment of arable fields and meadows. This may very well have been an intended strategy. The land of deserted farms was a resource for grazing but also for future expansion. By keeping it in a reasonably good shape not all the work once invested in the land was wasted.

In summary, the late-medieval crisis and in particular the population drop initiated by the Black Death of 1350 did not only result in profound and long-term societal changes, but also in environmental and ecological changes. These changes were not only passive consequences of the crisis – they also affected the course of the crisis through different feedback mechanisms, both positive and negative. This study has provided some insights into the environmental changes during the crisis and suggested some possible feedbacks. But still we have only glimpses of a reality that was certainly much more complex. To better understand social processes and agricultural strategies during the crisis we need more studies of the environmental consequences. This is true for the late-medieval crisis as well as for other crisis throughout human history.

Even though each societal crisis has its own historical context, many processes – both social and ecological – are similar. It may therefore be rewarding for future studies not to regard the late-medieval crisis as a unique catastrophe, but to compare it for instance with the sixth-century crisis. Each societal crisis has its own characteristics but is also part of larger picture of recurring periods of expansion and decline. To make comparisons with the present-day situation is more difficult but not impossible. In preindustrial societies a much larger proportion of the population than today worked with agriculture and had a more direct dependency on their local environment. Today, in the industrial world, few of us are directly involved in food production. This, however, does not make our dependency on the environment smaller. More than ever, human impact on the environment has serious consequences for society and any possible crisis in the future may lead to environmental change. Studies of past society-environment interactions will certainly not solve present-day or future problems, but provide historical examples of human strategies and ecological consequences and how they may be interrelated.

Notes

1   Crutzen 2002
2   IPCC 2013
3   Barker 2006; Goudie 2013
4   Williams 2006, 395ff, 475
5   Tainter 1988; Diamond 2005
6   Whitmore *et al.* 1990, 37; Redman 1999, 170
7   Malthus 1803. For an introduction to this discussion see for instance Moran 2010, 25ff
8   Wagner *et al.* 2014
9   Larsen *et al.* 2008; Gräslund & Price 2012
10 Näsman & Lund 1988; Widgren 2012; Lagerås 2013a
11 Andersen & Berglund 1994; Lagerås *et al.* 1995; Lagerås 1996; 2007
12 Williams 2000, 29; Rudel *et al.* 2005
13 For historical human diseases, see for instance Mähäläinen (ed.) 2006; for livestock epidemics during the fourteenth century, see Kershaw 1973
14 Österberg 1971
15 Diamond 2005
16 An important exception is America, where the ecological consequences of European conquest in the fifteenth and sixteenth centuries have gained increased attention during the last decades. Cf. Mann 2006, 350ff
17 Emanuelsson 2009, 225ff
18 Bernes 2011, 62ff
19 Competition between cattle and wild herbivores has been studied in modern populations (e.g. Stewart *et al.* 2002)
20 Myrdal 2012b, 183
21 Ruddiman 2003; 2005, 115ff

22 Claussen *et al*. 2005; Broecker & Stocker 2006; Olofsson & Hickler 2008
23 Ruddiman 2003, 284
24 Zillén *et al*. 2008; Zillén & Conley 2010
25 Redman 1999, 122
26 Myrdal 2003, 237; Vestbö-Franzén 2004, 225
27 Myrdal 2012a, 217; 2012b, 222
28 Emanuelsson 2009, 40, 232, with reference to Kjekshus 1977

8.

Studying the late-medieval crisis
– reflections on research perspectives

Lars Ersgård

In studying the late-medieval crisis, it may be simplest to look upon the phenomenon as decline, as just a matter of negative impact on society in a limited period. However, it is also possible to look upon the crisis from a broader perspective, following its consequences in a considerably larger context than exclusively the medieval. The purpose of the following is to cast some reflections on the archaeological results, presented in previous chapters, from such a perspective, primarily on the basis of the question of how the late-medieval crisis can be comprehended as a part of the development towards modern society.

Originally, Swedish research on the late-medieval crisis was focused on the question of whether this crisis had hit society at all and, if so, to what extent it had affected primarily the agrarian settlement in terms of desertion. Today no one denies the fact that the crisis was extensive, also in Sweden, with severe demographic consequences. In an explicit way it is analysed as a part of a dynamic, societal development. Janken Myrdal's model, referred to in the previous chapters, is the most pronounced example of such a perspective.[1] Based on historical materialism a dialectic focus on class struggles is the theoretical starting point of this model. The actions of the nobility in the initial phase of the crisis became an incentive to extensive class conflicts in the later part of the fourteenth century/beginning of the fifteenth, resulting in a more positive development at the end of the Middle Ages and finally in a new historical "synthesis" in the shape of the nation state of the sixteenth century.

Myrdal's perspective is the one of an economic historian, incorporating the crisis in a greater narrative of the Middle Ages as a socio-economic course of upturns and declines. Claiming the validity of all geographical contexts, grand narratives of this kind have become subject to criticism. For example, archaeologists working with late-medieval contexts of marginal woodlands in northern Sweden have claimed that the grand narrative of the late-medieval crisis is less representative of development in these areas.[2]

The purpose of the archaeological investigation presented in this book has not been to look upon the crisis from the perspective of central versus marginal area, neither to present a brand new narrative of the crisis. All grand narratives are characterised by a certain degree of simplification, probably necessary when explaining profound societal processes. However, here the aim has been to emphasise the complexity of the crisis, rather than telling a new overall story of the phenomenon. Using the potential of archaeology, this chapter endeavours to reveal new aspects of societal changes, focusing on the strategies people were forced to develop, dealing with their everyday lives during this harsh times, and the results of these choices in the longer term as well as the shorter.

Before he meaning and the consequences of this perspective are developed a brief European reference to Swedish development is presented. Hence a closer look is taken at late-medieval England, a country where the source materials concerning the crisis, the written as well as the archaeological, are abundant. However, the perspectives in English research have been somewhat different compared to Scandinavia.

The population in England, according to results of modern research, was probably reduced by at least 50% in the period 1350–1450, a decrease on par with the situation in Sweden in the corresponding period.[3] In many respects the development of the two countries shows several similarities. However, the picture of late-medieval England tends to appear as less dramatic compared with Sweden.

Facing major problems from 1348–50, caused by the great decrease of the population, the inhabitants of the English society "with remarkable resilience ... returned to work, and the whole system held together."[4] Some activities, like house construction and mining, stopped momentarily and were resumed later in the fourteenth century. Rebellions against increased tax burdens occurred but when they had settled, society seems to have adjusted to the new conditions engendered by a greatly reduced population.

The peasants gaining a major control of production was an important consequence of the demographic changes of fourteenth century.[5] It enabled increased freedom of action for the peasants, who were no longer just an anonymous group of "producers". Increasingly they could act more independently than before, enlarging their holdings in the countryside or acting as entrepreneurs in a market.

Archaeological study of late-medieval England has for a long time had its focus on agrarian settlement and its changes. Deserted villages and farmsteads in particular have been a dynamic field of research since the 1940s, archaeologists and historians having worked in close cooperation.[6] However, using deserted settlement as a primary source for studies of economy and society in the English countryside has been a matter of debate.[7] After all the deserted villages represent only a minority of all existing villages in the late Middle Ages.

Desertion has occurred to a greater or lesser degree during all periods and deserted villages have not, in the same way as in Sweden, become synonymous with the ravages of the late-medieval crisis. However, a major part originating from the time span 1350–1700, this phase has played a significant role in the discussion on the causes of desertion.[8]

Recent research has shown that only a minor part of desertion can be linked to the plagues of the mid-fourteenth century. Thus, there is no simple connection between the decrease of population and desertion. Rather, the causalities being complex, desertion appears as a gradual process.[9]

The late-medieval crisis in England stands out as a rather complex history, including major decrease of population and societal decline as well as elements of emancipation, new initiatives and expanding markets.[10] Will archaeology also help us to reveal a similar complexity in Sweden?

In the grand narrative of the late-medieval crisis in Sweden, the survival strategies of the nobility in the initial phase have been a decisive factor, directing social development and affecting society's ability of recovery in a negative way.[11] The peasants, being mostly an anonymous group of taxpayers in this early phase of the crisis, did not stand out as independent actors until the rebellions of the 1430s. However, using archaeology it will be possible to nuance this picture.

Through archaeology we can, in another way than with the written record alone, write a history "from below", reaching the single household and the strategies of everyday life. In a previous chapter of this book such histories have been told, concerning farmsteads in different parts of the country, their inhabitants facing new challenges after the plagues at the middle of the fourteenth century.

Responses to decline in the middle of the fourteenth century, as they have been observed in the archaeological record, were discussed in Chapter 5 in relation to the phasing out of the manorial system of the High Middle Ages. Being in dissolution around 1350, this system received its final death blow in the plagues.[12] Probably the consequences were the same as in England. The landowners leaving the direct control of production, the peasants at once gained a primary responsibility in the management of their holdings. Hence the later part of the fourteenth century must have meant, despite an immense diminishing of population and increasing tax burdens, a new freedom of action for the peasants, making it possible for them to develop their own strategies of survival and create new ways of cooperation. This freedom opened the way for specialisation of activities in the agrarian society, which had previously been organised within, and restricted by, a manorial system.

The development of the mining districts north of the Lake Mälaren stands out as an elucidative example. The advanced blast furnace technique had been well-established in these areas since the end of the twelfth century. However, it was not until it began to be organised as a collective enterprise of freeholders after 1350, that this mining activity could be developed and specialised, then becoming one of the economic mainstays of the new nation state in the sixteenth and the seventeenth centuries (Fig. 58). A full understanding of the transition from subordinated tenants to self-owning peasant miners is still lacking but probably it occurred in the later part of the fourteenth century. The peasant miners taking part in the rebellion of the 1430s, are no tormented losers in the wake of the big crisis but a well-organised group with a new social identity.

Specialisation and division of labour were central elements of west European societies in early modern times, the economy of the households increasingly being oriented towards a market.[13] By all accounts we see a beginning of this already in the late Middle Ages. Despite the loss of at least half of the population, people were able to turn the negative trend, increasing the productivity of households through specialisation. So, the decline at the middle of the fourteenth century included the downfall of a social system as well the start of a new one.

However, there is still another aspect of the crisis to reflect on – the cultural one. So far, a cultural perspective has been practically invisible in the research of the crisis, mostly being studied from a socio-economic point of view. In Chapter 5 significant regional differences of late-medieval Sweden were emphasised, differences hardly being comprehensible from other than a cultural perspective. Primarily, these differences have been about various approaches to the landscape, to the single farm and the towns. Essentially, the focus here has been directed towards the eastern and western parts of southern Sweden respectively.

The differences mentioned above were the result of cultural divergence being discernable at the earliest in the thirteenth century. This phenomenon was a decisive, continued movement

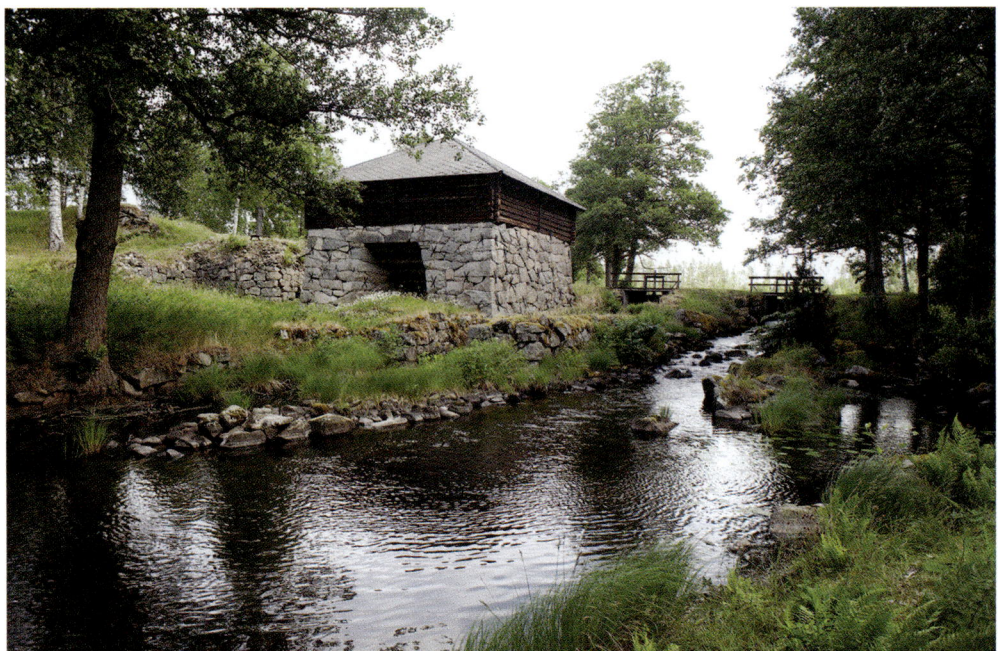

Fig. 58. Ruin of a blast furnace from the eighteenth century by the factory of Silvhytteå in the municipality of Hedemora, province of Dalarna (photo: Bengt A. Lundberg, Swedish National Heritage Board)

in society, which did not come to an end because of the late-medieval crisis. On the contrary, the latter strengthened the cultural differences, thus making it reasonable to discuss them in a wider historical context.

The previous discussion on the regional differences has primarily revolved around the following phenomena: mobility versus continuity of the settlement structure, the interaction between town and countryside as well as the relation between social forms of cooperation and proto-industrial activities. In the opinion of this author, the agrarian society of the west, as in the province of Halland, showed great spatial flexibility, adjusting settlement to a new orientation of production in the late Middle Ages. In the east people seem to have acted within a spatial structure, staying fixed since the High Middle Ages and further on in the time of the crisis.

In the eastern parts of Sweden a strong interaction between towns and countryside was a significant part of the survival strategies in the time of the crisis. However, in the west the late-medieval towns were of little importance for their surrounding countryside. On the contrary, the peasants of this region seem to have developed a trade of their own, independent of the towns.

In the east activities of a proto-industrial character were developed in the late Middle Ages, above all in the iron producing districts north of the Lake Mälaren, taking the form of villages of peasant miners. In the west no such activities were developed except for the southern part of Halland where proto-industrial iron making was established in the late Middle

Ages.[14] Specialised activities were developed in the west in the thirteenth and fourteenth centuries, however being restricted to the context of the single farmstead.

How is it possible to comprehend these regional contrasts in a wider perspective? In recent years Swedish historian Christer Winberg has presented the most profound study on Swedish regional characteristics, focusing mainly on the nineteenth and twentieth centuries.[15] Making some references towards earlier periods, he emphasizses "three formative phases" as particularly decisive in the regional development of the western and eastern parts of Sweden respectively.[16]

The first formative phase includes the thirteenth century, when political power was moved towards the eastern part of Sweden. Parallel to this change, extensive urbanisation took place in this part of the country, especially in the Mälaren valley area. The latter phenomenon did not affect the western parts to any significant extent.

The second phase started at the beginning of the seventeenth century, when Stockholm became the formal capital of the country and the administration of the realm together with all associated bureaucracy becoming concentrated in this town. The nobility also concentrated their interests in the eastern parts of Sweden, paving the way for a "de-feudalisation" of western Sweden and the emergence of a social class of freeholders in this region.

The third of the phases started at the end of the eighteenth century and the first half of the nineteenth century, when a class of freeholders was well-established in western Sweden. In the east the nobility strengthened its position through an intensification and rationalisation of the management of their estates. During this period, secularisation began in the east, whereas religious life in the west was characterised by the emergence of revivalist movements.

The remaining regional differences in the era of modernity stand out as an important conclusion.[17] Despite better communications between the regions and increased administrative and political centralisation, the differences became strengthened and deepened. Thus, an essential pattern becomes discernible, covering the time span from at least the thirteenth century to present times – a *longue durée*, to use the terminology of the French *Annales* school.

This is not the place for discussing the origins of the regional differences in the early Middle Ages. However, there is reason to reflect on the impact of the late-medieval crisis on the actual, cultural pattern. Contributing to a strengthening of the latter, did the crisis also contribute to the formation of modern Sweden?

When the peasants of western Sweden developed their strategies for survival in the era of the crisis, they acted within a context rather different from that of the eastern parts. Having never developed any closer dependence on nearby towns and their settlement never having been subject to any regulation, people were living in another cultural world than their counterparts in the east. A crucial element of this world was the single farmstead with its household, playing the role as the primary actor in the landscape. By all accounts the village played the corresponding role in the eastern parts.[18] No doubt this fact has been of very great importance for the development of an individual independence among the peasants of western Sweden, concerning not only of their acting in the landscape but also of their relation to kingdom and nobility.[19]

As clearest evidence, this was expressed in the seventeenth and eighteenth centuries when a group of freeholders became the dominant social stratum. A strong individual mentality, emanating from the single farmstead, supported this stratum. This mentality included a specific spirit of the small business owner, providing the basis for peasant trade as well as rural crafts, independent of the towns of the region. The later activity was developed to an extensive cottage industry, especially weaving, becoming characteristic of several parts of western Sweden in modern times. The first signs of such activities may already be discernible in the late Middle Ages.

In conclusion, there are reasons to understand the time of the late-medieval crisis as a highly formative phase towards modern society. This chapter has emphasised important elements of emancipation in the development of the crisis. However, it has been about an emancipation following different cultural pathways.

Through archaeology it has been possible to grasp different aspects of human actions in the later part of the fourteenth and in the fifteenth centuries. An utterly severe societal situation did not – despite the unimaginable loss of human lives – result only in feudal suppression but also in innovations. Taking new initiatives in their everyday lives, peasants and townsmen could form a basis for a new society. However, their acting must be considered in the light of varying cultural contexts, directing the development in different ways.

Thus, the picture of the late-medieval crisis will be a complex one, Sweden in this respect reminding us much of England. Probably the two countries reflect a common, West European development. The situation in Eastern Europe was partly another one. For example in Russia, there was no emancipation of the peasants, rather an increasingly fierce serfdom in the sixteenth and seventeenth centuries.[20]

This book has focused on the late-medieval crisis largely from the "small" perspective, i.e. the perspective of the single household and the single farmstead. At the same time it has discussed the late-medieval farmstead in a wider historical context, hopefully elucidating the links between past and present, between Middle Ages and modern times.

Notes

1   Myrdal 2012a, 234ff
2   Svensson *et al.* 2013
3   Dyer 2002, 235, 272; Palm 2001, 24f
4   Dyer 2002, 272
5   Dyer 2002, 265
6   Taylor 2010
7   Jones 2010, 8f; Lewis 2007, 134
8   Dyer 2010, 29
9   Dyer 2010, 44
10   Dyer 2010, 44
11   Myrdal 2012a, 234f
12   Cf. Ericsson 2012, 40
13   De Vries 2008, 71f; cf. Larsson 2009, 390f
14   Strömberg 2008
15   Winberg 2000
16   Winberg 2000, 118f
17   Winberg 2000, 120
18   Winberg 2000, 113
19   Winberg 2000, 84
20   Martin 2012, 293f

9.

Epidemics in a social context

Caroline Arcini

We live in the twenty-first century more than 600 years after the Black Death and epidemics are still a major concern. In spite of tremendous medical advances, like vaccine and antibiotics, epidemics pose a threat to individuals and society. Awareness is high and preventive measures and cures are developed to meet new epidemics and to keep pace with the fast evolution of new germs and diseases. This is always a challenge because new outbreaks never completely behave like their predecessors, partly due to the changing character of the infections themselves, but also due to changes in society, culture and human behaviour. These changes make it difficult to predict the impact of future epidemics and pandemics, and also, of course, to learn from the past. Still, historical studies reveal some general patterns and similarities, not the least in how people have responded to the threats of epidemics and how they have handled their fears and their losses, which provide valuable perspectives to recent epidemics and may contribute to better preparedness for new ones.

During the 1900s the world witnessed three pandemics, all caused by influenza viruses – the Spanish flu of 1918–20, the Asian flu of 1957 and the Hong Kong flu of 1967–68. The latter two killed 4 and 1 million, respectively, whereas the Spanish flu killed, incredibly, 50–100 million people globally (37,000 of them in Sweden; Fig. 59). No wonder the fear of epidemics is deeply rooted and rumours spread swiftly when new ones are approaching. Recent examples from Europe are SARS, avian flu and swine flu. How we as individuals respond depend on many factors, like the flow of information from authorities and predictions by medical experts through media.

As this book is being written there is an on-going epidemic in Africa, which to its cultural character has similarities with the plague. It is an outbreak of Ebola, a virus that causes a haemorrhagic fever. Since the first outbreak in 1976 there have been as many as 19 recurring outbreaks, the last ones with only 2 years apart. The on-going epidemic (2014) is regarded as the most serious ever and WHO classifies it as an international public health emergency. For the first time, people outside Africa have also been contaminated. Those infected were people nursing aid workers that were brought home for medical care.

Even though Ebola and plague are different in several respects there are similarities between them, not the least in how cultural customs and practices around the sick and the handling of the dead play an important role in the transmission and spread of the disease. In West Africa the custom of touching the body of the diseased at funerals may contribute

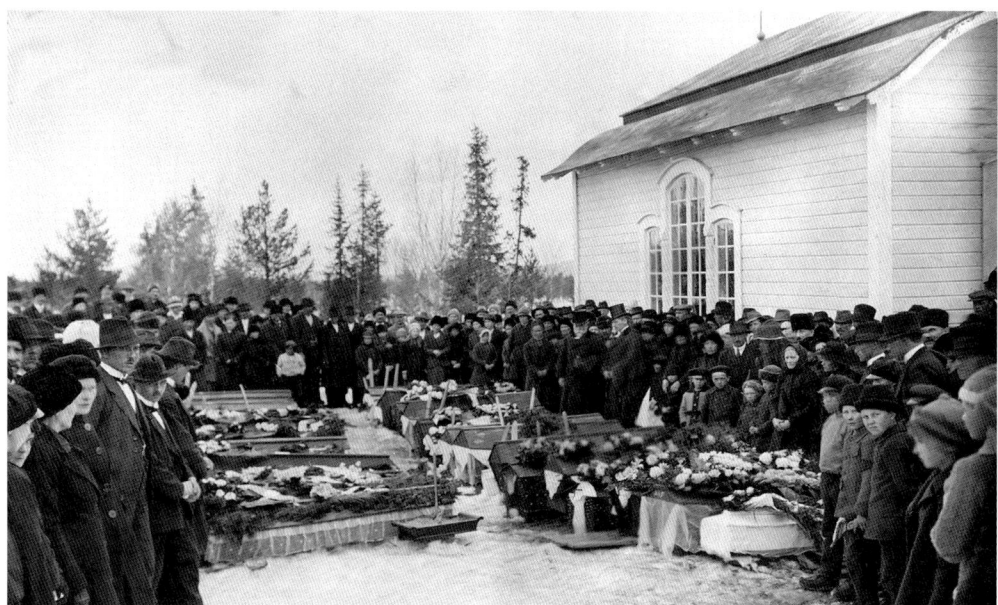

Fig. 59. Funeral for 51 victims of the Spanish flu, Arjeplog cemetery in northern Sweden, Easter Eve, 4 April 1920 (photo: Sandberg. From the photo archive at the Silver Museum in Arjeplog)

to the spread of the virus. Similarly, in the fourteenth century, the washing and wrapping of the dead, together with other customs, like the last rites and of course the gathering at funerals, probably contributed to the Black Death's fast conquest of Europe. In Sweden it was not until the last plague epidemic of 1710 that some of these customs were banned and special burial places for plague victims were established far from the churchyards. We know from written sources that these new regulations from the authorities were not well received by the people.

What also connects past and present epidemics, from the Black Death to Ebola, is of course the shock and tragedy for families and individuals. From parts of Europe chroniclers from the time give us a vivid picture of the horror of the Black Death, and there is no reason to doubt their testimony. To experience the death of near and loved ones was not unusual during the Middle Ages, and in particular infant mortality was very high, but the ravage of the plague and other major epidemics was something else.

In the Nordic countries written records from the Black Death are scarce, but church books from later plague epidemics give us insight into how individual families suffered when hit by the plague. For example, when the plague came to Sorby Magle Kirkerup parish on the island of Zealand in Denmark in January 1656, the effects for some families were disastrous. One couple hit hard was Franz Jensøn and Charen Hansdatter. Many years before Franz had lost his first wife and their two sons and surely he must have felt that he had already received his share of God's trials. Three weeks after his first wife died he had married Charen, and in the succeeding years they had five sons and 11 daughters. Then in 1656 came the plague. In 13 May one of their sons died and within less than 2 months the plague had taken all of their five sons and two of their daughters. The worst day must have been 24 May. They were about to bury one son and one daughter when suddenly their youngest son also died. They put him in the same coffin with his brother. How did Franz Jensøn and his wife recover from such a disaster? How did they manage to carry on? Of course they had no choice. There were still children to care for, and when Franz and Charen died, at 73 and 71 years old, three of their offspring were alive and well.

Even though the first strike of the Black Death in the fourteenth century may have been the most devastating, plague outbreaks haunted the European population for centuries. When the family of Franz and Charen were hit, plague had been more or less around for 300 years. It occurred periodically and always deceived behind the door. Some outbreaks lasted for only one or a few months, but sometimes the plague stayed and became a normal part of life. In London, for example, there were only 3 years without plague in the period 1604–66. This naturally held down population numbers and affected most parts of everyday life. Still, people did not surrender to the plague, which is reflected in the fact that many marriages were arranged even during the worst of outbreaks. In Sweden, church books from the plague years of 1710–13 show that betrothals and marriages began to increase well before the epidemic died out. Sometimes this hurry resulted in very short marriages when the new couples moved into contaminated houses.

In spite of the tragedies of individuals and families, several historians have concluded that the Black Death and the crisis, and in particular the drop in population numbers, resulted in improved living conditions for the survivors.[1] In addition, the crisis enabled social change, which in turn laid the foundation for the strong expansion that followed during the sixteenth century. Hence, the plague and similar historical disasters may have paved the way for progress and better living standards.[2] However awful it may sound, there seems to have been some truth in the old saying, 'one man's loss is another man's gain.' However, that this may not always be the case with pandemics is evident from the aftermath of the Spanish flu. Similar to the Black Death it caused the death of millions in a few years, but the societal reaction appears to have been very different. For instance, it did not lead to increased investments, higher wages or any migration of labour from less affected areas to the more severely affected.[3] On the contrary, unemployment increased, living standards deteriorated and the proportion of poor in the population increased.[4] Obviously we may expect different societal reactions to pandemics in different historical contexts. Also within the same pandemic there was variation, for instance between different areas and different social classes.

In Chapter 6 skeleton remains were used to study possible changes in living conditions in connection with the Black Death. Progress with this approach has been made in recent years, most noticeably by Sharon Dewitte, who studied conditions in a sub-population of medieval London. She showed that living conditions improved for the survivors and for succeeding generations, in the sense that they, on average, achieved an older age than before the plague.[5] In the study presented here, height was used as an indicator of living conditions. Height is frequently also used to study secular changes in modern society and therefore enables comparisons in a wider time perspective.[6]

The increase in stature noted after the Black Death was only temporary, and from the sixteenth century onwards stature gradually declined to reach a nadir in the mid-nineteenth century. Men in Sweden became several centimetres shorter than during the Middle Ages and actually as short as 6000 years ago.[7] After 1850, stature increased again. In the late nineteenth century it reached medieval levels and then continued to increase strongly throughout the twentieth century. The fastest increase in height in a short time is the one documented for post-war Japan, but also in Sweden and much of Europe body length increased dramatically during the same period. The modern increase in stature was due to improved living conditions and a change in diet, in Sweden particularly an increased consumption of milk. In order to compete with grain prices from America many Swedish farmers turned to animal husbandry and, with improved transport, fresh milk also reached the population in cities. Milk production and distribution was favoured by Pasteur's discovery and by the separator, which made dairy products easily accessible and cheap. Authorities saw increased milk consumption as an effective and inexpensive way to improve living condition and in the 1930s free milk was introduced in schools.[8] Hence, the connection between stature on the one side and living conditions and diet on the other is evident from modern times. Also the slight increase in height during the Late Middle Ages was certainly due to improved living conditions, but our study of stable isotopes showed no clear association to a change in diet. Note, however, that there may have been important dietary changes not reflected in the isotope values.

Human health has improved greatly in Europe and many other parts of the world during the last century. Many have experienced better living conditions due to access to more nutritious food, vaccines against various childhood diseases and flu, antibiotics against bacterial infectious diseases, better housing and sanitation, education and vacations. Although the risk of epidemics in Europe and the developed countries is still present, nowadays it is mainly in developing countries that epidemics pose a serious problem and occasionally lead to high mortality. This is true also for the plague. Isolated cases of plague also still occur each year in developed countries, in particular in the USA where it was first introduced in 1900 from Asia and where it is resident among wild rodents. But it is only in the developing countries, mainly in Africa but also in Asia and South America, that plague still leads to serious outbreaks. Most of them hit villages and small towns in poor, rural areas. Madagascar is one country that has been hit by recurring outbreaks of plague – bubonic as well as pneumonic – during the last few years. At present an on-going outbreak in the fall of 2014 has caused 40 deaths so far. If diagnosed early, bubonic plague can be successfully treated with antibiotics, and there is little danger of a new pandemic of plague. It is relatively easily stopped by access to antibiotics and insect control in infected areas, but locally, in poor countries, plague is still a feared and deadly disease.

Notes
1   Dyers 2002, 296; Benedictow 2004, 390; Myrdal 2012a, 229
2   Myrdal 2012a, 204
3   Karlsson *et al.* 2014
4   Karlsson *et al.* 2014
5   DeWitte 2014
6   Werner 2008
7   Bennike 1985
8   Martiin 2010, 226

10.

Summary of conclusions

The Black Death and the late-medieval crisis have been thoroughly studied and debated for half a century but still appear mysterious and elusive. Research has provided detailed insights and interpretations on several important aspects whereas others remain largely unexplored. Many question marks remain regarding sequences of events and causalities during the crisis and not the least regarding its consequences, both in a short-term and long-term perspective. Naturally, much of the causality will remain hidden to us, partly because of the fragmentary character of historical sources but most of all because of the complexity of the matter.

In this book we have taken a deeper look at some non-written sources and used analytical methods and perspectives from archaeology and the natural sciences. Our aim has been to provide new angles to some of the classical research questions formulated by historians and also to present new research perspectives. Similar to written records, the non-written records vary considerably in character, quantity and quality between different countries, regions and areas. This is true also for southern Sweden. For instance, most pollen records are from marginal uplands where peatlands are numerous and well-preserved, whereas most archaeological and osteological records are from densely populated lowlands where the preservation of skeletons is good and archaeological research activity has been high. Hence, different regions and different source materials and methods contribute in different ways. The results and interpretations presented in this book reflect this diversity and point to several interesting aspects of the crisis. Our primary conclusions can be summarised as follows:

- Pollen data show that there was widespread farm abandonment in the uplands in the wake of the Black Death and that the total land cover of arable land was approximately halved. Abandonment was a quick process that started immediately after 1350, i.e. the first strike of the plague. It was followed by reforestation, particularly in the highest parts of the uplands, where birch, oak, pine and spruce expanded. However, in other parts, the land of deserted farms was to a large degree kept open by grazing. As a consequence, the decrease of pastures was much smaller than the decrease of arable land, which indicates that animal husbandry gained in importance in relation to crop cultivation during the crisis. The first re-establishment of arable land after the crisis started in the late fifteenth century.
- The archaeological record gives evidence of farm abandonment, also in agricultural villages in the lowlands, and shows how crop cultivation was replaced or complemented

by other activities. People reacted quickly to the new circumstances. Different strategies to meet the crisis were soon developed at household level or by several households together. In Particular, non-agrarian activities exemplified by fish smoking and metal forging were expanded and reorganised, probably to meet labour shortage. As expected, building activities more or less stopped at 1350, which is evident from dendrochronological data from both upland and lowland areas. The same data also give evidence of woodland regeneration on abandoned land. Abandonment was not confined to the countryside but happened also in towns. But the development of towns during the crisis is complex and reveals examples also of new establishments and restructuring.

- The consequences of the crisis show regional differences. According to the pollen record abandonment was more widespread in upland areas than in lowlands, but the interpretation is tentative because the lowlands are still represented by very few data. A summary of different kinds of archaeological data indicates another spatial distinction, namely between the western and eastern parts of southern Sweden. It seems like not only environmental conditions, but also different settlement patterns and social organisation affected the course of the crisis. Furthermore, the crisis appears to have accentuated the cultural differences between these regions.

- The absence of mass graves indicates that the victims of the Black Death and of recurring outbreaks of plague during the late fourteenth century were buried in ordinary churchyards. Clusters of graves and double and triple graves identified at several churchyards in Sweden probably represent plague victims. It seems like the medieval population, as far as ever possible, held on to their religious customs and rituals and took care of their diseased, even during the worst of crisis. Special plague cemeteries were not established until the last plague of 1710–13.

- The widespread perception that living standards improved after the Black Death gets some support from the study of stature, which was based on a large number of medieval skeletons. Average stature increased slightly after 1350, both among men and women, but the increase is small and only statistically significant for women. Several authors suggest that people after the Black Death ate more meat and dairy products, but stable-isotope analyses of teeth from a churchyard in Lund revealed no dietary changes during the crisis. However, pollen data from the uplands indicated a relative increase in animal husbandry in the wake of the population drop, but this change may not necessarily have affected the consumption patterns in lowlands and towns. The contradictory results call for further research.

Together with the discussions presented throughout this book we hope that these conclusions show the great potential of the non-written records also when dealing with a research problem that has a long tradition of historical research. We have focused on source materials and methods that are familiar to us and tried to make the conclusions accessible for readers of different background and interests. With this approach we wanted to introduce historians to these materials, and at the same time introduce palaeoecologists and archaeologists to the intriguing and complex research problems of the late-medieval crisis. Hence, in several respects this is an introductory study. With continued research based on a diversity of source materials and perspectives, the study of the late-medieval crisis can develop into a truly interdisciplinary endeavour.

References

Abel, W. 1980. Agricultural fluctuations in Europe: from the thirteenth to the twentieth centuries. Methuen & Co, London (Reprinted by Routledge in 2013)

Adam av Bremen, Historien om Hamburgerstiftet och dess biskopar. Translated into Swedish by E. Svenberg. Profide et Christianissimo 6 (1984). Prorius, Stockholm

Alfsdotter, C. 2011. Att falla i god jord: en bioarkeologisk analys av massgrav 2 från sankt Mikaels kyrkogård i Lund. Unpublished examination paper in osteology. Lund University

Allen, L. H. & Uauy R. 1994. Guidelines for the study of mechanisms involved in the prevention or reversal of linear growth retardation in developing countries. *European Journal of Clinical Nutrition* 48 Suppl. 1, 212–216

Ambrose, S. H. & Norr, L. 1993. Experimental evidence for the relationship of the carbon isotope ratios of whole diet and dietary protein to those of bone collagen and carbonate. In: Lambert, J. B. & Grupe, G. (eds) *Prehistoric Human Bone: archaeology at the molcular level.* Springer, Berlin

Andersen, S. T. & Berglund, B. E. 1994. Maps for terrestrial non-tree pollen (NAP) percentages in north and central Europe 1800 and 1450 yr B.P. In: Frenzel, B. (ed.) *Evaluation of Land Surfaces Cleared from Forest in the Roman Iron Age and the Time of Migrating Germanic Tribes Based on Regional Pollen Diagrams*, 119–134. Paläoklimaforschung 12. Gustav Fischer Verlag, Stuttgart

Andersson, H. 1982. Städer i öst och väst – regional stadsutveckling under medeltiden. *Bebyggelsehistorisk tidskrift* 3, 55–67

Andersson, H. 1985. Västkustens medeltida städer – eller vem har nytta av städer. *Bebyggelsehistorisk tidskrift* 10, 38–44

Andersson, H. & Anglert, M. (eds) 1989. *By, huvudgård och kyrka: studier i Ystadsområdets medeltid.* Lund studies in medieval archaeology 5. Almqvist & Wiksell, Stockholm

Andrén, A. 1985. *Den urbana scenen: städer och samhälle i det medeltida Danmark.* Acta Archaeologica Lundensia, series in 8°, 13. Liber, Malmö

Andrén, A. 1986. I städernas undre värld. In: Andrén, A. (ed.) *Medeltiden och arkeologin: festskrift till Erik Cinthio*, 259–269. Lund studies in Medieval Archaeology 1. Lund University

Antonsson, H. 2009. The extent of farm desertion in central Sweden during the late medieval agrarian crisis: landscape as a source. *Journal of Historical Geography* 35, 619–641

Anund, J., Bergquist, U., Bäck, M. & Pettersson, K. 1992. A medieval cauldron foundry: craftsmanship and craftsmen in Pantern, Uppsala. In: Ersgård, L., Holmström, M. & Lamm, K. (eds) *Rescue and research: reflections of society in Sweden 700–1700 AD*, 221–251. Arkeologiska undersökningar, Skrifter 2. Riksantikvarieämbetet, Stockholm

Arcini, C. 1996. Ståtliga var järnåldersmännen från Albäcksbacken. In: Karsten, P. (ed.) *Carpe Scaniam: axplock ur Skånes förflutna*, 91–100. Riksantikvarieämbetet, Stockholm

Arcini, C. 1999. *Health and Disease in Early Lund: osteo-pathologic studies of 3,305 individuals buried in the first cemetery area of Lund 990–1536*. Archaeologica Lundensia 8. Dept of Community Health Sciences, Lund University

Arcini, C. 2007. Reconstructing daily life in past populations. In: Kaliff, A. (ed.) *Archaeology in the East and West: papers presented at the Sino-Sweden archaeology forum, Beijing in September 2005*, 261–274. Riksantikvarieämbetet, Stockholm

Arcini, C. 2008. Detta lämnar ingen oberörd. In: Fendin, T. (ed.) *Döden som straff: glömda gravar på galgbacken*, 68–103. Östergötlands läns museum, Linköping

Arcini, C. & Tagesson, G. 2005. Kroppen som materiell kultur: gravar och människor i Linköping genom 700 år. In: Kaliff, A. & Tagesson, G. (eds) *Liunga, Kaupinga: kulturhistoria och arkeologi i Linköpingsbygden*. Arkeologiska undersökningar, 282–319. Skrifter 60. Riksantikvarieämbetet, Stockholm

Arcini, C., Jacobsson, B. & Persson, B. 2006. *Pestbacken*. Riksantikvarieämbetet, Stockholm

Aston, T. H., Philpin, C. H. E. (eds) 1985. *The Brenner Debate: agrarian class structure and economic development in pre-industrial Europe*. Cambridge University Press

Åstrand, J. 2006. En medeltida skogsgård vid Markaryd: särskild arkeologisk undersökning av RAÄ 75, Markaryds socken, Sm. *Smålands Museum rapport 2006*: 45. Växjö

Åstrand, J. 2007. Den medeltida gården vid Markaryd. In: Hansson, M. (ed.) *Utmarker, gårdar och människor: om järnålder och medeltid i sydvästra Småland*, 55–85. Smålands museum, Växjö

Atkinson, M. D. 1992. *Betula pendula* Roth (*B. verrucosa* Ehrh.) and *B. pubescens* Ehrh. *Journal of Ecology* 80, 837–870

Bååth, K. 1983. Öde sedan stora döden var…: bebyggelse och befolkning i Norra Vedbo under senmedeltid och 1500-tal. Liber/Gleerup, Lund

Backe, M. 1988. Osteologisk rapport från Vreta kloster K:A, Vreta kloster Sn, Östergötland. In: Tagesson, G. (ed.) *Rapport, Arkeologisk undersökning samt osteologisk analys Vreta kloster kyrka, fornlämning 50, Vreta kloster socken Linköpings kommun Östergötland*. Östergötlands länsmuseum, Linköping

Bacot, A. W. 1914. A study of the bionomics of the common rat fleas and other species associated with human habitations, with special reference to the influence of temperature and humidity at various periods of the life cycle of the insect. *Journal of Hygiene* 13(Suppl.), 447–654

Barber, B. & Thomas, C. 2002. *The London Charterhouse*. MoLAS Monograph 10. Museum of London Archaeology Service, London

Barker, G. 2006. *The Agricultural Revolution in Prehistory: why did foragers become farmers?* Oxford University Press, Oxford

Bartholin, T. 1987. Dendrochronology in Sweden. In: Eronen, M. (ed.) *Dendrochronology around the Baltic*, 79–88. Annales Academiæ Scientarum Fennicæ. Series A. III Geologica–Geographica 145. Suomalainen Tiedeakatemia, Helsinki.

Bartholin, T. 1989a. Alla tiders träd. In: Aniansson, B. (ed.) *Forska på tvären*, 121–128. Naturvetenskapliga forskningsrådets årsbok 88/89

Bartholin, T. 1989b. Dendrokronologiske undersøgelser af Ystadområdets kirker. In: Andersson, H. & Anglert, M. (eds) *By, huvudgård och kyrka: studier i Ystadsområdets medeltid*, 211–219. Lund Studies in Medieval Archaeology 5. Almqvist & Wiksell, Stockholm

Bartholin, T. S. 1990. Dendrokronologi – og metodens anvendelsesmuligheter indenfor bebyggelsehistorisk forskning. *Bebyggelsehistorisk Tidskrift* 19, 43–61

Behre, K.-E. 1981. The interpretation of anthropogenic indicators in pollen diagrams. *Pollen et Spores* 23, 225–245.

Benedictow, O. 2004. *The Black Death 1346–1353: the complete history*. Boydell Press, Woodbridge

Benedictow, O. 2012. New perspectives in medieval demograhy: the medieval demographic system. In: Bailey, M. & Rigby, S. (eds) *Town and Countryside in the Age of the Black Death*, 3–42. Brepols, Turnhout

Bennike, P. 1985. *Paleopathology of Danish Skeletons: a comparative study of demography, disease and injury*. Akademisk Forlag, Copenhagen.

Berg, A. 2004. *Järnbruk och skog under 1000 år: vegetationshistorien kring sjön Kalven i Norbergs bergslag*. Examination paper. Department of Forest Ecology, Swedish University of Agricultural Sciences

Berglund, B. E. 1969. Vegetation and human influence in South Scandinavia during Prehistoric time. *Oikos Suppl.* 12, 9–28

Berglund, B. E. (ed.) 1991. The cultural landscape during 6000 years in southern Sweden: the Ystad Project. *Ecological Bulletins* 41. Copenhagen

Berglund, B., Eriksson, K., Holm, I., Karlsson, H., Karlsson, J., Pettersson, S., Sundberg, A., Ulfhielm, B., Welinder, S. 2009. The historical archaeology of the medieval crisis in Scandinavia. *Current Swedish Archaeology* 17, 55–78

Bergqvist, J. 2013. *Läkare och läkande: läkekonstens professionalisering i Sverige under medeltid och renässans* [English summary: Leeches and leechcraft: the professionalization of the art and craft of healing in Sweden during the Middle Ages and Renaissance]. Lund Studies in Historical Archaeology 16. Lund

Bernes, C. 2011. *Biodiversity in Sweden*. Monitor 22. Swedish Environmental Protection Agency, Stockholm

Beronius Jörpeland, L. 1992. The formation of occupation layers as an archaeological source. In: Ersgård, L., Holmström, M. & Lamm, K. (eds) *Rescue and Research: reflections of society in Sweden 700–1700 AD*, 00–00. Riksantikvarieämbete, Arkeologiska undersökningar, Skrifter 2. Stockholm

Beronius Jörpeland, L. & Bäck, M. 2003. "Skallerbohlet beläget widh häradz skilnaden ...". In: Anund, J. (ed.) *Landningsplats forntiden: arkeologiska fördjupningsstudier kring yngre stenålder, järnålder och historisk tid inom det område som tas i anspråk för den tredje landningsbanan vid Arlanda flygplats*, 177–214. Riksantikvarieämbetet, Arkeologiska undersökningar, Skrifter 49. Stockholm

Beronius Jörpeland, L. 2010. *Medeltida landsbygdsbebyggelse i Stockholms län*. Riksantikvarieämbetet UV Mitt, Rapport 2010: 8. Stockholm

Bielicki, T., Waliszko, Q., Hulanicka,B. & Kotlarz, K. 1986. Social class gradients in menacheal age in Poland. *Annals of Human Biology* 13, 1–11

Bisgaard, L. 2009. Danish plague patterns, 1360–1500. In: Bisgaard, L. & Søndergaard, L. (eds) *Living with the Black Death*, 85–111. University Press of Southern Denmark, Odense

Björ, J. 2005. St Mikael – de fattigas kyrka? En osteologisk analys och jämförande studie mellan skelettmaterial från S:t Mikael och Kv. Banken, Visby, Gotland. Unpublished examination paper in bioarchaeology. Högskolan Gotland, Visby

Björkman, L. 1996a. The late Holocene history of beech *Fagus sylvatica* and Norway spruce *Picea abies* at stand-scale in southern Sweden. *Lundqua Thesis* 39. Department of Quaternary Geology, Lund University

Björkman, L. 1996b. Long-term population dynamics of Fagus sylvatica at the northern limits of its distribution in southern Sweden: a palaeoecological study. *The Holocene* 6, 225–234

Björkman, L. 1997a. The history of *Fagus* forest in southwestern Sweden during the last 1500 years. *The Holocene* 7, 419–432

Björkman, L. 1997b. The role of human disturbance in the local late Holocene establishment of Fagus and Picea forests at Flahult, western Småland, southern Sweden. *Vegetation History and Archaeobotany* 6, 79–90

Björkman, L. 2000. *Pollenanalytisk undersökning av en torvmarkslagerföljd från Trälhultet i Biskopstorps naturreservat, Halmstads kommun*. Lundqua Uppdrag 29. Department of Quaternary Geology, Lund University

Björkman, L. 2003a. *Pollenanalytisk undersökning av en torvmarkslagerföljd från den arkeologiska undersökningslokalen "område 2" nordost om Köphult inför ombyggnaden av E4:an, delen länsgränsen till Strömsnäsbruk, Markaryds kommun*. Lundqua Uppdrag 48. Department of Quaternary Geology, Lund University

Björkman, L. 2003b. *Pollenanalytisk undersökning av en torvmarkslagerföljd från den arkeologiska undersökningslokalen "område 12/13" nordväst om Exhult inför ombyggnaden av E4:an, delen länsgränsen till Strömsnäsbruk, Markaryds kommun.* Lundqua Uppdrag 47. Department of Quaternary Geology, Lund University

Björkman, L. 2003c. *Pollenanalytisk undersökning av tre torvmarkslokaler från Öggestorps och Rogberga socknar inför ombyggnaden av Riksväg 31, delen Öggestorp–Åkarp, Jönköpings kommun.* Lundqua Uppdrag 45. Department of Quaternary Geology, Lund University

Björkman, L. 2005. *Pollenanalytisk undersökning av en torvmarkslagerföljd från Baggabygget i Rönnö naturreservat, Laholms kommun.* Lundqua Uppdrag 47. Department of Quaternary Geology, Lund University

Björkman, L. & Bradshaw, R. H. W. 1996. The immigration of Fagus sylvatica L. and Picea abies (L.) Karst. into a natural forest stand in southern Sweden during the last 2000 years. *Journal of Biogeography* 23, 235–244

Blomqvist, R. 1951. *Lunds historia: 1 Medeltiden.* Liber/Gleerup, Lund.

Boccaccio, G. 1353 [1995]. *The Decameron.* Penguin, London

Bogard, A., Fraser, R., Heaton, T. H. E., Vaiglova, P. Charles, M., Jones, G., Evershed, R. P., Styring, A. K., Andersen, N. H., Arbogast, R.-M., Bartosiewicz, L., Gardeisen, A., Kanstrup, M., Maier, U., Ninov, L., Schäfer, M. & Stephan, E. 2013. Crop manuring and intensive land management by Europe's first farmers. *Proceedings of the National Academy of Sciences* 110, 12589–12594

Bois, G. 1985. Against the neo-Malthusian orthodoxy. In: Aston, T. H. & Philpin, C. H. E. (eds) 1985. *The Brenner Debate: agrarian class structure and economic development in pre-industrial Europe*, 107–118. Cambridge University Press, Cambridge

Bolander, A. 2014. Smoke houses and entrepreneurship in two rural villages of medieval Scania, Örja and Skegrie. In: Svart Kristiansen, M. & Giles, K. (eds) *Dwellings, Identities and Homes: European housing culture from the Viking Age to Renaissance*, 185–194. Jutland Archaeological Society, Aarhus.

Bonnier, A.-C. 2008. Sockenkyrkorna under medeltiden. In: Dahlberg, M. & Franzén, K. (eds) *Sockenkyrkorna: kulturarv och bebyggelsehistoria*, 129–176. Riksantikvarieämbetet, Stockholm

Boserup, E. 1965. *The Conditions of Agricultural Growth: the economics of agrarian change under population pressure.* Allen & Unwin, London

Bradshaw, R. H. W. 1988. Spatially-precise studies of forest dynamics. In: Huntley, B. & Webb, T. III (eds) *Vegetation History*, 725–751. Kluwer, Dordrecht

Bradshaw, R. H. W., Holmqvist, B. H., Cowling, S. A. & Sykes, M. 2000. The effects of climate change on the distribution and management of *Picea abies* in southern Scandinavia. *Canadian Journal of Forest Research* 30, 1992–1998

Bragée, P. 2013. *A Palaeolimnological Study of the Anthropogenic Impact on Dissolved Organic Carbon in South Swedish Lakes.* Lundqua Thesis 71. Quaternary Sciences, Department of Geology, Lund University

Brenner, R. 1985. The agrarian roots of the European capitalism. In: Aston, T. H. & Philpin, C. H. E. (eds), *The Brenner Debate: agrarian class structure and economic development in pre-industrial Europe*, 213–327. Cambridge University Press

Broberg, B. 1992. The late-medieval towns of Sweden: an important research resource. In: Ersgård, L., Holmström, M. & Lamm, K. (eds) *Rescue and Research: reflections of society in Sweden 700–1700 AD.* Arkeologiska undersökningar, Skrifter 2. Rikantikvarieämbetet, Stockholm

Broecker, W. S. & Stocker, T. F. 2006. The Holocene CO2 rise: anthropogenic or natural? *EOS* 87, 27

Brooke, C. & Keir, G. 1975. *London 800–1216: the shaping of a city.* Francis Henry Wollaston Sheppard, London

Broström, A., Sugita, S. & Gaillard, M.-J. 2004. Pollen productivity estimates for reconstruction of past vegetation cover in the cultural landscape of Southern Sweden. *The Holocene* 14, 371–384

Broström, A., Nielsen, A. B., Gaillard, M.-J., Hjelle, K., Mazier, F., Binney, H., Bunting, J., Fyfe, R., Meltsov, V., Poska, A., Räsänen, S., Soepboer, W., von Stedingk, H., Suutari, H. & Sugita, S. 2008. Pollen productivity estimates of key European plant taxa for quantitative reconstruction of past vegetation: a review. *Vegetation History and Archaeobotany* 17, 461–478

Budd, P., Montgomery, J. Barreiro, B. & Thomas, R. G. 2000. Differential diagenesis of strontium in archaeological human dental tissues. *Applied Geochemistry* 15, 687–694

Campbell, B. M. S. 2006. The land. In: Horrox, R. & Ormrod, W. M. (eds) *A Social History of England, 1200–1500*, 179–237. Cambridge University Press, Cambridge

Campbell, B. M. S. 2012. Grain yields on English demesnes after the Black Death. In: Bailey, M. & Rigby, S. (eds) *Town and Countryside in the Age of the Black Death*, 121–174. Brepols, Turnhout

Cardell, A. Färsk fisk, var mans mat. In: Ericsson, G., Gardelin, G., Karlsson, M. & Magnell, O. (eds) Kv Blekhagen 10, 11, 12: arkeologisk undersökning 2003–2004. Unpublished report. Kulturens Museum, Lund

Carelli, P. 2001. *En kapitalistisk anda: kulturella förändringar i 1100-talets Danmark.* Lund studies in Medieval Archaeology 26. Almqvist & Wiksell, Stockholm

Carlsson, K. 2007. *Var går gränsen? Arkeologiska uttryck för religiösa och politiska aktörer i nuvarande Västsverige under perioden 1000–1300.* Lund Studies in Historical Archaeology 6. Lund University

Carlsson, T., Lindeblad, K. & Nielsen, A.-L. 2001. *Boplats och by: bebyggelseutveckling i Stora Ullevi 200-1600 e.Kr.* Riksantikvarieämbetet UV Öst, Rapport 2001: 5

Carmichael, A. G. 1986. *Plague and the Poor in Renaissance Florence.* Cambridge University Press, Cambridge

Chinn, S., Rona, R. J. & Price, C. E. 1989. The secular trend of height in primary schoolchildren in England and Scotland 1972–9 and 1979–86. *Annals of Human Biology* 16, 387–395

Christensen, P. 2009. Appearance and disappearance of the plague: still a puzzle? In: Bisgaard, L. & Søndergaard, L. (eds) *Living with the Black Death*, 11–21. University Press of Southern Denmark, Odense

Christophersen, A. 1978. Kvarteret S:t Peter i Lund. *Ale* 1978 (2), 17–32

Cinthio, M. 1992. Några daterings- och tolkningsproblem aktualiserade i samband med bearbetningen av gravar och kyrkogård tillhörande Trinitatiskyrkorna i Lund. *Meta* 1–2, 30–39

Cinthio, M. 2002. De första stadsborna: medeltida gravar och människor i Lund. Symposion, Stockholm/Stehag

Cipolla, C. M. 1976. *Public Health and Medical Profession in the Renaissance.* Cambridge University Press, Cambridge

Cipolla, C. M. 1981. *Fighting the Plague in Seventeenth-century Italy.* University of Wisconsin Press, Madison

Claussen, M., Brovkin, V., Calov, R., Ganopolski, A. & Kubatzki, C. 2005: Did humankind prevent a holocene glaciation? Comment on Ruddiman's hypothesis of a pre-historic anthropocene. *Climatic Change* 69, 409–417

Cohn, S. K. Jr. 2002. The Black Death: end of a paradigm. *American Historical Review* 107, 703–738

Cohn, S. K. Jr. 2003. *The Black Death transformed: disease and culture in early Renaissance Europe.* Arnold, London

Connelid, P. & Rosén, C. 1997. Agrarian settlement and landscape change in medieval Halland, South-West Sweden. In: Andersson, H., Carelli, P. & Ersgård, L. (eds) *Visions of the Past: trends and traditions in Swedish medieval archeology*, 23–42. Lund Studies in Medieval Archaeology 19/ Riksantikvarieämbetet, Arkeologiska undersökningar, Skrifter 24. Lund/Stockholm

Connelid, P. & Mascher, C. 2003. Hallands "vandrande landsbyar": vägar till den dolda medeltida och tidigmoderna agrarbebyggelsen. *Utskrift* 7, 100–127

Connelid, P. & Zedig, H. 2007. Medeltid vid Gamla Köpstad. *Nordisk bygd* 18, 15–20

Cox, G. & Sealy, J. 1997. Investigating identity and life histories: isotopic analysis and historical documentation of slave skeletons found on the Cape Town Foreshore, South Africa. *International Journal of Historical Archaeology* 1, 207–224

Cronon, W. 1983. *Changes in the Land: Indians, colonists, and the ecology of New England.* Hill and Wang, New York (1st revised edition published by Hill & Wang in 2003)

Crosby, A. W. 1972. *The Columbian Exchange: biological and cultural Consequences of 1492.*

Greenwood Press, Westport (Reprinted by Praeger in 2003)

Crutzen, P. J. 2002. Geology of mankind. *Nature* 415, 23

Dahlbäck, G. 1982. *Helgeandsholmen: 1000 år i Stockholms ström.* Liber, Stockholm

Dahlberg, M. & Franzén, K. (eds) 2008. *Sockenkyrkorna: kulturarv och bebyggelsehistoria.* Riksantikvarieämbetet, Stockholm

DeNiro, M. J. & Epstein, S. 1978. Influence of diet on the distribution of carbon isotopes in animals. *Geochimica et Cosmochimica Acta* 42, 495–506

DeNiro, M. J. & Epstein, S. 1981. Influence of diet on the distribution of nitrogen isotopes in animals. *Geochimica et Cosmochimica Acta* 45, 341–351

DeWitte, S. N. 2009. The effect of sex on risk of mortality during the Black Death in London, A.D. 1349–1350. *American Journal of Physical Anthropology* 139, 222–234

DeWitte, S. N. 2014. Health in post-Black Death London (1350–1538): age patterns of periosteal new bone formation in post-epidemic population. *American Journal of Physical Anthropology* 155, 260–267

DeWitte, S. N. & Wood, J. W. 2008. Selectivity of Black Death mortality with respect to pre-existing health. *Proceedings of the National Academy of Sciences* 105, 1436–1441

DeWitte, S. N. & Huges-Morey, G. 2012. Stature and frailty during the Black Death: the effect of stature on risk of epidemic mortality in London, A.D. 1348–1350. *Journal of Archaeological Science* 39, 1412–1419

Diamond, J. 2005. *Collapse: how societies choose to fail or succeed.* Viking, New York

Diamond, J. 2007. Easter Island revisited. *Science* 317, 1692–1694

Durhed, E. 2001. S:t Clemens och S:ta Gertrud: en analys av två medeltida kyrkogårdsmaterial i Visby. Unpublished examination paper in osteology. Högskolan på Gotland, Visby

Dyer, C. 1989. *Standards of Living in the Later Middle Ages: social change in England c. 1200–1520.* Cambridge University Press, Cambridge

Dyer, C. 2002. *Making a Living in the Middle Ages: the people of Britain 850–1520.* Yale University Press, New Haven/London

Dyer, C. 2010. Villages in crisis: social dislocation and desertion, 1370–1520. In: Dyer, C. & Jones, R. (eds) *Deserted Villages Revisited*, 28–45. University of Hertfordshire Press, Hatfield

Dyer, C. & Everson, P. 2012. The development of the study of medieval settlements, 1880–2010. In: Christie, N. & Stamper, P. (eds) *Medieval Rural Settlement: Britain and Ireland, AD 800–1600*, 11–30. Windgather Press, Oxford

Eckstein, D. 1984. *Dendrochronological Dating.* Handbooks for archaeologists 2. European Science Foundation, Strasbourg.

Edwards, K. J. 1991. Using space in cultural palynology: the value of the off-site pollen record. In: Harris, D. R. & Thomas, K. D. (eds) *Modelling Ecological Change: perspectives from neoecology, palaeoecology and environmental archaeology*, 61–73. Institute of Archaeology, University College London

Eliasson, P. & Hamilton, G. 1999. "Blifver ondt att förena sigh" – några linjer i den svenska skogslagstiftningen om utmark och skog. In: Pettersson, R. (ed.) *Skogshistorisk forskning i Europa och Nordamerika*, 47–106. Kungl. Skogs- och Lantbruksakademien, Stockholm

Emanuelsson, M. 2001. *Settlement and Land-use History in the Central Swedish Forest Region: the use of pollen analysis in interdisciplinary studies.* Silvestria 223. Swedish University of Agricultural Sciences, Umeå

Emanuelsson, U. 2009. *The Rural Landscapes of Europe: how man has shaped European nature.* Formas, Stockholm

Ericsson, A. 2012. *Terra medievalis: jordvärderingssystem i medeltidens Sverige.* Acta Universitatis Agriculturae Sueciae 81. Swedish University of Agricultural Sciences

Eriksson, G. 1996. Skogshistoria, kulturpåverkan och urskogsvärden I fem skogsreservat I Kronobergs län. Unpublished Master's Thesis, University of Umeå

Eriksson, O., Cousins, S. A. O. & Bruun, H. E. 2002. Land-use history and fragmentation of traditionally managed grasslands in Scandinavia. *Journal of Vegetation Science* 13, 743–748

Ersgård, L. 1986. Expansion och förändring i Uppsalas medeltida bebyggelse. In: Cnattingius, N. & Nevéus, T. (eds) *Från Östra Aros till Uppsala: en samling uppsatser kring det medeltida Uppsala*, 78–100. Uppsala stads historia 7. Riksantikvarieämbetet, Stockholm

Ersgård, L. 1988. *"Vår marknad i Skåne": bebyggelse, handel och urbanisering i Skanör och Falsterbo under medeltiden*. Lund Studies in Medieval Archaeology 4. Almqvist & Wiksell, Stockholm

Ersgård, L. 2001. Människan vid kusten: fiskebebyggelse från Skagerack till Bottenhavet under senmedeltid och början av nyare tid. In: Andrén, A., Ersgård, L. & Wienberg, J. (eds) *Från stad till land: en medeltidsarkeologisk resa tillägnad Hans Andersson*, 95–104. Lund Studies in Medieval Archaeology 29. Almqvist & Wiksell, Stockholm

Etter, H. & Schneider, J. 1982–83. Die Pest in Zürich. *Turicum* 4, 43-49

Eveleth, P. B. & Tanner, J. M. 1990. *Worldwide Variation in Human Growth*. 2nd edition. Cambridge University Press, Cambridge

Feldt, A.-C. & Tagesson, G. 1997. *Två gårdar i biskopens stad: om den arkeologiska undersökningen i kvarteret Brevduvan, Linköping 1987 och 1989*. Östergötland Fakta 3. Östergötlands länsmuseum, Linköping

Fjällström, M. 2013. Analys av stabila kol- och kväveisotoper av skelettmaterial från Lund, Skåne. Unpublished report

Framme, G. 1985. Ödegårdar i Vätte härad. Skrifter utgivna av Dialekt-, Ortnamns- och Folkminnesarkivet i Göteborg 1. Göteborg

Frank, R. W. Jr. 1995. The "hungry gap," crop failure, and famine: the fourteenth-century agricultural crisis and Piers Plowman. In: Sweeney, D. (ed.) *Agriculture in the Middle Ages: technology, practice, and representation*, 227–243, University of Pennsylvania Press, Philadelphia

Fredh, D. 2012. *The Impact of Past Land-Use Change on Floristic Diversity in Southern Sweden – A Quantitative Approach Based on High-Resolution Pollen Data*. Lundqua Thesis 66. Quaternary Sciences, Department of Geology, Lund University

Fredh, D., Broström, A., Zillén, L., Mazier, F., Rundgren, M., Lagerås, P. 2012. Floristic diversity in the transition from traditional to modern land-use in southern Sweden A.D. 1800–2008. *Vegetation History and Archaeobotany* 21, 439–452

Frei, K. M., Frei, R., Mannering, U., Gleba, M., Nosch, M. L. & Lyngstrøm, H. 2009. Provenance of ancient textiles: a pilot study evaluating the strontium isotope system in wool. *Archaeometry* 51, 252–276

Gadd, C.-J. 2011. The agricultural revolution in Sweden: 1700–1870. In: Myrdal, J. & Morell, M. (eds) *The Agrarian History of Sweden: from 4000 BC to AD 2000*, 118–164. Nordic Academic Press, Stockholm

Gaillard, M.-J., Birks, H. J. B., Emanuelsson, U., Karlsson, S., Lagerås, P. & Olausson, D. 1994. Application of modern pollen/land-use relationships to the interpretation of pollen diagrams – reconstruction of land-use history in South Sweden, 3000–0 BP. *Review of Palaeobotany and Palynology* 82, 47–73

Gaillard, M.-J., Sugita, S., Mazier, F., Trondman, A.-K., Broström, A., Hickler, T., Kaplan, J. O., Kjellström, E., Kokfelt, U., Kuneš, P., Lemmen, C., Miller, P., Olofsson, J., Poska, A., Rundgren, M., Smith, B., Strandberg, G., Fyfe, R., Nielsen, A. B., Alenius, T., Balakauskas, L., Barnekow, L., Birks, H. J. B., Bjune, A., Björkman, L., Giesecke, T., Hjelle, K., Kalnina, L., Kangur, M., van der Knaap, W. O., Koff, T., Lagerås, P., Latałowa, M., Leydet, M., Lechterbeck, J., Lindbladh, M., Odgaard, B. V., Peglar, S., Segerström, U., von Stedingk, H. & Seppä, H. 2010. Holocene land-cover reconstructions for studies on land cover-climate feedbacks. *Climate of the Past* 6, 483–499

Gauffin, S. 1979. Fagmon: ett ödesböle i Jämtland. In: Hemmendorff, O. (ed.) *Arkeologi i fjäll, skog och bygd: 2 Järnålder–medeltid*, 135–144. Fornvårdaren 24. Jämtlands läns museum, Östersund

Gauffin, S. 1981. Ödesbölet Svedäng, Alsens socken: rapport från en arkeologisk undersökning. Jämtlands läns museum, Östersund

Gejvall, N. 1960. *Westerhus: medieval population and church in the light of skeletal remains*. Kungl.

vitterhets-, historie- och antikvitetsakademien, Stockholm

Giesecke, T. & Bennett, K. D. 2004. The Holocene spread of *Picea abies* (L.) Karst. In Fennoscandia and adjacent areas. *Journal of Biogeography* 31, 1523–1548

Gissel, S., Jutikkala, E., Österberg, E., Sandnes, J. & Teitson, B. (eds) 1981. *Desertion and Land Colonization in the Nordic Countries c. 1300–1600: comparative report from the Scandinavian research project on deserted farms and villages.* Almqvist & Wiksell, Stockholm

Götmark, F. & Kiffer, Ch. 2014. Regeneration of oaks (*Quercus robur/Q. petraea*) and three other tree species during long-term succession after catastrophic disturbance (windthrow). *Plant Ecology* DOI 10.1007/s11258-014-0365-4

Goudie, A. 2013. *The Human Impact on the Natural Environment – past, present and future.* Wiley-Blackwell, Chichester

Grainger, I., Hawkins, D., Cowal, L. & Mikulski, R. 2008. *The Black Death Cemetery, East Smithfield, London.* MoLAS Monograph 43. Museum of London Archaeology Service, London

Grandin, L., Forenius, S. & Willim, A. 2008. *Smedjan på garden: arkeometallurgiska analyser av material från gården Vålle, Bohuslän, Lurs socken, Vålle 1:6, RAÄ 361.* Geoarkeologisk undersökning. Riksantikvarieämbetet UV Uppsala, Rapport 2008: 23

Gräslund, B. & Price, N. 2012. Twilight of the gods? The 'dust veil event' of AD 536 in critical perspective. *Antiquity* 86, 428–443

Grundberg, L. 2001. "Där som inga lagliga köpstäder äro..." – medeltida urbaniseringstendenser i ett norrländskt perspektiv. *Bebyggelsehistorisk tidskrift* 42, 75–102

Grundberg, L. & Hårding, B. 2003. *Arkeologisk undersökning av en medeltida begravningsplats och boplats från järnåldern, RAÄ 23 och 97, Torsåkers socken, Ångermanland, Del 1 och 2.* Länsmuseet Västernorrland, Rapport 2003: 4

Grupe, G., Price, T. D., Schörter, P., Söllner, F., Johnson, C. & Beard, B. 1997. Mobility of Bell Beaker people revealed by strontium isotope ratios of tooth and bone: a study of southern Bavarian skeletal remains. *Applied geochemistry* 12, 517–525

Gustafsson, M. E. R. & Franzén, L. G. 2000. Inland transport of marine aerosols in southern Sweden. *Atmospheric Environment* 34, 313–325

Gustafsson, A., Werdelin, L., Tullberg, B. S. & Lindenfors, P. 2007. Stature and sexual stature dimorfismus in Sweden from the 10th to the end of the 20th Century. *American Journal of Human Biology* 19, 861–870.

Haensch, S., Bianucci, R., Signoli, M., Rajerison, M., Schultz, M., Kacki, S., Vermunt, M., Weston, D. A., Hurst, D., Achtman, M., Carniel, E. & Bramanti, B. 2010. Distinct clones of *Yersinia pestis* caused the Black Death. *PloS Pathogens* 6(10), doi: 10.1371/journal.ppat.1001134

Hall, V. 2003. Vegetation history of mid- to western Ireland in the 2nd millennium A.D.: fresh evidence from tephra-dated playnological investigations. *Vegetation History and Archaeobotany* 12, 7–17

Hämäläinen, P. (ed.) 2006. *When Disease Makes History – Epidemics and Great Historical Turning Points.* Helsinki University Press, Helsinki

Hansson, A., Olsson, C., Storå, J., Welinder, S. & Zetterström, Å. 2005. *Agrarkris och ödegårdar i Jämtland.* Jamtli förlag, Östersund

Hårdh, B. & Larsson, L. 2007. *Uppåkra – Lund före Lund.* Årsboken 2007. Föreningen Gamla Lund, Lund

Harrison, D. 2000. *Stora döden: den värsta katastrof som drabbat Europa.* Ordfront, Stockholm

Hartzel, L. 2010. *Liv och död i det tidigmedeltida Västerås: en osteologisk analys av skelett från Kvarteret Johannes.* Fou rapport 8. Statens Historiska Museer, Stockholm

Hatton, T. J. 2014. How have Europeans grown so tall? *Oxford Economic Papers* 66, 349–372

Højrup, O. & Jensen, S. 1963. *Levnedsløb i Sørbymagle og Kirekrup kirkebøger 1646–1731.* Landbohistoriskt Selskab, Copenhagen

van Hoof, T. B., Bunnik, F. P. M., Waucomont, J. G. M., Kürschner, W. M. & Visscher, H. 2006. Forest re-growth on medieval farmland after the Black Death pandemic – implications for atmospheric CO_2 levels. *Palaeogeography, Palaeoclimatology, Palaeoecology* 237, 396–411

Hovanta, E. 1994. Dendrokronologisk bestämning av byggnader i Hälsingland (with English summary: Dendrochronological investigations of buildings in the province of Hälsingland). *Bebyggelsehistorisk tidskrift* 27, 133–142

Howland, M. R., Corr, L. T., Young, S. M. M., Jones, V., Jim, S., van der Merwe, N. J., Mittchell, A. D. & Evershed, R. P. 2003. Expression of the dietary isotope signal in the compound-specific δ^{13}C values of pig bone lipids and amino acids. *International Journal of Osteoarchaeology* 13, 54–65

Hult, O. T. 1916, Pesten i Sverige 1710. *Hygienisk Tidskrift* 8, 79–192

Hultberg, T., Brunet, J., Broström, A. &Lindbladh, M. 2010. Forest in a cultural landscape – the vegetation history of Torup in southernmost Sweden. *Ecological Bulletins* 53, 141–153

Hultkrantz, J. V. 1927. Über die Zuhahme der Körpegrösse in Sweden in den Jahren 1840–1926. Nova acta Regiae Societatis Scientiarum Upsaliensis, Series 4. Uppsala University

Hynynen, J., Niemistö, P., Viherä-Aarnio, A., Brunner, A., Hein, S., Velling, P. 2010. Silviculture of birch (*Betula pendula* Roth and *Betula pubescens* Ehrh.) in northern Europe. *Forestry* 83, 103–119

Ilmoni, I. 1846–1853. *Bidrag till historien om Nordens sjukdomar, Del 1–3*. Helsingfors

IPCC 2013. *Climate change 2013 – The physical science basis. Contribution of Working group I to the Fifth Assessment Report of the Intergovernmental Panel on Climate Change* [Stocker, T. F., Qin, D., Plattner, G.-K., Tignor, M., Allen, S. K., Boschung, J. Nauels, A., Xia, Y., Bex, V. & Midgley, P. M. (eds.)]. Cambridge University Press, Cambridge/New York

Iregren, E. 1973. Julita kloster, Södermanland. Unpublished report. Statens Historiska Museum, Stockholm

Iversen, J. 1941. Landnam i Danmarks stenalder. *Danm. Geol. Unders.* Ser. II 66, 1–68

Iversen, J. 1949. The influence of prehistoric man on vegetation. *Danm. Geol. Unders.* Ser. IV 3, 1–25

Jacobsson, B. 2002. Pestbacken: en begravningsplats för pestoffer från åren 1710 och 1711, Blekinge, Olofströms kommun, Jämshögs socken, Holje 5:68 och 5:69. Riksantivarieämbetet UV Syd Rapport 2002: 15

Johansson, E. (Ed.) 2002. *Periferins landskap: historiska spår och nutida blickfält i svensk glesbygd.* Nordic Academic Press, Stockholm

Jones, R. 2010. Contrasting patterns of village and hamlet desertion in England. In: Dyer, C. & Jones, R. (eds) *Deserted Villages Revisited*, 8–27. University of Hertfordshire Press, Hatfield

Jonsson, K. & Nordström, A. 2003. *En tidigkristen gravplats och medeltida kyrklämning: gravar och kyrkor i Sura 900-1800.* Kulturmiljöavdelningen Rapport A 2003: A16. Västmanland läns museum, Västerås

Karlsson, G. 1996. Plague without rats: the case of fifteenth-century Iceland. *Journal of Medieval History* 22, 263–284

Karlsson, S. & Risberg, J. 1996. Växthistoria och strandförskjutning i området kring Fjäturen och Gullsjön, södra Uppland. In: Johansson, Å. & Lindgren, C. (eds) *En introduktion till det arkeologiska projektet Norrortsleden, Uppland, Fresta och Täby socknar*, 71–126. Riksantikvarieämbetet UV Mitt, Dokumentation av fältarbetsfasen 2005: 1

Karlsson, M., Nilsson, T. & Pichler, S. 2014. The impact of the 1918 Spanish flu epidemic on economic performance in Sweden. An investigation into the consequences of an extraordinary mortality shock. *Journal of Health Economics* 36, 1–19

Karsvall, O. 2011. Utjordar and the question of deserted farms – a case study of the parish of Svanhals. *Bebyggelsehistorisk Tidskrift* 61, 22–38

Keene, D. 1984. A new study of London before the Great Fire. *Urban History Yearbook* 20, 11–21

Keene, D. 1989. Medieval London and its region. *London Journal* 14(2), 9–11

Kellgren, K. G. 1930. Pesten på Gotland 1710–12. *Karolinska Förbundet Årsbok* 1930, 76–105

Kershaw, I. 1973. The great famine and agrarian crisis in England 1315–1322. *Past and Present* 59, 3–50

Kimura, K. 1984. Studies on growth and development in Japan. *Yearbook of Physical Anthropology* 27, 179–214

Kinnaird, J. W. 1974. Effect of site conditions on the regeneration of birch (*Betula pendula* Roth and *B. pubescens* Ehrh.). *Journal of Ecology* 62, 467–472

Kjekshus, H. 1977. *Ecology Control and Economic Development in East African History*. University of California Press, Berkeley

Kjellström, A. 2003. Människorna i slaget: vad benen berättar. In: Syse, B. (ed.) *Långfredagsslaget: en arkeologisk historia*, 60–108. Upplandsmuseets skriftserie 3. Upplandsmuseet, Uppsala

Kjellström, A., Storå, J., Possnert, G. & Linderholm, A. 2009. Dietary patterns and social structures in medieval Sigtuna, Sweden, as reflected in stable isotope and trace element values in human skeletal remains. *Journal of Archaeological Science* 36, 2689–2699

Knudsen, L. G. 2009. The course of the mid-17th century plague epidemic in Denmark. In: Bisgaard, L. & Søndergaard, L. (eds) *Living with the Black Death*, 113–134. University Press of Southern Denmark, Odense

Koepke, N. & Baten, J. 2005. The biological standard of living in Europe during the last two millennia. *European Review of Economic History* 9, 61–95

Kohn, M. J., Schoeninger M. J. & Barker, W. W. 1999. Altered states: effects of diagenesis on fossil tooth chemistry. *Geochimica et Cosmochimica Acta* 18, 2737–2747

Kuh, D., Power, C. & Blane, D. 1997. Social pathways between childhood and adult health. In: Kuh, D. & Ben-Sclomo, Y. (eds) *A Life Course Approach to Chronic Disease*, 169–200. Oxford Medical Publications, Oxford

Lagerås, P. 1996. *Vegetation and Land-use in the Småland Uplands, Southern Sweden, During the last 6000 Years*. Lundqua Thesis 36. Dept of Quaternary Geology, Lund University

Lagerås, P. 2002. Skog, slåtter och stenröjning: paleoekologiska undersökningar i trakten av Stoby i norra Skåne. In: Carlie, A. (ed.) *Skånska regioner – tusen år av kultur och samhälle i förändring*, 363–411. Arkeologiska undersökningar, Skrifter 31. Riksantikvarieämbetet, Stockholm

Lagerås, P. 2007. *The Ecology of Expansion and Abandonment: medieval and post-medieval land-use and settlement dynamics in a landscape perspective*. Riksantikvarieämbetet, Stockholm

Lagerås, P. 2013a. Agrara fluktuationer och befolkningsutveckling på sydsvenska höglandet tolkade utifrån röjningsrösen. (English summary: Agricultural and population dynamics in the South-Swedish Upland interpreted from radiocarbon-dated clearance cairns) *Fornvännen* 108, 263–277

Lagerås, P. 2013b. Medieval colonisation and abandonment in the South Swedish Uplands: a review of settlement and land use dynamics inferred from the pollen record. *Archaeologia Baltica* 20, 77–90

Lagerås, P. & Bartholin, T. S. 2003. Fire and stone clearance in Iron Age agriculture: new insights inferred from the analysis of terrestrial macroscopic charcoal in clearance cairns in Hamneda. *Vegetation History and Archaeobotany* 12, 83–92

Lagerås, P., Jansson, K. & Vestbö, A. 1995. Land-use history of the Axlarp area in the Småland uplands, southern Sweden: palaeoecological and archaeological investigations. *Vegetation History and Archaeobotany* 4, 223–234

Lamb, H. H. 1982. *Climate, History and the Modern World*. 2nd edition. Routledge, New York/London

Larsen, L. B., Vinther, B. M., Briffa, K. R., Melvin, T. M., Clausen, H. B., Jones, P. D., Siggaard-Andersen, M.-L., Hammer, C. U., Eronen, M., Grudd, H., Gunnarson, B. E., Hantemirov, R. M., Naurzbaev, M. M. & Nicolussi, K. 2008. New ice core evidence for a volcanic cause of the A.D. 536 dust veil. *Geophysical Research Letters* 35, 1–5

Larsson, J. 2009. *Fäbodväsendet 1550–1920: ett centralt element i Nordsveriges jordbrukssystem*. Acta Universitatis Agriculturae Sueciae 2009: 51. Swedish University of Agricultural Sciences

Larsson, J. 2012. The expansion and decline of a transhumance system in Sweden, 1550–1920. *Historia Agraria* 56, 11–39

Larsson, L. 2007. The Iron Age ritual building at Uppåkra, southern Sweden. *Antiquity* 81, 11–25

Larsson, L-O. 1970. Kronans jordeböcker från 1500-talet och den senmedeltida ödegårdsprocessen: några synpunkter på terminologi och retrospektiv metod. *Historisk tidskrift* 1970(1), 24–76

Larsson, L.-O. 1975. *Det medeltida Värend: studier i det småländska gränslandets historia fram till 1500-talets mitt*. 2nd edition. Kronoberg läns hembygdsförbund, Växjö

Lee-Thorp, J. A., Sealy, J. C. & van der Merwe, N. J. 1989. Stable carbon isotope ratio differences between bone collagen and bone apatite, and their relationship to diet. *Journal of Archaeological Science* 16, 585–599

Lee-Thorp, J. A. & Sponheimer, M. 2003. Three case studies used to reassess the reliability of fossil bone and enamel isotope signals for paleodietary studies. *Journal of Anthropological Archaeology* 22, 208–216

Le Roy Ladurie, E. 1985. A reply to Robert Brenner. In: Aston, T. H. & Philpin, C. H. E. (eds) 1985. *The Brenner Debate: agrarian class structure and economic development in pre-industrial Europe*, 101–106. Cambridge University Press

Lewis, C. 2007. New avenues for the Investigation of currently occupied medieval rural settlement: preliminary observations from the Higher Education Field Academy. *Medieval Archaeology* 51, 133–163

Lilja, H., Jacobsson, B. & Arcini, C. 2001. *Svartbrödernas kyrkogård i Åhus. Arkeologisk undersökning 1996, fornlämning 23, Åhus sn, Skåne.* Kristianstad länsmuseum, Kristianstad

Lindbladh, M. 1998. *Long Term Dynamics and Human Influence in the Forest Landscape of Southern Sweden.* Silvestria 78. Swedish University of Agricultural Sciences

Lindbladh, M. & Bradshaw, R. H. W. 1998. The origin of present forest composition and pattern in southern Sweden. *Journal of Biogeography* 25, 463–477

Lindbladh, M., Niklasson & M., Nilsson, S. G. 2003. Long-time record of fire and open canopy in a high biodiversity forest in southeast Sweden. *Biological Conservation* 114, 231–243

Lindbladh, M., Brunet, J., Hannon, G., Niklasson, M., Eliasson, P., Eriksson, G. & Ekstrand, A. 2007. Forest history as a basis for ecosystem restoration – a multidisciplinary case study in a South Swedish temperate landscape. *Restoration Ecology* 15, 284–295

Lindbladh, M., Niklasson, M., Karlsson, M., Björkman, L. & Churski, M. 2008. Close anthropogenic control of Fagus sylvatica establishment and expansion in a Swedish protected landscape – implications for forest history and conservation. *Journal of Biogeography* 35, 682–697

Lindeblad. K. & Tagesson, G. 2004. *Stora Ullevi bytomt, Östergötland, S:t Lars socken, Linköpings stad, RAÄ 345, 423-1820-2003.* Arkeologisk slutundersökning. Riksantikvarieämbetet, Avdelningen för arkeologiska undersökningar UV Öst, Dokumentation av fältarbetsfasen 2004: 3.

Lindeblad, K. & Tagesson, G. 2005. Byn och staden: Stora Ullevi och Linköping. In: Kaliff, A. & Tagesson, G. (eds) *Liunga, Kaupinga: kulturhistoria och arkeologi i Linköpingsbygden*, 237–281. Arkeologiska undersökningar, Skrifter 60. Riksantikvarieämbetet, Stockholm

Lindkvist, T. 2010. Riksbildning och statsbildning: regionala variationer i det blivande Sverige. *Med hammare och fackla* 51, 14–40

Lindman, G. (ed.) 2004. *Gårdar från förr: nordbohuslänsk bebyggelsehistoria utifrån arkeologiska undersökningar av tre medeltida gårdar.* Arkeologiska undersökningar, Skrifter 56. Riksantikvarieämbetet, Stockholm

Linnæus, C. 1751 [reprint 1975]. *Skånska resa.* Wahlström & Widstrand, Stockholm

Livi Bacci, M. 2000. *The Population of Europe: a history.* Blackwell, Oxford

Ljung, J.-Å. 1991. Medeltida bebyggelse i Örebro: en kort sammanfattning främst utifrån undersökningarna i kvarteren Bromsgården och Tryckeriet 10. *Arkeologi i Sverige* (new series) 1. Riksantikvarieämbetet, Stockholm

Lovén, C. 1996. *Borgar och befästningar i det medeltida Sverige.* Kungl. Vitterhets-, historie- och antikvitetsakademien, Stockholm

Lütgert, S. A. 2000. Victims of the Great Famine or the Black Death? The archaeology of the mass graves found in the former graveyard of Holy Ghost Hospital, Lübeck (N. Germany), in the European context. *Hikuin* 27, 255–265

Magnell, O. 2006. Att befolka en stadsdel: pälsare i det medeltida kvarteret Blekhagen, Lund. *META* 2006(4), 19–33

Magnusson, G. 1985. Lapphyttan: an example of medieval iron production. In: *Medieval Iron in Society: papers presented at the symposium in Norberg, May 6-10, 1985.* Jernkontoret/ Riksantikvarieämbetet, Stockholm

Magnusson, G. 2010. Medeltida järnhantering: en europeisk översikt. *Med hammare och fackla* 51, 103–130

Magnusson, L. & Isacson, M. 1988. Proto-industrialisering: en förutsättning för den industriella revolutionen? *Bebyggelsehistorisk tidskrift* 16, 5-8

Malm, G. 1984. Uppsala domkyrka: en kortfattad murverksanalys. *META* 1984, 3–4.

Malthus, T. R. [1803] 2003. *An Essay on the Principle of Population*. W. W. Norton, New York

Mann, C. C. 2006. *1491 – New revelations of the Americas before Columbus*. Vintage, New York

Martiin, C. 2010. Swedish milk, a Swedish duty: dairy marketing in the 1920s and 1930s. *Rural History* 21, 213–232

Martin, J. 2012. Russia. In: Kitsikopoulos, H. (ed.) *Agrarian Change and Crisis in Europe, 1200–1500*, 292–329. Routledge, New York/London

Martin, R., Saller, K. 1957. *Lehrbuch der Anthropologie in Systematischer Darstellung*. Band I, 3. Aufl. Gustav Fischer Verlag, Stuttgart

Maurer, A.-F., Galer, S. J. G., Knipper, C., Beierlein, L., Nunn, E. V., Peters, D., Tutken, T., Alt, K. W. & Schone, B. R. 2012. Preservation vs. anthropogenic contamination of natural bioavailable strontium in Saxony-Anhalt, Germany, with implications for isoscapes in past migration studies. *Science of the Total Environment* 433, 216–229

Mazier, F., Broström, A., Bragée, P., Fredh, D., Stenberg, L., Thiere, G., Sugita, S. & Hammarlund, D. 2015. Two hundred years of land-use change in the South Swedish Uplands: comparison of historical map-based estimates with pollen-based reconstruction using the Landscape Reconstruction Algorithm with historical maps. *Vegetation History and Archeobotany* 24: 555–570

McAnany, P. A. & Yoffee, N. (eds) 2010. Q*uestioning Collapse: human resilience, ecological vulnerability, and the aftermath of empire*. Cambridge University Press, Cambridge

Menander, H. & Arcini, C. 2013. Dominikankonventet S:t Olof. In: Hedvall, R., Lindeblad, K. & Menander, H. (eds) *Borgare, bröder och bönder: arkeologiska perspektiv på Skänninges äldre historia,* 191–227 Riksantikvarieämbetet, Stockholm

Meyer, H. E. & Selmer. R. 1999. Income, educational level and body height. *Annals of Human Biology* 26(3), 219–223

Mills, C. M. & Crone, A. 2012. Dendrochronological evidence for Scotland's native timber resources over the last 1000 years. *Scottish Forestry* 66, 18–33

Moberg, A., Sonechkin, D. M., Holmgren, K., Datsenko, N. M., Karlén, W. 2005. Highly variable Northern Hemisphere temperatures reconstructed from low- and high-resolution proxy data. *Nature* 433, 613–617

Moe, D. 1991. Hustad, Arstad and Naustad: a vegetational study of three farms in Saltne, North Norway. *Norsk Geografisk Tidskrift* 45, 11–24

Moore, P. D., Webb, J. A. & Collinson, M. E. 1991. *Pollen Analysis* (2nd edition). Blackwell, Oxford

Moran, E. F. 2010. *Environmental Social Science: human-environment interactions and sustainability*. Wiley-Blackwell, Chichester

Moseng, O. G. 2009. Climate, ecology and plague: the second and the third pandemic reconsidered. In: Bisgaard, L. & Søndergaard, L. (eds) *Living with the Black Death*, 23–45. University Press of Southern Denmark, Odense

Myrdal, J. 1999. *Jordbruket under feodalismen 1000-1700*. Det svenska jordbrukets historia. Natur och kultur, Stockholm

Myrdal, J. 2003. *Digerdöden, pestvågor och ödeläggelse: ett perspektiv på senmedeltidens Sverige*. Runica et Mediævalia, Stockholm.

Myrdal, J. 2006. The forgotten plague: the Black Death in Sweden. In Hämäläinen, P. (ed.) *When Disease Makes History – Epidemics and Great Historical Turning Points*, 141–186. Helsinki University Press, Helsinki

Myrdal, J. 2009. The Black Death in the North: 1349–1350. In: Bisgaard, L. & Søndergaard, L. (eds) *Living with the Black Death*, 63–82. University Press of Southern Denmark, Odense

Myrdal, J. 2011. Farming and feudalism, 1000–1700. In: Myrdal, J. & Morell, M. (eds) *The Agrarian History of Sweden: from 4000 BC to AD 2000*, 72–117. Nordic Academic Press, Stockholm

Myrdal, J. 2012a. Scandinavia. In: Kitsikopolous, H. (ed.) *Agrarian Change and Crisis in Europe, 1200–1500*, 204–249. Routledge, New York/London

Myrdal, J. 2012b. *Boskapsskötseln under medeltiden: en källpluralistisk studie*. Nordiska museets handlingar 139. Nordiska museets förlag, Stockholm

Myrdal, J. & Söderberg, J. 1991. *Kontinuitetens dynamik: agrar ekonomi i 1500-talets Sverige*. Acta Universitatis Stockholmiensis, Stockholm Studies in Economic History 15. Almqvist & Wiksell, Stockholm

Näsman, U., Lund, J. (eds.) 1988. *Folkevandringstiden i Norden: en krisetid mellem ældre og yngre jernalder*. Aarhus Universitet, Aarhus

Nordberg, M. 1996. I *kung Magnus tid – Norden under Magnus Eriksson: 1317–1374*. Bonnier, Stockholm

Norman, P. 1993. Medeltida utskärsfiske: en studie av fornlämningar i kustmiljö. Nordiska museets Handlingar 116. Stockholm

Nyborg, E. 2009. The Black Death as reflected in Scandinavian art and architecture. In: Bisgaard, L. & Søndergaard, L. (eds) *Living with the Black Death*, 187–206. University Press of Southern Denmark, Odense

O'Connell, T. C., Kneale, C. J., Tasevska, N. & Kuhnle, G. G. C. 2012. The diet-body offset in human nitrogen isotopic values: a controlled dietary study. *American Journal of Physical Anthropology* 149, 426–434

Olausson, M. 1989. Kyrklägdan: en tusenårig gårdshistoria. In: Hemmendorff, O. (ed.) *Arkeologi i fjäll, skog och bygd: 2 Järnålder–medeltid*. Fornvårdaren 24. Jämtlands läns museum, Östersund

Olofsson, J &, Hickler, T. 2008. Effects of human land-use on the global carbon cycle during the last 6,000 years. *Vegetation History and Archaeobotany* 17, 605–615

Olsson, I. U. 1991. Accuracy and precision in sediment chronology. *Hydrobiologia* 214, 25–34

Österberg, E. 1971. *Gränsbygd under krig: ekonomiska, demografiska och administrativa förhållanden i sydvästra Sverige under och efter nordiska sjuårskriget*. Bibliotheca Historica Lundensis 26. Gleerup, Lund

Österberg, E. 1977. *Kolonisation och kriser: bebyggelse, skattetryck, odling och agrarstruktur i västra Värmland ca 1300–1600*. Bibliotheca Historica Lundensis 43. Gleerups, Lund

Österberg, E. 1981a. Methods, hypotheses and study areas. In: Gissel, S., Jutikkala, E., Österberg, E., Sandnes, J. & Teitson, B. (eds) *Desertion and Land Colonization in the Nordic countries c. 1300–1600: comparative report from the Scandinavian research project on deserted farms and villages*, 26–77. Almqvist & Wiksell, Stockholm

Österberg, E. 1981b. Ödegårdar i medeltidens Norden: rapport från ett forskningsprojekt. *Bebyggelsehistorisk tidskrift* 2, 62–67

Palm, L. Andersson 2001. *Livet, kärleken och döden: fyra uppsatser om svensk befolkningsutveckling 1300–1850*. Department of History, Gothenburg University.

Persson, B. 2001. *Pestens gåta: farsoter i det tidiga 1700-talets Skåne*. Studia Historica Lundensia 5. Nordic Academic Press, Lund

Persson, O. & Persson, E. 1983. *The Löddeköpinge Investigation V: report on the anthropmetrics of the skeletons from the early medieval cemetery in Löddeköpinge (Scania, S. Sweden)*. Institute of Archaeology, Report Series 19. Lund University

Persson, O. & Persson, E. Rapport om skelettmaterialet från Tygelsjö. Malmö Museum S10: 011. Unpublished report

Pettersson Jensen, I.-M. 2012. *Norberg och järnet: bergsmännen och den medeltida industrialiseringen*. Jernkontorets bergshistoriska skriftserie 46. Stockholm

Pihlman, A. & Kostet, J. 1986. Åbo (fi. Turku). Medeltidsstaden 3. Åbo landskapsmuseum

Ponting, C. 2007. *A New Green History of the World: the Environment and the Collapse of Great Civilisations*. Vintage, London

Poska, A., Saarse, L., Koppel, K., Nielsen, A. B., Avel, E., Vassiljev, J., Meltsov, V. 2014. The Verijärv area, South Estonia over the last millennium: a high resolution quantitative land-cover reconstruction based on pollen and historical data. *Review of Palaeobotany and Palynology*, 207: 5–17

von Post, L. 1967. Forest tree pollen in South Swedish peat bog deposits. *Pollen et Spores* 9, 375–401

Postan, M. M. 1972. *The Medieval Economy and Society: an economic history of Britain in the Middle Ages.* Weidenfeld & Nicolson, London

Postan, M. M., Hatcher, J. 1985. Populations and class relation in feudal society. In: Aston, T. H. & Philpin, C. H. E. (eds) 1985. *The Brenner Debate: agrarian class structure and economic development in pre-industrial Europe*, 64–78. Cambridge University Press

Poulton, R. & Woods, H. 1984. *Excavations on the Site of the Dominican Friary at Guildford in 1974 and 1978.* Surrey Archaeological Society 9, Guildford

Preinitz, L. 1987. Pesten i Stockholm 1710–1711. *Sydsvenska Medicinhistoriska Sällskapets Årsskrift* 24, 157–179

Price, T. D. (ed.) 1989. *The Chemistry of Prehistoric Human Bone.* Cambridge University Press, Cambridge

Price, T. D. 2013. Human mobility at Uppåkra: a preliminary report on isotopic proveniencing. In: Hårdh, B. & Larsson, L (eds) *Studies at Uppåkra: an Iron Age city in Scania, Sweden*, 157–169. Institute of Archaeology, Lund University, Lund

Price, T. D., Grupe, G. & Schröter, P. 1994. Reconstruction of migration patterns in the Bell Beaker Period by stable strontium isotope analysis. *Applied Geochemistry* 9, 413–417

Price, T. D., Bentley, R. A., Lüning, J., Gronenborn, D. & Wahl, J. 2001. Prehistoric human migration in the Linearbandkeramik of Central Europe. *Antiquity* 75, 593–603

Price, T. D., Burton, J. H. & Bentley, A. R. 2002. The characterisation of biologically available strontium isotope ratios for the study of prehistoric migration. *Archaeometry* 44, 117–135

Price, T. D., Frei, K. M., Dobat, A., Lynnerup, N. & Bennike, P. 2011. Who was in Harold Bluetooth's army? Strontium isotope investigation of the cemetery at the Viking Age fortress at Trelleborg, Denmark. *Antiquity* 85, 476–489

Raab, B. & Vedin, H. 1995. *National Atlas of Sweden: climate, lakes and rivers.* Almqvist & Wiksell, Stockholm.

Raihle, J. 1990. Datering av profana timmerhus från medeltiden i Jämtland och Härjedalen [with English summary: Secular medieval log buildings in the provinces of Jämtland and Härjedalen]. *Bebyggelsehistorisk tidskrift* 20, 27–38

Ranåker, M. 2009. Flerpersonsgravar under medeltid: Västerhus kyrkogård belyst av andra begravningsplatser. In: Iregren, E., Alexandersen, V. & Redin, L. (eds) *Västerhus: kapell, kyrkogård och befolkning*, 26–39. Kungliga Vitterhets-, Historie- och Aktikvitetsakademien, Stockholm

Redman, C. L. 1999. *Human Impact on Ancient Environments.* University of Arizona Press, Tucson

Regner, E. 2005. *Den reformerade världen: monastisk och materiell kultur i Alvastra kloster från medeltid till modern tid.* Stockholm Studies in Archaeology 35. Stockholm University

Ringberg, B. 1988. Late Weichselian geology of southernmost Sweden. *Boreas* 17, 243–263

Rosén, C. 2009. *Vålle – en gårdstomt och smedja i norra Bohuslän. Bohuslän, Lur socken, Vålle 1:6, fornlämning 361.* Riksantikvarieämbetet UV Väst, Rapport 2009: 15

Rosén, C. 2013. Människor, gårdar, landskap: att leva på en gård i Västsverige under den tidigmoderna tiden. Riksantikvarieämbetet, Stockholm

Rosén, C. in press. Urbanism and the very small town: a case study from western Sweden. In: Cornell, P. (ed.) Urban variation – utopia, planning and practice. The Early Modern Town 2. GOTARC C. University of Gothenburg

Ruddiman, W. F. 2003. The anthropogenic greenhouse era began thousands of years ago. *Climatic Change* 61, 261–293

Ruddiman, W. F. 2005. *Plows, Plagues, and Petroleum: how humans took control of climate.* Princeton University Press, Princeton/Oxford

Rudel, T. K., Coomes, O. T., Moran, E., Achard, F., Angelsen, A., Xu, J. & Lambin, E. 2005. Forest transitions: toward a global understanding of land use change. *Global Environment Change* 15, 23–31

Sandklef, A. 1973. *Allmogesjöfart på Sveriges västkust 1575–1850*. Institutet för västsvensk kulturforskning, Skrifter 10. Gleerup, Lund

Sandnes, J. 1981. Settlement developments in the Late Middle Ages (approx. 1300–1540). In: Gissel, S., Jutikkala, E., Österberg, E., Sandnes, J. & Teitson, B. (eds) *Desertion and Land Colonization in the Nordic Countries c. 1300–1600: comparative report from the Scandinavian research project on deserted farms and villages*, 78–114. Almqvist & Wiksell, Stockholm

Schmidt Sabo, K. 2001. *Vem behöver en by? Kyrkheddinge, struktur och strategi under tusen år*. Arkeologiska undersökningar, Skrifter 38. Riksantikvarieämbetet, Stockholm

Schmidt Sabo, K. (ed.) 2013. Örja 1:9, Skåne, Landskrona kommun, Örja socken, Örja 1:9, fornlämningarna Örja 9, 35, 40, 41 & 42, Dnr 3.1.1.-04741-2009. Riksantikvarieämbetet, UV Rapport 2013: 68

Schoeninger, M. J., De Niro, M. J. & Tauber, H. 1983. Stable nitrogen isotope ratios of bone collagen reflect marine and terrestrial components of prehistoric human diet. *Science* 220, 1381–1383

Schoeninger, M. J. & De Niro, M. J. 1984. Nitrogen and carbon isotopic composition of bone collagen from marine and terrestrial animals. *Geochimica et Cosmochimica Acta* 48, 625–639

Schuenemann, V. J., Bos, K., Dewitte, S., Schmedes, S., Jamieson, J., Mittnik, A., Forrest, S., Coombes, B. K., Wood, J. W, Earn, D. J. D., White, W., Krause, J. & Poinar, H. N. 2011. Targeted enrichment of ancient pathogens yielding the pPCP1 plasmid of *Yersinia pestis* from victims of the Black Death. *Proceedings of the National Academy of Science* 108, E746–752

Schwarcz, H. P. & Schoeninger, M. J. 1991. Stable isotope analyses in human nutritional ecology. *Yearbook of Physical Anthropology* 34, 283–321

Scott, S. & Duncan, C. 2001. *Biology of Plagues: evidence from historical populations*. Cambridge University Press, Cambridge

Scott, S. & Duncan, C. 2004. Return of the Black Death: the world's greatest serial killer. Wiley, Chichester

Segerström, U. 1990. The natural Holocene vegetation development and the introduction of agriculture in northern Norrland, Sweden: studies of soil, peat and especially varved lake sediments. PhD Thesis. Department of Ecological Botany, University of Umeå

Sellevold, B. J., Hansen, U. L. & Balslev Jørgensen, J. 1984. *Prehistoric Man in Denmark: a study in physical anthropology. Vol. 3. Iron Age man in Denmark*. Nordiske fortidsminder, Series B 8. Copenhagen

Seppänen, L. in press. Continuity or change? Medieval frames and foundations for the early modern town of Turku. In: Cornell, P. (ed.) Urban variation – utopia, planning and practice. The Early Modern Town 2. GOTARC C. University of Gothenburg

Shimazaki, H., & Shinomoto, S. 2010. Kernel bandwidth optimization in spike rate estimation. *Journal of Computational Neuroscience* 29, 171–182

Signoli, M., Seguy, I., Biraben, J.-N., Dutour, O. & Belle, P. 2002. Paleodemography and historical demography in the context of an epidemic: plague in Provence in the eighteenth century. *Population* 57, 829–854

Sillen, A., Sealy, J. C., & Van der Merwe, N. J. 1998. Chemistry and paleodietary research: no more easy answers. *American Antiquity* 54, 504–512

Sjögren, K.-G., Price, T. D. & Ahlström, T. 2009. Megaliths and mobility in south-western Sweden: investigating relations between a local society and its neighbours using strontium isotopes. *Journal of Anthropological Archaeology* 28, 85–101

Sjögren, K.-G. & Price, D. T. 2013. A complex Neolithic economy: isotope evidence for the circulation of cattle and sheep in the TRB of western Sweden. *Journal of Archaeological Science* 40, 690–704

Sjøvold, T. 1990. Estimation of stature from long bones utilizing the line of organic correlation. *Human Evolution* 5, 431–447

Sjøvold, T. 1982. Skelettfynden. In: Dandanell, B. (ed.) *Tusen år på kyrkudden: Leksands kyrka, arkeologi och byggnadshistoria*, 165–178. Dalarnas fornminnes- och hembygdsförbunds skrifter 25. Dalarnas Museum, Falun

Skansjö, S. 1983. *Söderslätt genom 600 år: bebyggelse och odling under äldre historisk tid*. Skånsk senmedeltid och renässans. Skriftserie utgiven av Vetenskaps-societeten i Lund 11. Gleerup, Lund

Sköld, E., Lagerås, P., Berglund, B. E. 2010. Temporal cultural landscape dynamics in a marginal upland area: agricultural expansions and contractions inferred from palynological evidence at Yttra Berg, southern Sweden. *Vegetation History and Archaeobotany* 19, 121–136

Skyllberg, E. 2003. Näveberg – en sörmländsk bergslag. *Bebyggelsehistorisk tidskrift* 43, 63–72

Slack, P. 1985. *The Impact of Plague in Tudor and Stuart England*. Routledge & Kegan Paul, London

Söderberg, J. 2007. Prices and economic change in medieval Sweden. *Scandinavian Economic History Review* 55, 128–152

Stebich, M., Brüchmann, C., Kulbe, T., Negendank, J. F. W. 2005. Vegetation history, human impact and climate change during the last 700 years recorded in annually laminated sediments of Lac Pavin, France. *Review of Palaeobotany and Palynology* 133, 115–133

Steckel, R. 1995. Stature and standard of living. *Journal of Economic Literature* 33, 1903–1940

Stewart, K. M., Bowyer, R. T, Kie, J. G., Cimon, N. J., Johnson, B. K. 2002. Temporospatial distributions of elk, mule deer and cattle: resource partitioning and competitive displacement. *Journal of Mammalogy* 83, 229–244

Stibeus, M. 1986. Piksborg, inte bara en fogdeborg: ett medeltida gränsfäste i Finnveden. Unpublished examination paper in medieval archaeology. Lund University

Stiernman, S. A. 1775. Samling utaf kongl. brev, stadgar och förordningar, etc. angående Sweriges rikes commerce, politic och economie uti gemen; ifrån år 1523 in till närwarande tid. Del 6. Kungliga Rådet, Stockholm

Stone, R. & Appleton Fox, N. 1996. *A View from Hereford's Past: a report on the archaeological excavation in Hereford Cathedral Close in 1993*. Logaston Press, Hereford

Stoklund, B. 2000. *Bondefiskere og strandsiddere: studier over de store sæsonfiskerier 1350–1600*. Landbohistorisk Selskab, Copenhagen

Strömberg, B. 2008. *Det förlorade järnet: dansk protoindustriell järnhantering*. Riksantikvarieämbetet, Stockholm

Sugita, S. 2007. Theory of quantitative reconstruction of vegetation I: pollen from large sites REVEALS regional vegetation composition. *The Holocene* 17, 229–241

Svensson, E. 1998. *Människor i utmark*. Lund Studies in Medieval Archaeology 21. Lund University

Svensson, E., Pettersson, S., Nilsson, S., Boss, L. & Johansson, A. 2012. Resilience and medieval crisis at five rural settlements in Sweden and Norway. *Lund Archaeological Review* 18, 89–106

Tagesson, G. 2002. *Biskop och stad: aspekter av urbanisering och sociala rum i medeltidens Linköping*. Lund Studies in Medieval Archaeology 30. Lund University

Tainter, J. A. 1988. *The Collapse of Complex Societies*. Cambridge University Press, Cambridge

Takahasi, E. 1984. Secular trend in milk consumption and growth in Japan. *Human Biology* 56, 427–437

Takaishi, E. 1994. Secular changes in growth of Japanese children. *The International Journal of Pediatric Endocrinology* 7, 163–173

Tanner, J. M., Hayashi, T., Preece, M. A. & Cameron, N. 1982. Increase in length of leg relative to trunk in Japanese children and adults from 1957 to 1997: comparison with British and with Japanese Americans. *Annals of Human Biology* 9, 411–23

Tanner, J. M. 1987. Growth as a mirror of the condition of society: secular trends and class distinctions. *Acta Paedriatrica Japonica* 29(1), 96–103

Taylor, C. 2010. The origins and development of deserted village studies. In: Dyer, C. & Jones, R. (eds) *Deserted Villages Revisited*, 8–27. University of Hertfordshire Press, Hatfield

Thomas, R. 2007. Maintaining social boundaries through the consumption of food in medieval England. In: Twiss, K. (ed.) *The Archaeology of Food and Identity*, 130–151. Occasional Publication 34. Center for Archaeological Investigations, Carbondale

Thordeman, B. 1939. *Armour from the Battle of Wisby 1361.* Kungliga Vitterhets Historie och Antikvitets Akademien, Stockholm

Thun, T. 2005. Norwegian conifer chronologies constructed to date historical timber. *Dendrochronologia* 23, 63–74

Trondman, A.-K., Gaillard, M.-J., Mazier, F., Sugita, S., Fyfe, R., Nielsen, A. B., Twiddle, C., Barratt, P., Birks, H. J. B., Bjune, A. E., Björkman, L., Broström, A., Caseldine, C., David, R., Dodson, J., Dörfler, W., Fischer, E., van Geel, B., Giesecke, T., Hultberg, T., Kalnina, L., Kangur, M., van der Knaap, P., Koff, T., Kuneš, P., Lagerås, P., Latalowa, M., Lechterbeck, J., Leroyer, C., Leydet, M., Lindbladh, M., Marquer, L., Mitchell, F., Odgaard, B. V., Peglar, S. M., Persson, T., Poska, A., Rösch, M., Seppä, H., Veski, S. & Wick, L. 2014. First pollen-based quantitative reconstructions of Holocene regional vegetation cover (plant functional types and land-cover types) in Europe suitable for climate modelling. *Global Change Biology* doi, 10.1111/gcb.12737

Twigg, G. 1984. *The Black Death: a biological reappraisal.* Batsford, London

Uppsala. Medeltidsstaden 3. 1976. Riksantikvarieämbetet och Statens Historiska Museer, Stockholm

Vejde, P. G. 1938 Om pesten i Småland 1710-11. *Hylten-Cavallius-föreningen Årsbok* 1938, 161–195

Vestbö-Franzén, A. 2004. *Råg och rön: om mat, människor och landskapsförändringar i norra Småland, ca 1550–1700* [English abstract: Research on rye – food, humans and structural changes in the agrarian landscape of northern Småland 1550–1700]. Jönköpings läns museum, Jönköping

Vretemark, M. 1997. *Från ben till boskap: kosthåll och djurhållning med utgångspunkt i medeltida benmaterial från Skara. Part I.* Skrifter från Skaraborgs länsmuseum 25. Skaraborg

Vretemark, M. 2010. De medeltida Skaraborna. In: Vretemark, M. & Borrman, H. (eds) *S:t Per i Skara: om liv och död i den medeltida staden,* 95–100. Skrifter från Västergötlands museum 37. Västergötlands museum, Skara

Vretemark. M & Axelsson T. In press. *Varnhem innan munkarna kom.* Skrifter från Västergötlands museum

de Vries, J. 2008. *The Industrious Revolution: consumer behavior and the household economy, 1650 to the present.* Cambridge University Press, Cambridge

Wagner, D. M., Klunk, J. *et al.* 2014. *Yersinia pestis* and the Plague of Justinian 541–543 AD: a genomic analysis. *The Lancet Infectious Diseases* 14, 319–326

Wand, M. P. & Jones, M. C. 1995. *Kernel Smoothing.* Chapman & Hall/CRC, London

Weimarck, G. 1953. *Studier över landskapets förändring inom Lönsboda, Örkeneds socken, nordöstra Skåne.* Gleerup, Lund

Weise, S. 2009. The medieval cemetery S:t Jörgen in Malmö: a paleodemographic analysis. Anthropological Department, Institute of Forensic Medicine, University of Southern Denmark. PhD Thesis

Werdelin, L., Myrdal, J. & Sten, S. 2002. Patterns of stature variation in medieval Sweden. *Hikuin* 27, 293–306

Werner, B. 2005. Growth in Sweden: surveillance of growth patterns and epidemiological monitoring of secular changes in height and weight among children and adolescents. Karolinska Institutet, Stockholm. PhD Thesis

Whitmore, T. M., Turner II, B. L., Johnson, D. L., Kates, R. W., Gottschang, T. R. 1990. Long-term population change. In: Turner II, B. L., Clark, W. C., Kates, R. W., Ruchards, J. F., Matthews, J. T. & Meyer, W. B. (eds.) *The Earth as Transformed by Human Action,* 25–39. Cambridge University Press, Cambridge

WHO 1983. *Measuring Change in Nutritional Status: guidelines for assessing the nutritional Impact of supplementary feeding programmes for vulnerable groups.* WHO, Geneva

Widgren, M. 2007. Precolonial landesque capital: a global perspective. In: Hornborg, A., McNeill, J. R. & Martinez-Alier, J. (eds) *Rethinking Environmental History: world-system history and global environmental change,* 61–77. Altamira Press, Lanham

Widgren, M. 2012. Climate and causation in the Swedish Iron Age: learning from the present to understand the past. *Geografisk Tidsskrift/Danish Journal of Geography* 112, 126–134

Wienberg, J. 1993. *Den gotiske labyrinth: middelalderen og kirkerne i Danmark*. Lund Studies in Medieval Archaeology 11. Lund University

Williams, M. 2000. Dark ages and dark areas: global deforestation in the deep past. *Journal of Historical Geography* 26, 28–46

Williams, M. 2006. *Deforesting the Earth: from prehistory to global crisis – an abridgmen*t. University of Chicago Press, Chicago/London

Winberg, C. 2000. *Hur Västsverige blev västsvenskt*. Humanistiska fakulteten Göteborgs universitet. University of Gothenburg

Woodbridge, J., Fyfe, R., Law, B. & Haworth-Johns, A. 2012. A spatial approach to upland vegetation change and human impact: the Aber Valley, Snowdonia. *Environmental Archaeology* 17, 80–94

Yeloff, D. & van Geel, B. 2007. Abandonment of farmland and vegetation succession following the Eurasian plague pandemic of 1347–52. *Journal of Biogeography* 34, 575–582

Yeloff, D., van Geel, B, Broekens, P., Bakker, J. & Mauquoy, D. 2007. Mid- to late-Holocene vegetation and land-use history in the Hadrian's Wall region of northern England: the record from Butterburn Flow. *The Holocene* 17, 527–538

Zillén, L. & Conley, D. J. 2010. Hypoxia and cyanobacteria blooms - are they really natural features of the late Holocene history of the Baltic Sea? *Biogeosciences* 7, 2567–2580

Zillén, L., Conley, D. J., Andrén, T., Andrén, E. & Björck, S. 2008. Past occurrences of hypoxia in the Baltic Sea and the role of climate variability, environmental change and human impact. *Earth-Science Reviews* 91, 77–92

Author presentations

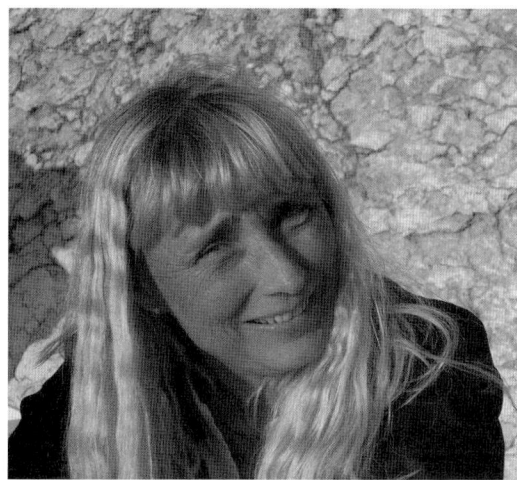

Caroline Arcini. Doctor in medical science at Lund University. Holds a position at the National Historical Museums in Sweden. Her thesis *Health and disease in the early Lund* (1999) represents one of her main research interests which is the reconstruction of living conditions in past populations using osteological materials and methods. Among previous articles are *Lacunae to fill: combining palaeopathological and documentary research in investigations of individuals from a post-medieval Swedish cemetery* (2008)

caroline.ahlstrom.arcini@shmm.se

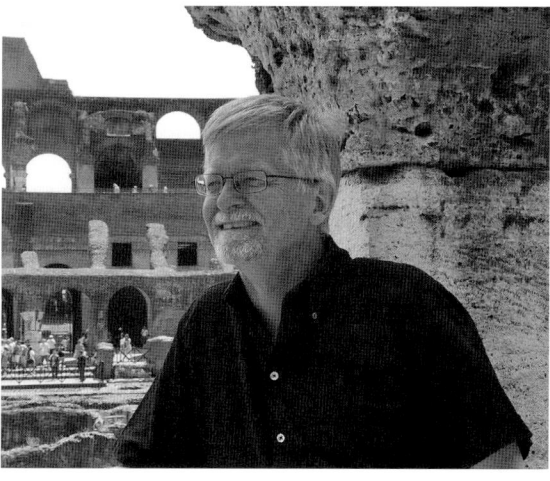

Lars Ersgård. Associate Professor in medieval archaeology. Researcher at the Department of Archaeology and Ancient History at Lund University. Main research interests are medieval and post-medieval urbanisation, the process of Christianisation and the pre-industrial, cultural landscape in a long term perspective.

lars.ersgard@ark.lu.se

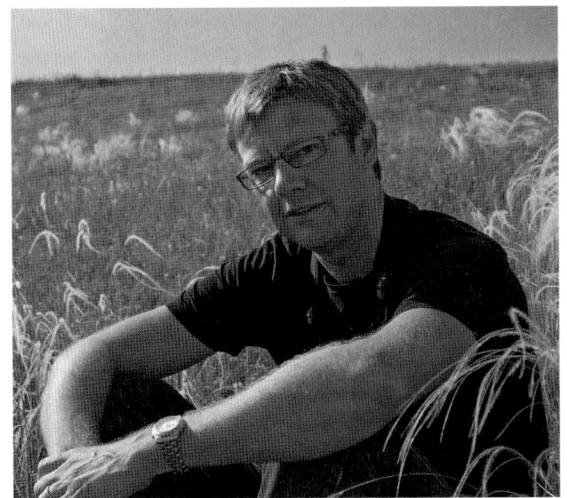

Per Lagerås. Associate Professor in agrarian history at the Swedish University of Agricultural Sciences and Doctor in Quaternary geology at Lund University. Holds a position at the National Historical Museums in Sweden. Main research interests are vegetation history, cultural landscape development and human-environment interactions. Among his previous books are *The Ecology of Expansion and Abandonment* (2007).

per.lageras@shmm.se

Appendix 1. Pollen sites

Pollen sites used in the study presented in Chapter 4. Numbers in the left column refer to the maps in Figure 5.

1 Skeakärret
N 56° 11' 25", E 13° 51' 3", 42 m a.s.l.
Small peatland (0.2 ha). Included in the present study were 20 pollen-analysed levels representing AD 680–present. The chronology for this time span was based on 6 AMS radiocarbon dates. Original publication by Lagerås 2002.

2 Torup
N 55° 33' 37", E 13° 12' 13", 50 m a.s.l.
Very small peatland (0.01 ha). Included in the present study were 25 pollen-analysed levels representing AD 255–1945. The chronology for this time span was based on 5 AMS radiocarbon dates. Original publication by Hultberg *et al.* 2010.

3 Häggenäs
N 55° 53' 34", E 13° 36' 4", 70 m a.s.l.
Very small peatland (0.03 ha). Included in the present study were 36 pollen-analysed levels representing AD 355–present. The chronology for this time span was based on 5 AMS radiocarbon dates. Original publication by Lindbladh *et al.* 2007.

4 Skärsgölarna
N 57° 0' 34", E 16° 7' 4", 77 m a.s.l.
Small peatland (0.5 ha). Included in the present study were 30 pollen-analysed levels representing AD 1–present. The chronology for this time span was based on 6 AMS radiocarbon dates. Original publication by Lindbladh *et al.* 2003.

5 Östra Ringarp
N 56° 16' 0", E 13° 18' 53", 100 m a.s.l.
Recently overgrown small lake (quagmire) (2 ha). Included in the present study were 32 pollen-analysed levels representing AD 1–present. The chronology for this time span was based on 7 AMS radiocarbon dates. Original publication by Lagerås 2007.

6 Grisavad
N 56° 16' 37", E 13° 19' 59", 100 m a.s.l.
Peatbog (7 ha). Coring close to the edge. Included in the present study were 38 pollen-analysed levels representing AD 1–present. The chronology for this time span was based on 6 AMS radiocarbon dates. Original publication by Lagerås 2007.

7   Bocksten   N 57° 7' 4", E 12° 33' 37", 110 m a.s.l.
                             Very small fen (0.05 ha). The site is called Bocksten A in the original publication.
                             Included in the present study were 71 pollen-analysed levels representing AD 1–
                             present. The chronology for this time span was based on 4 conventional
                             radiocarbon dates. Original publication by Björkman 1997a.

8   Yttra Berg   N 57° 4' 51", E 12° 48' 39", 110 m a.s.l.
                             Peatbog (3 ha). Included in the present study were 15 pollen-analysed levels
                             representing AD 1–present. The chronology for this time span was based on 5
                             AMS radiocarbon dates. Original publication by Sköld *et al.* 2010.

9   Trälhultet   N 56° 48' 27", E 12° 54' 31", 117 m a.s.l.
                             Peatland (4 ha). Coring close to the edge. Included in the present study were 33
                             pollen-analysed levels representing AD 1–present. The chronology for this time
                             span was based on 4 AMS radiocarbon dates. Original publication by Björkman
                             2000.

10   Exhult   N 56° 29' 26", E 13° 39' 3", 118 m a.s.l.
                             Large peatbog (240 ha) but with coring close to the edge. Included in the present
                             study were 58 pollen-analysed levels representing AD 1–present. The chronology
                             for this time span was based on 5 AMS radiocarbon dates. Original publication
                             by Björkman 2003b.

11   Köphult   N 56° 25' 18", E 13° 33' 11", 120 m a.s.l.
                             Large peatbog (165 ha) but with coring close to the edge. Included in the present
                             study were 35 pollen-analysed levels representing AD 110–present. The
                             chronology for this time span was based on 5 AMS radiocarbon dates. Original
                             publication by Björkman 2003a.

12   Rosts Täppa   N 56° 19' 32", E 13° 26' 21", 122 m a.s.l.
                             Small Peatbog (1 ha). Coring close to the edge. The site was called Värsjö
                             Utmark in the original publication. Included in the present study were 37 pollen-
                             analysed levels representing AD 1–present. The chronology for this time span
                             was based on 5 AMS radiocarbon dates. Original publication by Lagerås 2007.

13   Bjärabygget   N 56° 21' 31", E 13° 28' 24", 123 m a.s.l.
                             Large peatbog (>100 ha) but with coring close to the edge. Included in the
                             present study were 53 pollen-analysed levels representing AD 1–present. The
                             chronology for this time span was based on 4 AMS radiocarbon dates. Original
                             publication by Lagerås 2007.

14   Baggabygget   N 56° 35' 16", E 13° 23' 55", 140 m a.s.l.
                             Very small fen (0.05 ha). Included in the present study were 21 pollen-analysed
                             levels representing AD 65–present. The chronology for this time span was based
                             on 4 AMS radiocarbon dates. Original publication by Björkman 2005.

15   Råshult   N 56° 27' 16", E 14° 33' 16", 140 m a.s.l.
                             Small peatland (0.2 ha). The site was called Råshult In-field in the original
                             publication. Included in the present study were 20 pollen-analysed levels
                             representing AD 955–present. The chronology for this time span was based on 5
                             AMS radiocarbon dates. Original publication by Lindbladh & Bradshaw 1998.

16	Siggaboda	N 56° 27' 16", E 14° 33' 16", 140 m a.s.l. Very small peatland (0.01 ha). Included in the present study were 78 pollen-analysed levels representing AD 1–present. The chronology for this time span was based on 5 conventional radiocarbon dates. Original publication by Björkman & Bradshaw 1996.
17	Flahult	N 56° 58' 8", E 13° 50' 9", 180 m a.s.l. Small peatland (0.3 ha). Included in the present study were 40 pollen-analysed levels representing AD 1–present. The chronology for this time span was based on 4 conventional radiocarbon dates. Original publication by Björkman 1997b.
18	Lindhultsgöl	N 57° 8' 43", E 14° 28' 4", 212 m a.s.l. Small lake (8 ha). Included in the present study were 45 pollen-analysed levels representing AD 1000–present. The chronology for the time span AD 1–present was based on 2 AMS radiocarbon dates and 5 time markers in the Pb-content of the sediment. Also ^{210}Pb was used for dating the upper part of the sequence. Original publications by Fredh 2012; Bragée 2013.
19	Öggestorpsdalen	N 57° 43' 0", E 14° 21' 47", 218 m a.s.l. Small peatbog (2 ha). Included in the present study were 24 pollen-analysed levels representing AD 1–present. The chronology for this time span was based on 4 AMS radiocarbon dates. Original publication by Björkman 2003c.
20	Åbodasjön	N 57° 5' 9", E 14° 28' 57", 221 m a.s.l. Lake (53 ha). Included in the present study were 44 pollen-analysed levels representing AD 1000–present. The chronology for this time span was based on 3 AMS radiocarbon dates and 4 time markers in the Pb-content of the sediment. Also ^{210}Pb was used for dating the upper part of the sequence. Original publications by Fredh 2012 and Bragée 2013.
21	Store Mosse	N 57° 43' 23", E 14° 15' 33", 222 m a.s.l. Peatbog (45 ha). Coring close to edge. Included in the present study were 34 pollen-analysed levels representing AD 1–present. The chronology for this time span was based on 5 AMS radiocarbon dates. Original publication by Björkman 2003c.
22	Storasjö	N 56° 55' 53", E 15° 16' 5", 252 m a.s.l. Very small peatland (0.02). Included in the present study were 31 pollen-analysed levels representing AD 685–present. The chronology for this time span was based on 5 AMS radiocarbon dates. Original publication by Eriksson 1996.
23	Skärpingegöl	N 57° 9' 5", E 14° 43' 24", 255 m a.s.l. Very small lake lake (1 ha) Included in the present study were 30 pollen-analysed levels representing AD 755–present. The chronology for this time span was based on 3 AMS radiocarbon dates and time markers in the Pb-content of the sediment. Also ^{210}Pb was used for dating the upper part of the sequence. Unpublished data by Daniel Fredh.
24	Bråtamossen	N 57° 40' 35", E 14° 30' 18", 284 m a.s.l. Peatbog (5 ha). Coring close to the edge. Included in the present study were 26 pollen-analysed levels representing AD 110–present. The chronology for this time span was based on 6 AMS radiocarbon dates. Original publication by Lagerås *et al.* 1995.

25   Mattarp   N 57° 29' 29", E 14° 37' 16", 325 m a.s.l.
                           Very small peatland (0.05 ha). Included in the present study were 56 pollen-
                           analysed levels representing AD 1–present. The chronology for this time span
                           was based on 4 conventional radiocarbon dates. Original publication by
                           Björkman 1996b.

26   Fjäturen   N 59°27'41", E 17° 59' 26", 6 m a.s.l.
                           Lake (49 ha). Included in the present study were 28 pollen-analysed levels
                           representing AD 1–present. The chronology for this time span was based on 6
                           AMS radiocarbon dates. Original publication by Karlsson & Risberg 1996.

27   Kalven   N 60° 5' 3", E 15° 53' 30", 130 m a.s.l.
                           Lake (18 ha). Included in the present study were 41 pollen-analysed levels
                           representing AD 550–present. The chronology was based on varve counting
                           (annually laminated sediments). Original publication by Berg 2004.

28   Kassjön   N 63°55'32", E 20°0'35", 84 m a.s.l.
                           Lake (22 ha) Included in the present study were 33 pollen-analysed levels
                           representing AD 1–present. The chronology was based on varve counting
                           (annually laminated sediments). Original publication by Segerström 1990.

Appendix 2. Osteological stature data

Stature data used in Chapter 6. Numbers in the left column refer to the map in Figure 41.

Women

	Place, Church, Urban/Rural	Dating	n	Femur Mean (mm)	Stature Min. (cm)	Stature Max. (cm)	Stature Mean (cm)	Stature SD (cm)
1	Ystad, Lilla Tvären, U	c. 1150–1270	1				166.0	
2	Trelleborg, S:t Nicolai, U	c. 1300–1400	8		158.0	169.0	163.2	4.3
3	Tygelsjö,* R	c. 1100	5		154.7	164.7	160.9	3.9
4	Malmö, S:t Jörgen, U	c. 1320–1530	110	430	149.6	179.9	163.2	5.9
5	Tottarp, R	c. 1300–1400	3	410	156.2	159.5	157.8	1.6
6	Lund, S:t Andreas, U	c. 1000–1100	9	414	151.0	167.0	158.9	5.5
6	Lund, S:t Andreas, U	c. 1200–1300	28	419	149.6	170.1	160.2	5.3
6	Lund, S:t Andreas, U	c. 1200–1536	25	420	147.9	167.8	160.5	5.3
6	Lund, S:t Mikael, U	c. 1050–1300	11	417	147.8	167.8	159.6	5.5
6	Lund, S:t Mikael, U	c. 1300–1536	13	419	153.8	167.4	160.2	4.5
6	Lund, S:t Mikael, U	c. 1500–1525	0					
6	Lund, S:t Mårten, U	c. 1000–1100	7		155.0	174.0	162.3	9.8
6	Lund, S:t Mårten, U	c. 1200–1300	4		161.0	169.0	164.2	3.6
6	Lund, S:t Mårten, U	c. 1300–1536	14		155.0	173.0	162.3	5.9
6	Lund, S:t Stefan,* U	c. 1050–1536	336	421	144.1	178.2	159.5	6.3
6	Lund, Trinitatis, U	c. 990–1100	148	422	138.8	179.4	160.9	6.2
6	Lund, Trinitatis, U	c. 1100–1300	97	420	146.2	173.6	160.4	5.5
6	Lund, Trinitatis, U	c. 1300–1350	44	424	152.3	174.4	161.4	4.8
6	Lund, Trinitatis, U	c. 1350	32	417	147.8	168.3	159.6	4.8
6	Lund, Trinitatis, U	c. 1350–1536	31	423	154.1	168.3	161.2	3.7
7	Löddeköpinge,* R	c. 1050–1200	135	412	142.6	173.6	156.5	5.9
8	Landskrona, Helgeandshuset, U	c. 1300–1531	2	418	156.5	163.0	159.8	4.6
8	Landskrona, S:t Olof, U	c. 1100–1536	9	414	152.8	165.9	158.8	4.8
9	Helsingborg, S:t Clemens, U	c. 1050–1536	72	420	145.7	173.8	160.4	5.6
9	Helsingborg, S:t Nicolai, U	c. 1269–1536	72	429	151.7	178.8	162.9	5.4
9	Helsingborg, S:t Petri, U	c. 1050–1536	79	426	147.3	174.6	162.0	6.0
9	Helsingborg, Slottsvången	c. 1500–1600	0					
10	Åhus, U	c. 1243–1536	35	428	149.4	171.5	162.6	4.9
11	Laholm, Lagaholm, U	c. 1050–1450	3	417	158.6	161.2	159.6	4.9
12	Nya Lödöse, U	c. 1500–1620	19	435	154.4	173.6	164.4	6.0
13	Skara, S:t Per, U	c. 1100–1530	49	420	150.7	174.1	160.4	5.2

14	Varnhem, R	c. 1000–1300	35	423	141.7	169.9	161.3	5.6
15	Sverkersgården, R	c. 1100	3	409	157.3	157.8	157.6	0.3
16	Örberga, R	c. 1000–1300	9	419	147.5	169.1	160.2	6.9
17	Klosterstad, R	c. 1050–1536	21	425	151.5	172.5	161.6	5.2
17	Vadstena, Galgberget	c. 1550–1600	0					
18	Skänninge, S:t Olof, U	c. 1237–1536	37	428	153.3	173.8	162.8	5.3
19	Vreta, R	c. 1100–1600	16		151.0	165.0	160.4	4.2
20	Linköping, Domkyrkof., U	c. 1100–1400	9	417	155.4	165.9	159.7	3.5
21	Landeryd, R	c. 1250–1536	3	399	152.5	157.8	154.8	2.7
22	Visby, Korsbetningen	1361	0					
22	Visby, Kv. Banken, Allhelgona, U	c. 1100–	4	415	155.2	163.0	159.1	3.4
22	Visby, S:t Clemens, U	c. 1100–1531	1	424			161.5	
22	Visby, S:t Gertrud, U	c. 1400–1450	3	446	165.7	170.3	167.2	3.0
22	Visby, S:t Mikael, U	c. 1235–1531	10	400	151.5	173.8	161.5	7.4
23	Stockholm, Helgeandsholmen, U	c. 1320–1531	65	415	148.1	171.3	159.1	4.9
24	Sigtuna, U	c. 980–1300	57	428	149.5	181.2	162.4	6.1
24	Sigtuna, U	c. 1300–1530	1	397			154.3	
25	Västerås, unknown church, U	c. 1100–1200	4	409	147.9	162.5	157.5	6.6
26	Sura, U	c. 900–1300	1	430			163.0	
27	Långfredagsslaget, U	1520	0					
27	Uppsala, Kv. Kroken, U	c. 1300–1500	17	410	148.8	165.1	157.9	4.8
27	Viby–Julita, U	c. 1160–1527	0					
28	Leksand, R	c. 1050–1350	22	428	153.8	168.3	162.5	4.4
29	Västerhus, R	c. 1050–1350	75	425	143.2	174.5	161.8	6.8
30	Björned, R	c. 900–1200	0				163.0	

* Measure from M2 used for calculation of stature.

Men

	Place, Church, Urban/Rural	Dating	n	Femur Mean (mm)	Stature Min. (cm)	Stature Max. (cm)	Stature Mean (cm)	Stature SD (cm)
1	Ystad, Lilla Tvären, U	c. 1150–1270	1				177.0	
2	Trelleborg, S:t Nicolai, U	c. 1300–1400	5		169.0	178.0	172.6	3.8
3	Tygelsjö,* R	c. 1100	56		161.0	189.0	173.7	5.5
4	Malmö, S:t Jörgen, U	c. 1320–1530	205	467	155.4	195.9	172.8	6.0
5	Tottarp, R	c. 1300–1400	4	460	167.1	175.1	170.8	3.4
6	Lund, S:t Andreas, U	c. 1000–1100	14	447	161.1	177.0	167.6	4.4
6	Lund, S:t Andreas, U	c. 1200–1300	40	458	159.9	184.3	170.4	5.7
6	Lund, S:t Andreas, U	c. 1200–1536	36	461	155.4	182.8	171.1	6.3
6	Lund, S:t Mikael, U	c. 1050–1300	15	460	163.6	180.4	170.5	5.4
6	Lund, S:t Mikael, U	c. 1300–1536	10	465	157.8	183.6	172.3	8.8
6	Lund, S:t Mikael, U	c. 1500–1525	6	468	165.4	183.0	173.0	6.0
6	Lund, S:t Mårten, U	c. 1000–1100	13		153.0	185.0	169.6	9.8
6	Lund, S:t Mårten, U	c. 1200–1300	12		163.0	184.0	175.0	10.8
6	Lund, S:t Mårten, U	c. 1300–1536	12		166.0	182.0	175.6	4.6
6	Lund, S:t Stefan,* U	c. 1050–1536	424	461	145.1	193.4	171.8	7.4
6	Lund, Trinitatis, U	c. 990–1100	205	464	151.5	187.8	172.1	7.0
6	Lund, Trinitatis, U	c. 1100–1300	125	461	157.3	188.8	171.3	6.4
6	Lund, Trinitatis, U	c. 1300–1350	55	465	159.1	184.5	172.4	5.9
6	Lund, Trinitatis, U	c. 1350	43	467	157.5	192.0	172.8	8.2
6	Lund, Trinitatis, U	c. 1350–1536	31	459	156.2	199.9	170.7	8.7

7	Löddeköpinge,* R	*c.* 1050–1200	189	448	147.9	186.0	167.7	8.0
8	Landskrona, Helgeandshuset, U	*c.* 1300–1531	3	477	171.5	182.2	175.5	5.9
8	Landskrona, S:t Olof, U	*c.* 1100–1536	5	454	157.5	174.6	169.3	6.8
9	Helsingborg, S:t Clemens, U	*c.* 1050–1536	68	464	157.3	189.2	171.9	6.6
9	Helsingborg, S:t Nicolai, U	*c.* 1269–1536	181	473	155.7	190.7	174.5	6.6
9	Helsingborg, S:t Petri, U	*c.* 1050–1536	104	469	160.3	187.5	173.2	5.9
9	Helsingborg, Slottsvången	*c.* 1500–1600	7		166.0	184.3	172.0	6.9
10	Åhus, U	*c.* 1243–1536	73	469	162.0	189.6	173.3	6.2
11	Laholm, Lagaholm, U	*c.* 1050–1450	3	462	165.9	174.9	171.5	1.4
12	Nya Lödöse, U	*c.* 1500–1620	36	470	162.8	185.4	173.5	5.7
13	Skara, S:t Per, U	*c.* 1100–1530	40	461	160.4	185.1	171.1	5.2
14	Varnhem, R	*c.* 1000–1300	45	468	160.4	189.9	173.0	7.2
15	Sverkersgården, R	*c.* 1100	5	467	162.5	180.7	172.8	6.6
16	Örberga, R	*c.* 1000–1300	3	467	171.5	173.6	172.8	1.2
17	Klosterstad, R	*c.* 1050–1536	27	464	159.6	184.1	172.1	5.8
17	Vadstena, Galgberget	*c.* 1550–1600	8	470	166.5	180.1	173.5	4.9
18	Skänninge, S:t Olof, U	*c.* 1237–1536	82	472	155.2	191.0	173.9	6.7
19	Vreta, R	*c.* 1100–1600	12		166.0	186.0	174.4	7.7
20	Linköping, Domkyrkof., U	*c.* 1100–1400	29	460	158.3	189.9	170.8	7.4
21	Landeryd, R	*c.* 1250–1536	3	448	160.4	180.1	167.6	10.9
22	Visby, Korsbetningen	1361	365	456	157.5	189.9	172.0	6.3
22	Visby, Kv. Banken, Allhelgona, U	*c.* 1100–	2	459	167.5	174.0	170.7	4.6
22	Visby, S:t Clemens, U	*c.* 1100–1531	3	478	167.0	182.1	175.7	7.84
22	Visby, S:t Gertrud, U	*c.* 1400–1450	4	458	165.7	174.9	170.3	3.8
22	Visby, S:t Mikael, U	*c.* 1235–1531	14	471	156.4	188.5	173.9	7.7
23	Stockholm, Helgeandsholmen, U	*c.* 1320–1531	158	458	156.5	192.0	170.3	5.9
24	Sigtuna, U	*c.* 980–1300	136	466	159.4	186.0	172.5	5.4
24	Sigtuna, U	*c.* 1300–1530	10	467	159.4	179.8	172.8	6.1
25	Västerås, unknown church, U	*c.* 1100–1200	4	461	164.4	180.0	171.2	6.9
26	Sura, U	*c.* 900–1300	9	455	162.5	177.5	169.5	5.1
27	Långfredagsslaget, U	1520	34	470	163.0	185.7	173.6	5.8
27	Uppsala, Kv. Kroken, U	*c.* 1300–1500	21	456	151.7	181.8	169.9	6.7
27	Viby-Julita, U	*c.* 1160–1527	5	467	167.3	175.9	172.7	4.4
28	Leksand, R	*c.* 1050–1350	9	463	161.7	179.6	171.8	6.7
29	Västerhus, R	*c.* 1050–1350	62	468	160.4	188.8	173.1	6.4
30	Björned, R	*c.* 900–1200	2	449	161.3	174.9	168.1	9.6

* Measure from M2 used for calculation of stature.

Site locations and references

	Province	Place, Church, Urban/Rural	Type	Data source*
1	Scania	Ystad, Lilla Tvären, U	parish	Arcini this study
2	Scania	Trelleborg, S:t Nicolai, U	parish	Arcini this study
3	Scania	Tygelsjö,* R	parish	O. Persson & E. Persson unpubl.
4	Scania	Malmö, S:t Jörgen, U	sanctuary	J. Boldsen, C. Ödman unpubl.
5	Scania	Tottarp, R	parish	Arcini this study
6	Scania	Lund, S:t Andreas, U	parish	Arcini this study
6	Scania	Lund, S:t Mikael, U	parish	Arcini this study
6	Scania	Lund, S:t Mikael, U	executed individuals	Alfsdotter 2011
6	Scania	Lund, S:t Mårten, U	parish	Arcini this study
6	Scania	Lund, S:t Stefan,* U	parish	Arcini this study
6	Scania	Lund, Trinitatis, U	parish	Arcini this study
6	Scania	Lund, Trinitatis, U	monastery+parish	Arcini this study
7	Scania	Löddeköpinge,* R	parish	Persson & Persson 1983
8	Scania	Landskrona, Helgeandshuset, U	sanctuary	Arcini this study
8	Scania	Landskrona, S:t Olof, U	parish	Arcini this study
9	Scania	Helsingborg, S:t Clemens, U	parish	Arcini this study
9	Scania	Helsingborg, S:t Nicolai, U	convent+parish	Arcini this study
9	Scania	Helsingborg, S:t Petri, U	parish	Rolf Jonsson unpubl.
9	Scania	Helsingborg, Slottsvången	execution place	Arcini this study
10	Scania	Åhus, U	convent+parish	Arcini this study
11	Halland	Laholm, Lagaholm, U	parish	Arcini this study
12	Västergötland	Nya Lödöse, U	parish	M. Vretemark unpubl.
13	Västergötland	Skara, S:t Per, U	parish	Vretemark 2010
14	Västergötland	Varnhem, R	monastery+parish	Vretemark & Axelsson in press.
15	Östergötland	Sverkersgården, R	parish	Arcini this study
16	Östergötland	Örberga, R	parish	Arcini this study
17	Östergötland	Klosterstad, R	parish	Arcini this study
17	Östergötland	Vadstena, Galgberget	execution place	Arcini this study
18	Östergötland	Skänninge, S:t Olof, U	convent+parish	Arcini this study
19	Östergötland	Vreta, R	monastery+parish	Backe 1988
20	Östergötland	Linköping, Domkyrkof., U	parish	Arcini this study
21	Östergötland	Landeryd, R	parish	Arcini this study
22	Gotland	Visby, Korsbetningen	military massgrave	Arcini, Drenzel, Åkesson this study
22	Gotland	Visby, Kv. Banken, Allhelgona, U	parish	B. Sigvallius unpubl.
22	Gotland	Visby, S:t Clemens, U	parish	Durhed 2001
22	Gotland	Visby, S:t Gertrud, U	parish	Durhed 2001
22	Gotland	Visby, S:t Mikael, U	parish	Björ 2005
23	Södermanland	Stockholm, Helgeandsholmen, U	sanctuary	J. Sjögren unpubl.
24	Uppland	Sigtuna, U	parish	Kjellström this study
25	Västmanland	Västerås, unknown churcha, U	parish	Hartzel 2010
26	Västmanland	Sura, U	parish	Jonsson & Nordström 2003
27	Uppland	Långfredagsslaget, U	military massgrave	Kjellström 2003
27	Uppland	Uppsala, Kv. Kroken, U	parish	B. Sigvallius unpubl.
27	Uppland	Viby-Julita, U	monastey+parish	Iregren 1973
28	Dalarna	Leksand, R	parish	Sjøvold 1982
29	Jämtland	Västerhus, R	parish	Gejvall 1960
30	Ångermanland	Björned, R	parish	Grundberg & Hårding 2003

* All data compiled for this study by Arcini

Appendix 3. Isotope data

Detailed isotope data used in Chapter 6.

Inv. no.	Grave no.	Yrs AD	Sex	Age	Tooth element	$\delta^{13}C$ (‰)	$\delta^{15}N$ (‰)	$^{87}Sr/^{86}Sr$	Femur (mm)
KM 71839	26	990–1100	M	Adult	I1, mandible	-19.57	9.11	0.709558	425.0
KM 71839	27	990–1100	F	Adult	I1, mandible	-20.28	10.69	0.713853	455.5
KM 71839	29	990–1100	M	Adult	I1, mandible	-19.72	8.21	0.710397	427.0
KM 71839	42	990–1100	F	Adult	M1, maxilla	-19.79	8.10	0.711364	376.0
KM 66166	93	990–1100	F	Adult	M1, mandible			0.717150	
KM 71839	104	990–1100	M	Adult	M1, mandible	-19.64	11.07	0.709347	428.0
KM 66166	112	990–1100	M	Adult	M1, mandible	-19.55	11.6	0.709681	450.0
KM 71839	122	990–1100	M	Adult	I1, mandible	-19.16	13.97		409.0
KM 71839	168	990–1100	M	Adult	I1, mandible	-20.87	11.03		512.0
KM 71839	178	990–1100	F	Adult	I, mandible	-20.31	10.66	0.709394	389.0
KM 71839	188	990–1100	F	Adult	M1, mandible	-19.53	9.16	0.711598	428.5
KM 71839	192	990–1100	F	Adult	I2, mandible	-19.72	10.78	0.708170	419.0
KM 71839	204	990–1100	M	Adult	I2, mandible	-20.22	8.25	0.714325	460.0
KM 71839	238	990–1100	M	Adult	M1, maxilla	-20.36	9.28		503.5
KM 71839	239	990–1100	F	Adult	I1, mandible	-20.47	9.44	0.708691	404.0
KM 71839	252	990–1100	F	Adult	M1, mandible	-20.57	9.82	0.708809	386.0
KM 71839	272	990–1100	M	Adult	C, mandible	-19.44	12.40	0.709242	452.0
KM 66166	280	990–1100	F	Adult	M1, maxilla	-20.12	10.10	0.709027	455.5
KM 66166	282	990–1100	M	Adult	I2, mandible	-19.52	8.13	0.710371	421.0
KM 71839	299	990–1100	F	Adult	M1, maxilla	-20.37	9.77	0.711638	377.5
KM 66166	322	990–1100	M	Adult	I2, mandible	-18.84	11.60	0.711032	423.5
KM 66166	366	990–1100	M	Adult	I2, maxilla	-19.49	10.47	0.711144	510.0
KM 71839	482	1350/1370–1536	M	Adult	I1, mandible	-19.81	11.55	0.711039	474.0
KM 71839	507	1350/1370–1536	F	Adult	I, mandible	-19.58	12.02		443.5
KM 71839	540	1350/1370	F	Adult	I, mandible	-19.58	11.69	0.711475	399.0
KM 71839	561	1350/1370	F	Adult	I2, maxilla	-19.03	12.24		439.5
KM 71839	564	1350/1370	F	Adult	F, mandible	-20.16	12.72	0.710946	415.0
KM 71839	606	1300–1350	M	Adult	I, mandible	-19.12	12.47	0.709519	427.5
KM 71839	634	1300–1350	M	Adult	I, mandible	-19.67	10.75		496.0
KM 71839	661	1300–1350	F	Adult	M1, mandible	-19.03	12.38		445.0
KM 71839	697	1100–1300	M	Adult	M1, maxilla	-20.14	11.64	0.710732	417.0
KM 71839	754	1350/1370	M	Adult	M1, maxilla	-19.60	12.20	0.710539	419.5
KM 71839	757	1350/70–1536	F	Adult	M1, mandible	-19.58	12.95		408.0

Inv. no.	Grave no.	Yrs AD	Sex	Age	Tooth element	δ¹³C (‰)	δ¹⁵N (‰)	⁸⁷Sr/⁸⁶Sr	Femur (mm)
KM 71839	787	1350/1370	F	Adult	I, mandible	-19.31	10.94		427.5
KM 71839	792	1350/1370	M	Adult	I2, maxilla	-20.20	11.77	0.710914	413.5
KM 71839	800	1350/1370	F	Adult	I1, mandible	-19.27	11.34	0.710414	430.5
KM 71839	806	1350/1370	F	Adult	I2, maxilla	-20.17	12.04	0.710435	405.5
KM 71839	809	1350/1370–1536	F	Adult	C, mandible	-19.46	10.98	0.714923	408.5
KM 71839	827	1350/1370	F	Adult	I1, maxilla	-20.12	10.66	0.711638	442.0
KM 71839	856	1300–1350	F	Adult	M1 mandible	-20.15	11.64		440.0
KM 71839	865	1350/1370	M	Adult	MI, maxilla	-18.82	11.89	0.711289	424.5
KM 71839	869	1300–1350	F	Adult	M1, mandible	-20.11	12.13	0.710915	396.0
KM 71839	887	1350/1370	F	Adult	I2, maxilla	-19.90	12.55	0.711319	430.0
KM 71839	898	1100–1300	M	Adult	I1, maxilla	-20.08	11.63	0.711128	432.0
KM 71839	908	1300–1350	M	Adult	M1, maxilla	-20.78	11.13	0.714525	506.5
KM 71839	914	1100–1300	F	Adult	I2, mandible	-19.86	12.38	0.710353	391.0
KM 71839	927	1100–1300	F	Adult	I, mandible	-19.38	11.78	0.710334	455.0
KM 71839	1054	1100–1300	M	Adult	I, mandible	-19.78	13.10	0.711700	408.0
KM 71839	1059	1350/1370–1536	M	Adult	F, mandible	-20.18	12.30	0.709656	467.5
KM 71839	1082	990–1100	F	Adult	I, mandible	-18.72	12.26	0.711018	450.0
KM 71839	1103	990–1100	M	Adult	M1, maxilla	-19.69	10.91	0.710246	451.0
KM 71839	1115	1100–1300	M	Adult	I, mandible	-20.12	11.55		495.5
KM 71839	1140	1100–1300	M	Adult	I, mandible	-19.06	12.92	0.711306	413.5
KM 71839	1160	1350/1370	M	Adult	I, mandible	-19.37	11.56	0.710819	478.5
KM 71839	1161	1350/1370–1536	M	Adult	M1, mandible	-20.58	12.29	0.711083	443.5
KM 71839	1167	1350/1370–1536	M	Adult	I, mandible	-20.03	11.01	0.711909	518.5
KM 71839	1178	1350/70	M	Adult	M1, mandible	-20.36	12.81		446.0
KM 71839	1197	1350/1370–1536	F	Adult	I, mandible	-20.61	10.61	0.713411	396.5
KM 71839	1200	1300–1350	F	Adult	M1, maxilla	-20.03	12.11		401.5
KM 71839	1231	1300–1350	F	Adult	I, mandible	-20.23	12.09		400.0
KM 71839	1239	1100–1300	M	Adult	I, mandible	-18.82	13.29		498.5
KM 71839	1256	1350/1370	M	Adult	I, mandible	-20.19	11.06	0.711287	505,0
KM 71839	1278	1300–1350	F	Adult	I2, maxilla	-19.10	12.37	0.711068	444.5
KM 71839	1312	1350/1370	M	Adult	I, mandible	-20.24	12.17	0.711730	511.5
KM 71839	1327	1300–1350	F	Adult	I, mandible	-20.05	12.99		403.5
KM 71839	1352	1300–1350	M	Adult	M1, mandible	-20.94	11.84	0.711182	504.0
KM 71839	1381	1100–1300	F	Adult	I, mandible	-19.78	11.73	0.710558	444.0
KM 71839	1386	990–1100	M	Adult	I, mandible	-20.26	12.37	0.712669	504.0
KM 71839	1409	1100–1300	M	Adult	C, mandible	-19.32	10.52	0.711254	494.0
KM 71839	1421	1100–1300	M	Adult	I1, maxilla	-19.19	11.59		420.0
KM 71839	1444	1100–1300	F	Adult	I, mandible	-19.50	12.61	0.710509	381.0
KM 71839	1450	990–1100	M	Adult	I2, mandible	-20.94	11.79	0.712991	483.0
KM 71839	1456	1100–1300	F	Adult	M1, mandible	-19.06	13.02		399.5
KM 71839	1469	1100–1300	F	Adult	I, mandible	-20.54	14.57	0.719124	381.0
KM 71839	1472	1100–1300	M	Adult	I, mandible	-20.48	10.65	0.714108	492.5
KM 71839	1492	1100–1300	F	Adult	I, mandible	-19.72	12.22		444.5
KM 71839	1504	990–1100	F	Adult	M1, mandible	-21.52	10.73	0.718381	428.0
KM 71839	1512	990–1100	F	Adult	I, mandible	-19.34	12.70	0.711235	387.5
KM 71839	1600	1350/1370–1547	F	Adult	M1, mandible	-21.00	11.38	0.716129	439.0
KM 71839	1611	1300–1350	F	Adult	I, mandible	-19.75	11.18	0.713604	441.0
KM 71839	1632	1350–1370	F	Adult	I, mandible	-19.39	12.18		413.0
KM 71839	1638	1350–1370	M	Adult	I, mandible	-20.05	12.09		495.0
KM 71839	1667	1100–1300	M	Adult	I, mandible	-19.86	12.90		495.0
KM 71839	1711	1100–1300	M	Adult	I, mandible	-20.64	11.53	0.710211	519.0
KM 71839	1771	1350/1370–1536	M	Adult	I1, mandible	-19.20	13.22	0.710743	472.5

Inv. no.	Grave no.	Yrs AD	Sex	Age	Tooth element	$\delta^{13}C$ (‰)	$\delta^{15}N$ (‰)	$^{87}Sr/^{86}Sr$	Femur (mm)
KM 71839	1789	1350/1370–1536	F	Adult	I, mandible	-19.82	12.74		440.0
KM 71839	1795	1350/1370–1536	F	Adult	M1, mandible	-20.54	11.08	0.712418	435.0
KM 71839	1810	1350–1370	F	Adult	M2, mandible	-18.78	12.35		374.0
KM 71839	1827	1100–1300	M	Adult	I, mandible	-19.84	12.82		436.0
KM 71839	1904	1350/1370–1536	F	Adult	I2, maxilla	-19.87	12.38	0.710965	428.0
KM 71839	2032	1100–1300	M	Adult	I, mandible	-19.39	12.48		419.0
KM 71839	2101	1100–1300	M	Adult	I, mandible	-20.30	11.16		475.5
KM 71839	2224	1300–1350	M	Adult	I, mandible	-19.48	12.25	0.710779	510.0
KM 71839	2225	1300–1350	F	Adult	I, mandible	-19.59	12.84	0.710253	439.5
KM 71839	2508	1100–1300	F	Adult	I, mandible	-19.67	10.54		423.0
KM 71839	2518	1100–1300	F	Adult	I, mandible	-18.27	13.53	0.710882	454.0
KM 71839	2530	1300–1350	F	Adult	I, mandible	-20.16	11.17	0.712548	407.0
KM 71839	2552	1300–1350	M	Adult	I, mandible	-19.80	12.50	0.711311	434.5
KM 71839	3006	1100–1300	F	Adult	I, mandible	-22.30	12.33	0.711059	390.0
KM 71839	3006	1100–1300	M	Adult	I2, mandible	-19.85	12.20	0.714218	423.0
Domkyrka	28734	990–1100	M	Adult	I2, mandible	-20.53	10.74	0.710543	479.0
KM 71839	2031	990–1100	F	Adult	C, mandible	-19.05	12.24		
Domkyrka	28736	990–1100	F	Adult	I2, mandible			0.712669	373.5